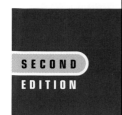

SECOND
EDITION

PHARMACISTS
TALKING WITH
PATIENTS

A GUIDE TO PATIENT COUNSELING

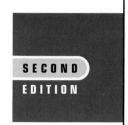

PHARMACISTS TALKING WITH PATIENTS

A GUIDE TO PATIENT COUNSELING

SECOND EDITION

Melanie J. Rantucci, BScPhm, MScPhm, PhD

Pharmacist Consultant, President
MJR Pharmacy Communications
White Rock, British Columbia
Canada

.Lippincott Williams & Wilkins

a Wolters Kluwer business

Philadelphia · Baltimore · New York · London
Buenos Aires · Hong Kong · Sydney · Tokyo

Acquisitions Editor: David Troy
Managing Editor: Meredith Brittain
Marketing Manager: Marisa O'Brien
Production Editor: Jennifer D.W. Glazer
Designer: Doug Smock
Compositor: International Typesetting and Composition
Printer: R.R. Donnelley—Crawfordsville
Cartoon Artist: Bot Roda
Bottom cover photo courtesy of ActiveAndAble.com

351 West Camden Street
Baltimore, MD 21201

530 Walnut Street
Philadelphia, PA 19106

Printed in the United States of America.

First Edition, 1997

Library of Congress Cataloging-in-Publication Data

Rantucci, Melanie J.
    Pharmacists talking with patients : a guide to patient counseling /
Melanie J. Rantucci. -- 2nd ed.
      p. ; cm.
    Includes bibliographical references and index.
    ISBN 0-7817-6330-4
    1. Pharmacist and patient. 2. Health counseling. 3. Communication
in pharmacy. I. Title.
    [DNLM: 1. Pharmacy--methods. 2. Counseling--methods. 3. Phar–
maceutical Services. QV 704 R213p 2006]
    RS56 .R36 2006
    362.17'82--dc22

    2005032336

To purchase additional copies of this book, call our customer service department at **(800) 638-3030** or fax orders to **(301) 223-2320.** International customers should call **(301) 223-2300.**

Visit Lippincott Williams & Wilkins on the Internet: http://www.LWW.com. Lippincott Williams & Wilkins customer service representatives are available from 8:30 am to 6:00 pm, EST.

06 07 08 09 10
1 2 3 4 5 6 7 8 9 10

The title "Pharmacists Talking with Patients" embodies the patient-centered approach of this text. In this second edition, discussion of many theoretical and practical issues and presentation of realistic situations will help pharmacy students and pharmacists become effective and efficient patient counselors.

Organizational Philosophy

Pharmacists Talking with Patients, Second Edition, progresses logically through the following steps: Preparing pharmacists for counseling patients by helping them to understand what counseling is, explaining what patients need, recommending how to structure the counseling session, specifying what tools and techniques can be used to make counseling more efficient and effective, enumerating the skills used in counseling, and, finally, describing how to implement counseling. The text is structured around six main objectives, described below.

Objective 1: To Understand Why Pharmacists Need to Become Adept in Patient Counseling

With the advent of premanufactured pharmaceuticals, an expanded role for dispensary assistants, and the concept of pharmaceutical care, the technical side of pharmacy has diminished for the community pharmacist, and its more social aspects have become increasingly important. Although pharmacists have always made an effort to know their clientele, and the public has traditionally seen pharmacists as a source of health information, a greater emphasis is now being placed on the pharmacist–patient interaction. In addition, various jurisdictions require pharmacists to provide patient counseling to differing degrees.

Although it is now generally well accepted by pharmacists that patient counseling is part of their role, they are not always as actively involved in this process as they should be. Chapter 1 discusses the benefits of patient counseling: By becoming active in patient counseling, pharmacists can simultaneously derive personal satisfaction and benefit their profession and their business.

Objective 2: To Be Able to Describe and Define Patient Counseling

The pharmacist is in an ideal position to ensure that drugs are used in the safest and most effective way possible, to assist patients in managing their disease states and medications, and to encourage appropriate self-care with nonprescription drugs. In addition, because people trust pharmacists as educated and approachable health professionals, they often present them with a variety of nonmedication–related questions concerning such issues as birth control or alcohol abuse. However, pharmacists often view their task as providing a list of instructions and warnings to patients about medications rather than as engaging in a socially interactive and psychological process.

Chapter 2 discusses the meaning of the term *patient counseling* and the goals of counseling from the perspective of both the pharmacist and the patient.

Objective 3: To Describe How People Feel About Being Ill and Using Medication

In their day-to-day practices, pharmacists need to be able to use their pharmaceutical and therapeutic knowledge to help their patients receive the maximum benefit from the medications they provide. To do this, they must understand patients and their needs regarding medication use. Chapters 3 and 4 discuss how people feel about being ill and using medication, why they may be nonadherent in their use of medication, what may motivate them to change their behavior, and in what ways they may need the pharmacist's help.

Objective 4: To Demonstrate the Use of Techniques Involved in Patient Counseling

To become efficient and effective in patient counseling, the pharmacist needs to become adept at using various techniques. Chapter 5 outlines protocols for proceeding with the various types of counseling encounters. To further assist pharmacists in counseling patients, Chapter 6 reviews methods and techniques for providing educational material, and it details the various resources that are available.

An important aspect of patient counseling is the relationship that develops between the patient and the pharmacist. Chapter 7 discusses this relationship and selected communication skills necessary for effective patient counseling.

Although patient counseling primarily involves a relationship between the pharmacist and the patient, contemporary pharmacy practice also involves interacting with other individuals. Chapter 7 therefore includes a discussion about interactions with peers, particularly other health professionals, illustrating how the techniques used in patient counseling can also enhance our relationships within the health care team.

Objective 5: To Identify and Deal with Special Situations

Each patient is an individual, and patients with certain conditions, medications, or social situations have greater needs. Elderly patients, patients with disabilities, those with communication difficulties, patients with terminal conditions, and those in situations such as unwanted pregnancy, drug and alcohol abuse, and psychological problems all require special consideration. Chapter 8 discusses issues involving counseling these patients and how pharmacists can tailor counseling to address these patients' unique needs. In addition, situations that can be very difficult and stressful for pharmacists, such as conflict and dealing with medication incidents, are discussed in Chapter 8.

Objective 6: To Be Able to Provide Counseling in Everyday Practice

Although most pharmacists have the desire to counsel patients, they often find the process difficult to implement. Chapter 9 deals with challenges faced by pharmacists in counseling and ways in which they can be overcome.

The appendices contain additional useful information to help implement patient counseling. Because the wording pharmacists use to gather information and to express facts and concepts can be critical in patient counseling, Appendix A includes sample dialogues that can serve as a helpful guideline for pharmacy students and pharmacists. And because pharmacists must be able to efficiently document their actions in patient counseling—such as medication history interviewing, pharmaceutical opinions and recommendations to other health care providers, and nonprescription drug counseling—examples of useful forms are provided in Appendix B.

Pedagogical Features

Nearly every chapter includes helpful pedagogical features that will aid the pharmacy student and pharmacist.

- **Chapter Objectives**: At the request of pharmacy educators who have used the first edition in pharmacy courses, each chapter now begins with a *list of objectives* and proceeds logically to accomplish them.
- **Case Studies**: *Pharmacist–patient dialogues* bring to life concepts that are under discussion. A description of the situation and a dialogue are accompanied by a discussion of the problems that the dialogue illustrates. An alternative dialogue usually follows, with a brief explanation of the changes to the dialogue that make it more effective.
- **Visual Learning**: *New cartoons and photographs* encapsulate and clarify important concepts. In addition, pharmacy students and pharmacists can use the helpful forms in the book to query patients and track their progress.
- **Tables**: *Tables* synthesize useful information in an easy-to-reference format. Where appropriate, tables have been added to summarize useful information.
- **Reflective Questions**: Also in response to requests from faculty, *reflective questions* have been added at the end of each chapter to help readers think about the material in the chapter as it relates to particular patients and situations, or in terms of their own practices.

Content That Is New to the Second Edition

The second edition incorporates a number of changes from the first edition. Many concepts discussed in the first edition have been further researched and in some cases implemented and evaluated, so the text reflects this updated and expanded information. This edition also includes sections about concepts that have become important in the field in the last few years, such as the therapeutic alliance between health professionals and patients, and collaborative working relationships between pharmacists and physicians. The second edition also discusses cultural and literacy issues, because pharmacists have come to better understand the impact of these concerns in health care and how to deal with them. And because gathering information is an important aspect of pharmacy practice today, more forms have been added to Appendix B, "Forms to Assist in Patient Counseling."

Finally, the revised text addresses issues in a manner that should apply to pharmacists in all countries where patient counseling services are being implemented, including not only North America, but also Australia, New Zealand, Great Britain, Scandinavia, and countries where the first edition has been translated, including Japan and Spain.

Summary

The main goal of this book is to help pharmacy students and pharmacists become effective and efficient patient counselors. In doing so, they will not only help their patients, but also gain more satisfaction from their careers.

Pharmacy students and pharmacists often find it difficult to incorporate patient counseling into their everyday practices. After reading and studying the topics covered in this book, readers should be better able to do this through achieving the objectives previously described. The discussion of many theoretical and practical issues and, where appropriate, the presentation of realistic situations as case studies will help pharmacy students and pharmacists become aware of the various elements that will make them effective and efficient patient counselors.

For pharmacy students, this book will provide an overview of patient counseling. This book is not intended to provide a complete education in this topic, simply because patient counseling cannot be learned solely from reading a book. This book should be used in conjunction with more comprehensive training in basic communication skills and further discussion of topics in social and administrative pharmacy.

All readers should practice the skills and concepts presented in this book to become more adept. Readers should identify the skills they already possess and the areas in which they must focus their development of new skills.

Pharmacists should draw on their own strengths and wealth of experience to interpret the concepts presented in this book in terms of their own needs. Just as each patient and each situation is unique, so too is each pharmacist and each practice setting. In addition, certain jurisdictions require pharmacists to provide various levels of patient counseling. Pharmacists must decide for themselves how patient counseling, as discussed in this book, can fit into their own practices and what adjustments need to be made to allow for its inclusion. They also must review pharmacy regulations in their particular jurisdiction along with the material presented here, and they should follow whichever is more stringent.

All pharmacists have the potential to counsel patients—they have the knowledge, the opportunity, and the inherent ability to communicate. The concepts presented in this book will help pharmacy students and pharmacists to become aware of their own strengths and identify areas that they need to focus on to become more effective in counseling their patients. The goal of *Pharmacists Talking with Patients*, Second Edition, ultimately is to help improve patient care as well as make the role of pharmacists even more valuable in the health care system.

CLASSROOM TEACHING TOOLS

For faculty adopting the book, the Classroom Teaching Tools—including role-playing workshops, student assignments, practice examination questions, and points to consider in student's answers to the reflective questions in the text—can be accessed at http://connection.lww.com/rantucci.

ACKNOWLEDGMENTS

I would like to thank Dr. Jeff Taylor, College of Pharmacy and Nutrition, University of Saskatchewan, Saskatoon, Saskatchewan, Canada and Michelle Deschamps, MSc.Phm., French Lake, New Brunswick, Canada for suggesting updates and new references to the first edition and contributing to the development of objectives and reflective questions.

The patient-counseling situations presented at intervals throughout this book were adapted from articles written by this author, printed in the regular pharmacy column "On Counselling" in the Canadian pharmacy journal *Pharmacy Practice*, published by Rogers Publishing Limited, a division of Rogers Media Inc.

CONTENTS

CHAPTER **5**   The Counseling Session

CHAPTER **6**   Information Provision and Educational Methods and Resources

CHAPTER **7**   Human Interactions and Counseling Skills in Pharmacy

CHAPTER **8** Tailoring Counseling to Meet Individual Patient Needs and Overcome Challenges

CHAPTER **9** Implementing Patient Counseling as a Pharmacy Service

APPENDIX **A** Suggested Dialogues for Counseling

APPENDIX **B** Forms to Assist in Patient Counseling

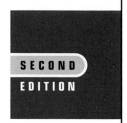

PHARMACISTS TALKING WITH PATIENTS

A GUIDE TO PATIENT COUNSELING

The Role of Patient Counseling in Pharmacy

CHAPTER 1

Objectives

After completing the chapter, the reader should be able to

1. describe the potential benefits of patient counseling to the patient.
2. describe the potential benefits of patient counseling to the pharmacist.
3. discuss how patient counseling may be seen as a service to the public and private and government insurers.
4. describe how patient counseling fits in with the pharmaceutical care model.
5. discuss the challenges faced by pharmacists in patient counseling.

Pharmacists today are aware that the practice of pharmacy has evolved over the years to include not only preparation and dispensing of medication to patients, but also interaction with patients and other health care providers throughout the provision of pharmaceutical care. Although from 1922 to 1969 pharmacists were prohibited from discussing therapies with their patients, recent changes to standards and legislation have made the provision of information a responsibility.[1] The Pharmacist Practice Activity Classification (PPAC) developed in 1998 by the American Pharmaceutical Association describes pharmacists' activities, including many tasks that involve patient interaction, such as interviewing the patient, obtaining patient information, educating the patient, providing verbal and written information, discussing, demonstrating, face-to-face patient contact, and patient counseling.[2]

In the practice philosophy of pharmaceutical care, pharmacists are responsible directly to the patients they serve.[3] From this patient-centered view, patient counseling improves patient care. From the pharmacist's point of view, it is integral to providing competitive and professional pharmacy services. It is evident that patient counseling and patient–pharmacist interaction are key to the pharmacist's role today.

PATIENT COUNSELING TO IMPROVE PATIENT CARE

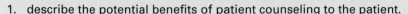

The most important role of patient counseling is to improve the quality of life and provide quality care for patients. The occurrences of so-called "drug misadventures"[4] (adverse effects, side effects, drug interactions, and errors in the use of medication) and nonadherence to treatment programs reduce quality of life and interfere with quality care. In addition, the high costs of health care today call for interventions to minimize waste and to maximize benefits of medical treatments.

As evidence of this need, more than 200 studies and estimates of medication use by nonhospitalized patients suggest that 50% of patients will use their medications incorrectly.[5] According to a report by the Department of Health and Human Services (DHHS) in 1990, 48% of the US population, and 55% of the elderly, fail to adhere in some way to their medication regimens.[6] In addition, one study reported that 32% of patients who were instructed by their doctors to have their prescriptions refilled failed to do so.[7] As further evidence of this, it has been calculated that, of the 25,815 prescriptions that could possibly be refilled in the average independent community pharmacy in 1988, only 14,681 were dispensed.[8] In other words, every second or third patient who receives a prescription is likely to use it incorrectly!

Although not all nonadherence is of consequence, studies show that 25% of patients will use a medication in a way that poses a threat to their health.[5] Nonadherence may result in prolonging or increasing the severity of an illness. It may also result in the physician's assuming—on the basis of poor response to the medication— that the illness was misdiagnosed, leading to more tests and possibly additional medication. A review of the literature determined that 5.5% of hospital admissions can be attributed to drug therapy nonadherence.[9]

Pharmacists can have a significant impact on these figures through patient counseling. According to the DHHS report "Medication Regimens: Causes of Noncompliance," lack of information about drugs is one of the four most significant variables that have the most bearing on reasons why the elderly may fail to comply with their medication regimens.[6] Many studies have demonstrated the effectiveness of pharmacist provision of information and reminders. For example, a study in Memphis, Tennessee, found adherence rates of 84.7% for patients receiving a high level of information about an antibiotic drug, compared with 63% for patients receiving less information.[6] Another study improved adherence to cardiac, antihypertensive, and oral hypoglycemic medications by 49% through a prescription reminder system.[8]

In addition to problems with adherence, patients may suffer adverse drug reactions. Since 1969, approximately 400,000 adverse reactions have been reported to the U.S. Food and Drug Administration, and in 1987, 20% of the cases resulted in either death or hospitalization.[4] Furthermore, occurrences of adverse reactions are substantially underreported; as few as 10% are reported.[3,4] A report by the American Association of Retired Persons indicates that 40% of elderly Americans taking prescription drugs experience adverse effects.[4] Patients may be spared some of these problems if they are made aware of the early signs of adverse drug reactions to report, and if pharmacists inquire about ongoing therapy, allowing early detection and treatment.

In addition to nonadherence and adverse drug reactions, through patient counseling pharmacists can bring to light many other drug-related problems such as untreated indications, improper drug selection, subtherapeutic dosage, overdosage, drug interactions, and drug use without indication.[3]

It has recently been acknowledged by the health care community that adverse events caused by errors in patient care and treatment are a huge problem contributing to prolonged hospital stays, increased illness and suffering, and loss of confidence in the health care system.[10] The U.S. Institute of Medicine report, "To Err is Human:

Building a Safer Health System," focusing on the quality of health care in America, estimated in 1999 that as many as 100,000 Americans die in hospitals annually from adverse events (more than car accidents, breast cancer, or AIDS).[10] The landmark Harvard Medical Practice Study, a population-based study of iatrogenic injury in hospitalized patients in New York State in 1984, found that 3.7% of patients suffered an injury that prolonged stay or caused disability, and 69% of the injuries were due to errors. Drugs accounted for 19.4% of the injuries and 45% of those were due to medication errors.[11] In another study of hospital admissions, 6.5 adverse drug events (ADEs include adverse reactions and errors) and 5.5 potential ADEs were found per 100 admissions with 28% due to errors. Errors were identified in more than one stage in 21% of the ADEs, with the most occurring in prescribing and administration stage.[12] Studies in community dispensary settings find estimates of medication errors ranging from 1.5% to 4% of prescriptions filled for ambulatory patients.[13] Systems analysis of medication errors conclude that contributing factors are multifactorial and involve immediate causes stemming from situational factors at the time the drug is provided to the patient, while others involve latent conditions related to the drug provision system from manufacture and regulatory systems to the patient.[14] Causes include failed communication, lack of patient education, incorrect drug administration, dispensing processes and drug distribution, and knowledge level of pharmacist, patient, and prescriber. These could all be identified and prevented through patient counseling. Patient education (both verbal and written) has been identified by the Institute for Safe Medication Practices as the most important error-prevention strategy.[15]

These medication use problems may result not only in increased risks for the patient, but also in extra time and expense. In a California study, the cost of hospitalization of elderly patients suffering from adverse drug reactions was found to be $340.1 million.[1] The cost of nonadherence to drug therapy has been estimated as 20 million lost work days and $1.5 billion in lost earnings annually, as well as $8.5 billion in unnecessary hospital expenditures in 1986—approximately 1.7% of all health care expenditures that year.[8,9] Overall, the annual cost of drug-related morbidity and mortality in the United States was estimated in 1995 by Johnson and Bootman to be $45.6 billion in direct health care costs.[16] In addition, the cost of preventable adverse events (everything that can go wrong with a patient in the health care system that is an unplanned and undesired harmful occurrence such as adverse reactions and medical errors) was estimated to be between $17 billion and $19 billion including lost income, disability, and medical expenses according to the report, "To Err is Human."[10] With costs in health care escalating each year, for the individual and for health plan sponsors in government and the private sector it is important that pharmacists become involved in patient counseling.

In addition to reducing drug-related morbidity and its subsequent costs to the individual and society, patient counseling may benefit patients in a number of other ways concerning improved outcomes and satisfaction with care. Patients may want reassurance that a medication is safe and effective. They may also need additional explanation about their illnesses that they did not receive from their physicians because they were too rushed, too upset, or too embarrassed to ask. Effective physician–patient communication has been found in many studies to improve patient outcomes.[17] Quality of communication in history-taking and during discussion of the management plan has been found to improve emotional health, symptom resolution, function, physiologic measures (i.e., blood pressure and blood sugar level), and pain control.[17] But physician–patient communication is often hurried and not thorough enough in regard to drug therapy issues.[18] Pharmacist–patient communication can make up for limited physician–patient communication, and could improve patient outcomes.

Patients find communication, interpersonal sensitivity, and partnership with their health care providers to improve satisfaction; they are consequently more likely to adhere to medical advice and to recall medical information provided.[19,20]

Counseling can further assist patients with self-care. Although many conditions are self-treatable, patients often need help in determining which symptoms are appropriate to self-treat and which need the attention of a physician. Nonprescription-drug misuse has been reported in the literature, with rates varying from 15% to 66% of study groups.[21–23] Self-treatment, when appropriate, can reduce the need for and costs of more formal care. As with prescription counseling, pharmacist counseling for nonprescription medications can benefit patients both medically and financially.

Finally, patients may benefit from counseling by pharmacists in non-medication–related situations. There appears to be a gap in the social and health care system regarding access to treatment. Patients are often unsure where to go for help with a variety of problems ranging from family planning to emotional problems. As available and approachable health professionals, pharmacists can fill this gap and help patients locate the appropriate social and health care services. Pharmacists in ambulatory care are often the first contact with the health care system, and as such can coordinate services for the patient and family, as well as provide continuity of care.[24] They are also ideally situated to provide public health services such as smoking cessation and weight loss counseling and counseling on preventing or coping with disease conditions.

These many benefits of patient counseling to patient care can be summarized in the words of a report released in 1990 by the US government office of DHHS, stating that "clinical pharmacy services add value to patient care not only in improvement in clinical outcomes and enhanced patient compliance, but also in reduction in health care utilization costs associated with adverse drug reactions."[25]

The material in this section is summarized in Table 1-1.

TABLE 1-1   Patient Counseling to Improve Patient Care

1. Reduces errors in using medication
2. Reduces noncompliance
3. Reduces adverse drug reactions
4. Improves outcomes
5. Increases satisfaction with care
6. Assists with self-care
7. Can provide referral for assistance with non-drug–related situations (e.g., family planning and emotional problems)
8. Reduces health care costs to individual, government, and society
9. Is an integral part of providing patient-centred pharmaceutical care

---

PROVIDING PROFESSIONAL PHARMACY SERVICES THROUGH PATIENT COUNSELING

Pharmacists have a professional obligation to counsel patients for many reasons including legal, personal, professional, and economic.

From the legal standpoint, the Omnibus Budget Reconciliation Act of 1990 (OBRA-'90) in the United States required pharmacists to provide patient counseling for Medicaid patients.[26] Congress outlined the items to be included in patient counseling as a minimum, but it was left up to each state to legislate specific regulations regarding patient counseling.[26] Since then, boards of pharmacy in 36 states have extended the OBRA-'90 mandate to require counseling for all patients.[27]

Regulations may change with time and in different jurisdictions, and each pharmacist should consult his or her respective pharmacy governing body to determine the final rules or compliance requirements where they practice. Most US jurisdictions require counseling be done by a pharmacist, although some states allow a designate to make "an offer to counsel" or do not address the question.[28-30] Laws in different jurisdictions also vary in scope and stringency on issues such as use of written information, and whether patients receiving refill prescriptions as well as those receiving new prescriptions need to be counseled.[30] A few states make the regulation mandatory only for certain patient groups such as Medicaid patients, but societal and professional pressures require that all patients be counseled. Legal challenges could be made based on the concept of different standards of care being established.[29] Therefore, even in jurisdictions where counseling is mandated only for certain patient groups, all patients should be included.

Historically, most courts have held that pharmacists do not have a duty to counsel or warn patients of potential dangers regarding their drug therapy when a prescription is proper on its face and neither the physician nor the drug manufacturer has indicated that warnings need to be given.[29] Other cases have held that pharmacists have a duty to warn patients in certain situations.[29] Complying with state requirements can be expected to reduce the risk of legal repercussions from consulting and to put pharmacists in a better position to defend themselves should a patient make a claim, particularly if actions involving patient counseling are documented.[31]

Pharmacists' involvement in patient counseling can also benefit pharmacists professionally. The technical and mechanical functions of pharmacists may easily be replaced in the future. We are seeing many changes in the pharmaceutical arena: drug-delivery systems such as implants; the use of computer, automated dispensing, robotics, and other potential types of automation; and new roles for pharmacy technicians.[31] In addition, nurses have already established roles in providing pharmacy services and in counseling patients, and computerized order entry systems assist physicians in selecting drugs and identifying drug-related problems.[31] Unless pharmacists become involved in all aspects of pharmaceutical care, including patient counseling, they in effect perform the role of technicians, thereby diminishing their professional status.[32]

At the same time, pharmacists are striving to be recognized by patients and other health professionals as important players in the health care team, that is, the team's experts in the field of drugs. Standards of practice for the profession of pharmacy by the American Pharmaceutical Association and other pharmacy organizations, as well as guidelines for patient counseling by these organizations, promote the role of pharmacists in patient counseling.

Apart from legal and professional inducements to counsel patients, pharmacists have a personal stake in patient-counseling involvement. A diminishing professional status affects pharmacists' self-worth and job satisfaction, which have been found to be related to clinical and professional aspects of the job.[33] In general, pharmacists report that counseling and patient education are the greatest sources of job satisfaction, and that they want to spend more time advising and counseling.[33,34] Pharmacists believe that there are advantages to patient counseling and that it increases their professional satisfaction.[35] Patient counseling offers pharmacists a chance to demonstrate professional capabilities and to use the knowledge that they have gained through many years of study.[31] Whereas dispensing tasks alone can be repetitive and unfulfilling, personal interaction can add variety and interest to the pharmacist's job. And there is the personal satisfaction of helping another person, particularly in helping that person to regain or maintain health.

However, the discrepancy between practice expectations and reality is often distressing to pharmacists, who feel frustrated at not fully using their knowledge. In fact, some studies have found that pharmacists who did not want to counsel patients were more satisfied with their jobs than pharmacists who wanted to counsel, likely because they were unable to do so in their existing circumstances.[36]

An additional personal benefit for pharmacists' involvement in patient counseling involves job stress. A pharmacist's job can be very stressful at times, primarily as a result of dealing with clients who are often ill and under stress themselves.[36] Through discussion with the patient during counseling, the pharmacist can come to understand the patient's position and gain his or her cooperation, ultimately reducing the level of stress of both patient and pharmacist.[36]

From the economic and business points of view, in an environment of tough competition, patient counseling can be seen as an extra service with the potential to entice customers. It has been observed that "because pharmaceutical products are virtually identical, the only manner in which pharmacies can differentiate themselves is by the services they provide."[37] A 1992 survey found that a quarter of patients thought a pharmacist should talk to them personally about their prescriptions every time a prescription is filled, one third thought the pharmacist should talk to them if they ask, and a further third reported the pharmacist should talk to them when they think it is necessary.[38] In general, patients have low knowledge and expectations of patient counseling offered by pharmacists, and a reluctance to ask pharmacists questions.[39] However, when made aware of the counseling role of pharmacists, patients are more likely to recognize this role, and when provided with more intense services, e.g., in an office-based practice versus a traditional pharmacy, patrons express higher expectations.[39,40] Although not all patients may expect patient counseling, it can be expected that there are segments of the population that would give preference to a pharmacy that provided this. Indeed, there is ample evidence that the public wants more comprehensive pharmacotherapeutic information, in particular information about side effects and interactions with other drugs as well as information on interactions between drugs and alcohol and how to use medicines.[41]

The growing competition in pharmacy with preferred provider organizations, mail-order, managed-care pharmacies, and international pharmacies serves to emphasize the economic need for pharmacists to enhance the value of personal contact with patients through patient counseling.[31]

TABLE 1-2	Providing Professional Pharmacy Services through Patient Counseling

1. Provides compliance with pharmacy legislations, standards, and regulations
2. Affords legal protection, since pharmacists may be held accountable for injury resulting from insufficient information provided to the patient
3. Maintains professional status as part of primary care and health care team
4. Increases job satisfaction and reduces stress
5. Is an added service to meet patient demand and aid in market competition
6. Increases revenue through payment for counseling services and reduces loss resulting from unfilled or un-refilled prescriptions
7. Is an integral part of providing pharmaceutical care

Earlier studies indicated that consumers would be willing to pay for patient-counseling services when the information presented is tailored to the individual needs of the patient and is provided in a private or semiprivate setting.[42] Since the institution of legislation requiring counseling in many jurisdictions, specific consulting services such as smoking cessation, diabetic or asthma counseling have become more appropriate to promote as additional services for a fee, particularly to pharmaceutical and insurance companies who recognize the sometimes long-term cost-saving benefits.[43]

Patient counseling can also help pharmacists reduce the amount of revenue lost as a result of unfilled or un-refilled prescriptions. Unfilled and un-refilled prescriptions were estimated to represent a loss of approximately 100 million prescriptions annually in 1987.[7] A 1992 survey of consumers found that 8.7% of the respondents do not fill their initial prescriptions, with a potential value of $2.8 billion or $1,000 per week for the average pharmacy.[38] In 1990 it was determined that in the average pharmacy, 11,134 prescriptions that are eligible for renewal each year are not refilled, and a 50% increase in refill compliance by verbal reinforcement and reminders could increase net profit by $26,805 (based on an average prescription price of $16.60, and expenses of 13% of sales).[8]

The material in this section is summarized in Table 1-2.

PATIENT COUNSELING AND PHARMACEUTICAL CARE

Provision of patient counseling by the pharmacist is necessary to practice within the model of pharmaceutical care. The American Society of Health System Pharmacists' guidelines on pharmacist-conducted patient counseling state that pharmacist-conducted patient counseling is a component of pharmaceutical care.[44]

The role of patient counseling in the model of pharmaceutical care is not limited to the provision of patient information. Indeed, patient counseling is interwoven throughout the pharmaceutical care model and is necessary throughout the process. Strand et al. refer to pharmaceutical care as an integrated patient-specific model of pharmacy practice and assert that to deliver pharmaceutical care the pharmacist must see the patient, explain the proposed relationship, discuss the various choices, obtain information, and seek cooperation, trust, and permission.[45] Each step in the pharmaceutical care process as described by Strand et al. requires patient–pharmacist interaction: Establishing the pharmacist–patient relationship; collecting and interpreting patient information; listing and ranking drug-related problems; determining desired pharmacotherapeutic goals; determining feasible alternatives; selecting and individualizing the most appropriate treatment regimen; designing a drug-monitoring plan; implementing the decisions about drug use; designing a monitoring plan to achieve desired therapeutic goals and following up to determine the success of treatment.

Particularly in the community pharmacy setting, consulting with the patient is the main source of information necessary for the pharmacist to provide pharmaceutical care. Through patient counseling, the pharmacist is able to develop a working relationship, to gather the necessary facts, and to determine the patient's needs and wishes. The patient is able to contribute to identifying problems and can play a role in deciding desired outcomes and goals, identifying solutions and options, treatment regimens, and in developing an individual plan. Through regular discussions with the patient, the pharmacist can ensure that the patient carries out the plan and that the plan is successful from both the pharmacist's and patient's points of view. Thus, patient counseling is an integral part of pharmaceutical care.

CHALLENGES IN PATIENT COUNSELING

It is evident from this discussion that patient counseling is a prime role for pharmacists for the benefit of patients and for the professionalism of the pharmacist. In spite of all the compelling reasons from the pharmacist's and patient's viewpoints of the need for patient counseling, many pharmacists are still not engaging in this critical role.[46] A review of research by De Young concludes that the quantity and quality of pharmacist–patient communication has improved little over the last 25 years.[47] Although pharmacists have favorable views of patient counseling and are accessible, they interact on average with about half of patients with new prescriptions for 1 minute or less.[47] It has been suggested that there are a number of reasons for this (to be discussed further in Chapter 9), but the root may be in policies, procedures, and implementation programs to motivate and assist pharmacists.[46] In addition, the quality of the pharmacist–patient relationship and the content and style of the communication may be crucial to improving the quality and quantity of patient counseling and satisfaction of pharmacists and patients with patient counseling.[48,49] The following chapters will investigate these issues.

REFLECTIVE QUESTIONS

1. How can patient counseling minimize medication errors?
2. How can patient counseling improve patients' satisfaction?
3. How do the recent trends in health care technology affect the need for patient counseling?
4. List three ways that patient counseling can improve pharmacists' job satisfaction.
5. List three mechanisms by which patient counseling can provide increased competitive advantages for pharmacies.

REFERENCES

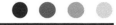

1. De Young M. A review of the research on pharmacists' patient-communication views and practices. Am J Pharm Ed. 1996;60(Spring):60–76.
2. Pharmacist Practice Activity Classification. American Pharmacists Association, 1998. Available at: www.aphanet.org/lead/practiceclass.html (accessed October 14, 2004).
3. Hepler C, Strand L. Opportunities and responsibilities in pharmaceutical care. Am J Hosp Pharm. 1990;47(3):533–554.
4. Manasse Jr. H. Medication use in an imperfect world: Drug misadventuring as an issue of public policy, Part 1. Am J Hosp Pharm. 1989;46(5):929–943.
5. Sackett D, Snow J. The magnitude of compliance and noncompliance. In: Haynes R, Taylor D, Sackett D, eds., Compliance in Health Care. The Johns Hopkins University Press, Baltimore, MD, 1979. p. 11–22.
6. Kessler D. A challenge for American pharmacists. Am Pharm. 1992;NS32(1):33–36.
7. Schering Laboratories. The forgetful patient: The high cost of improper patient compliance. Schering Report no. 9. Schering Laboratories, Kenilworth, NJ, 1987.
8. Jackson R, Huffman Jr. D. Patient compliance: The financial impact on your practice. NARD J. 1990;112(7):67–71.
9. Sullivan SD, Kreling DH, Hazlet TK. Noncompliance with medication regimens and subsequent hospitalization: A literature analysis and cost of hospitalization estimate. J Res Pharm Econ. 1990;2(2):19–34.
10. Kohn LT, Corigan JM, Donaldson M, eds. To Err is Human: Building a Safer Health System. National Academy of Medicine. National Academy Press, Washington, DC, 1999. Available at: www.nmap.edu/html/to_err_is_human/ (accessed October 20, 2004).
11. Brennan TA, Leape LL, Laird N, et al. Nature of adverse events in hospitalized patients. Results of the Harvard Medical Practice Study II. 1991, N Engl J Med. 324(6):377–384.
12. Leape LL, Bates DW, Cullen DJ, et al. Systems analysis of adverse drug events. JAMA. 1995;274(1):35–43.
13. Flynn EA, Barker K. Medication Errors Research. In: Cohen M, ed., Medication Errors: Causes, Prevention and Risk Management. American Pharmacists Association, Jones and Bartlett, Boston, MA, 2000. p. 6.1–6.30.
14. Leape LL. A Systems Analysis Approach to Medical Error. In: Cohen M, ed., Medication Errors: Causes, Prevention and Risk Management. American Pharmacists Association, Jones and Bartlett, Boston, MA, 2000. p. 2.1–2.10.
15. ISMP Medication Safety Alert! Community/Ambulatory Care Edition. 2004;3(9):4.
16. Johnson JA, Bootman JL. Drug-related morbidity and mortality: A cost of illness model. Arch Intern Med. 1995;155:1949–1956.
17. Stewart M. Effective physician-patient communication and health outcomes: A review. Can Med Assoc J. 1995;152(9):1423.
18. Sleath B, Roter D, Chewning B, et al. Asking questions about medication—analysis of physician-patient interactions and physician perceptions. Med Care. 1999;37(11):1169–1173.
19. Hall JA, Roter DL, Katz NR. Meta-analysis of correlates of provider behavior in medical encounters. Med Care. 1988;26:657–675.
20. Roter DL, Hall JA, Merisca R, et al. Effectiveness of interventions to improve patient compliance: A meta-analysis. Med Care. 1998;36:1138–1161.
21. Wilkinson I, Darby D, Mant A. Self-care and self-medication: An evaluation of individuals' health care decisions. Med Care. 1987;25(10):965–978.
22. Salerno E, Ries D, San J, et al. Self-medication behaviors. Fla J Hosp Pharm. 1985;5(7): 13–28.
23. Shimp L, Ascione F, Glazer H, et al. Potential medication-related problems in non-institutionalized elderly. DICP. 1985;19(10):766–772.

24. Plein J. Pharmacy's paradigm: Welcoming the challenges and realizing the opportunities. Am J Pharm Ed. 1992;56(4):283–287.
25. Kusserow RP. The Clinical Role of the Community Pharmacist. Report of the Office of the Inspector General. U.S. Government Printing Office, Washington, DC, 1990. p. 1–7.
26. Martin S. What you need to know about OBRA-'90. Am Pharm. 1993;NS33(1):26–28.
27. National Association of Boards of Pharmacy. 1999–2000 Survey of Pharmacy Law, Park Ridge, IL, 1999.
28. Anonymous. APhA surveys states on counseling laws. Am Pharm. 1993;NS33(3):23–24.
29. Ginsberg D, Bair T. States put Medicaid law into practice. Drug Topics. 1993;137(1): 18–20, 23.
30. Nichol MB, Michael LW. Critical analysis of the content and enforcement of mandatory consultation and patient profile laws. Ann Pharmacother. 1992;26:1149–1155.
31. Portner T, Fitzgerald Jr. WJ. OBRA-'90: Turning a challenge into an opportunity. Am Pharm. 1993;NS33(3):67–75.
32. Strand LM, Cipolle RJ, Morley PC. Pharmaceutical Care: An Introduction. Current Concepts. The UpJohn Co., Kalamazoo, MI, 1992. p. 15.
33. Anderson-Harper H, Berger B, Noel R. Pharmacists' predisposition to communicate, desire to counsel and job satisfaction. Am J Pharm Ed. 1992;56(4):252–258.
34. Chi J. Inside today's pharmacist 1992. Part 1: Career and work place. Drug Topics. 1992;136(6):47, 51–52, 57.
35. Meade V. APhA survey looks at patient counseling. Am Pharm. 1992;NS32:27–29.
36. Rybka-Miki C. Reducing stress in pharmacy practice. On Continuing Practice. 1989;16(2): 31–34.
37. Malone D, Rasciti K, Gagnon JP. Consumers' evaluation of value-added pharmacy services. Am Pharm. 1993;NS33(3):48–56.
38. Anonymous. Schering Report XIV, Improving Patient Compliance: Is There a Pharmacist in the House? Schering Laboratories, Kenilworth, NJ, 1992.
39. Schommer J. Patient' expectations and knowledge of patient counseling services that are available from pharmacists. Am J Pharm Ed. 1997;61(1):402–406.
40. Mackowiak JI, Manasse HR. Expectations for ambulatory services in traditional and office-practice pharmacies. Am J Hosp Pharm. 1984;41:1140–1146.
41. Airakisinen M, Vainio K, Koistinen J, et al. Do the public and pharmacists share opinions about drug information. Int J Pharm. 1994;8(4):168–171.
42. Carroll N. Consumer demand for patient oriented services in community pharmacies: A review and comment. J Soc Admin Pharm. 1985;3(2):64–69.
43. Anonymous. Pharmacist's letter. 1992;8(9):49.
44. Anonymous. ASHP guidelines on pharmacy-conducted patient counseling. Am J Hosp Pharm. 1993;50(3):505–506.
45. Strand L, Guerrero R, Nickman N, et al. Integrated patient-specific model of pharmacy practice. Am J Hosp Pharm. 1990;47(3):550–554.
46. Svarstad B, Bultman D, Mount J. Patient counseling provided in community pharmacies: Effects of state regulation, pharmacist age, and busyness. J Am Pharm Assoc. 2004;44: 22–29.
47. De Young M. A review of the research on pharmacists' patient-communication views and practices. Am J Pharm Ed. 1996;60(2):60–76.
48. Deschamps M, Dyck A, Taylor J. What are we saying? Content and organization of patient counseling by community pharmacists. Can Pharm J. 2003;136(6):30–35.
49. Worley M, Schommer J. Pharmacist-patient relationships: Factors influencing quality and commitment. J Soc Admin Pharm. 1999;16(3/4):157–173.

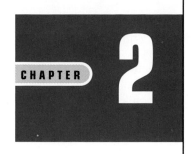

CHAPTER 2

The Definition and Goals of Patient Counseling in Pharmacy

Objectives

After completing the chapter, the reader should be able to

1. differentiate between the terms *patient counseling, consulting,* and *patient education.*
2. list the counseling and education goals of patient counseling in pharmacy.
3. describe the differences between the various models of patient–provider relationships.
4. describe the adult educational approach of andragogy as applied to patient counseling.
5. define patient counseling in pharmacy.

When pharmacists talk about patient counseling, they are often referring to a variety of activities. Each pharmacist may have a different idea of what patient counseling involves. To some, it is simply the provision of drug information; to others, it is the education of the patient about his or her medication and illness; to still others, patient counseling involves a broader range of helping activities. Before proceeding with further discussion about counseling, it is important to clarify what counseling means and what goals we hope to achieve.

THE MEANING OF COUNSELING

The words *counseling, consulting,* and *patient education* are often used interchangeably by pharmacists, but they actually connote different activities and approaches. The word *counsel* is defined in the dictionary as giving advice, but it also implies mutual discussion and an exchange of opinions.[1,2] To *consult* means to seek advice, and suggests almost exclusively receiving advice rather than exchanging information. *Education* involves a slightly different sphere of interaction: It is defined in the dictionary as "instruction and development to impart skills and knowledge."[1,2]

The theories underpinning the professional fields of counseling and education offer more comprehensive explanations of these terms. In counseling theory, for example, counseling is considered similar, in many ways, to psychotherapy.[3] Counseling and psychotherapy involve the same activities, but place emphasis on different areas.

Both involve listening, questioning, evaluating, interpreting, supporting, explaining, informing, advising, and ordering. However, the main emphasis in psychotherapy is on listening, whereas in counseling the emphasis is equally on listening and informing.[3]

In educational theory, education connotes much more than simply imparting knowledge. It may be defined as "progressive changes of a person affecting knowledge, attitudes, and behavior as a result of instruction and study."[4] Education involves processes through which people develop their abilities, and enrich their knowledge, and which help bring about changes in their attitudes or behavior.[5]

From this semantic discussion, it may be seen that the activity that pharmacists refer to as "patient counseling" involves counseling in the psychological sense, as well as activities that aim to educate patients. It encompasses theories of counseling and education in varying degrees, depending on the situation and the needs of the patient.

THEORETICAL ROOTS OF PATIENT COUNSELING

Because a large component of patient counseling is counseling in the psychological sense, it is useful to understand some of the roots of counseling theory.

Behavioral Theory

An important basis of counseling theory is the theory of behavior drawn from the work of B.F. Skinner, who suggested that behavior that is reinforced (rewarded) is repeated and, conversely, behavior that is not reinforced or that is actually punished is not repeated.[6]

A broader approach is cognitive behavior modification.[6] It assumes that it is not the experience alone that is the cause of behavior, it is the individual's underlying cognition of the experience (conceptions, ideas, meanings, beliefs, thoughts, inferences, expectations, predictions, or attributions).[7] These cognitions vary from individual to individual and are acquired throughout the course of life through experiences.[7]

Through counseling, by persuasion and argument, the individual's false assumptions, irrational conclusions, and misconceptions will be changed so that he or she thinks, feels, and behaves on a more rational basis.[7]

Thus, when explaining to the patient the reasons behind medication instructions and the ways in which the medication will treat the condition, the pharmacist attempts to change the patient's thoughts about the usefulness of the medication, and the importance of adherence. This change in the patient's thoughts is expected to result in a behavioral change with regard to taking medication.

Behavior therapy is the source of some of the patient education methods that will be described in Chapters 4 and 6, such as self-monitoring, demonstration (modeling), and practice (behavior rehearsal).

Theories of Health Behavior

Theories of health behavior are also important to the development of counseling skills used in patient counseling. There have been many attempts to analyze why patients behave the way they do when they are ill and need to take medication. Theories of health behavior suggest that patients' perceptions about the severity and possible outcomes of their conditions, the effectiveness and benefits of medication use, and various triggers to taking medication may be critical elements in patient medication use. This will be discussed further in Chapter 3.

These theories indicate that patient counseling involves not only an exchange of information, but should also involve an attempt to change the patient's health beliefs. Behavior change will be discussed further in Chapter 4.

Humanist Approaches to Counseling

The humanist school of psychology considers people's thoughts and feelings in addition to behaviors.[8] When pharmacists counsel patients they should acknowledge that patients are not only behaving (acting) due to external controls of stimulus and reward, but also thinking and feeling. When a patient is nonadherent, not only is he or she acting by not taking his or her medication, but is also doing so because of thoughts and feelings about the illness and medication use. As a result, pharmacists' counseling should take the patient's feelings and thoughts into consideration.

The person-centered approach to counseling, developed by Carl Rogers, is part of humanistic psychology and is one of the greatest influences on the field of counseling.[7] This approach to counseling is based on the idea that people will naturally grow and develop their capacities (self-actualization). A person is able to solve his or her own problems in a relationship with a helping person who is nonjudgmental and where the person feels cared for, genuinely and unconditionally.[8]

From this perspective, the pharmacist helps patients get the most benefit from their therapy by helping them feel capable of controlling their own medication use—in other words, by helping them identify and solve their own problems in this area. This echoes the concepts in pharmaceutical care of patient-centered care.

A key element of Carl Roger's patient-centered helping approach is the pharmacist's genuine feelings of warmth and concern for patients and his or her trust in their abilities to solve their own problems.[8] This is exemplified in part by the pharmacist spending the necessary time with each patient and by the pharmacist's helping attitude during the interaction.

An Eclectic Counseling Theory

A counseling approach described by Gerard Egan seems to synthesize many of the above theories of counseling.[7] The focus of the theory is the process of helping. It is assumed that people are responsible for their own behavior and situation, and that they are essentially capable of solving their own problems.[7] In fact, people cannot solve other people's problems for them; they can only help them do so. The aim of counseling is therefore to help people manage their problems more effectively.[7]

The process of helping described by Egan involves three stages: Clarifying the problem (to explore the individual's viewpoint of the problem); setting goals (achieving an overview of the individual's problems and setting goals to overcome them); and facilitating action (to help the person plan ways of achieving the goals set, to carry out the goals, and to evaluate the outcomes).[7] Again this seems to echo the concepts of pharmaceutical care.

The helping process suggested by Rogers and by Egan's eclectic counseling theory will be further elaborated later in this chapter.

Treatment Decision-Making Models

In the field of medicine, there are a number of models of treatment decision making that describe the relationship between the patient and physician. Although for many health problems there is only one correct course of action, for some conditions there are several options that may have different outcomes in terms of the patient's quality of life and cost-benefits.[9,10] There are actually four different models that describe the ways in which treatment decisions are made: Paternalistic, informed decision making, professional-as-agent, and shared decision making as shown in Table 2-1.[9]

The traditional model has been paternalistic, where it is assumed that the doctor knows best, so that he or she selects the treatment with little patient involvement or consideration of the patient's values or preferences.

The polar opposite of this would be an informed decision-making model whereby the patient alone would make decisions when provided with all necessary technical information. The clinician's role is to provide information to support the patient's decision.

A third model, the professional-as-agent model, is probably closest to the current idea of patient-centered practice; it incorporates the patient's preferences but assumes that only the doctor has sufficient technical knowledge to make a final decision.

TABLE 2-1 Models of Decision Making	
Model Type	**Characteristics**
Paternalistic	Assumes doctor knows best
	Doctor selects treatment
	Patient involvement limited to giving consent
	No consideration of patients' values or preferences
Informed decision making	Patient alone will make decision when provided with all necessary technical information
	Clinician's role is to provide information to support patient in decision
Professional-as-agent	Assumes only doctor has sufficient technical knowledge to make final decision
	Recognizes importance of incorporated patient's preferences
	Final decision made by clinician
Shared decision making	Patient and clinician engage in the decision-making process
	Information and values are shared
	Uses physician's technical knowledge and experience and patient's experience, culture, and preferences

Sources: Coulter A. Partnerships with patients: the pros and cons of shared clinical decision making. J Health Serv Res Policy. 1997;2(2):112–121. Stevenson F, Barry C, Britten N, et al. Doctor-patient communication about drugs: the evidence for shared decision making. Soc Sci & Med. 2000;50:829–840.

More recently there has been a movement to a shared clinical decision-making model in which both the patient and clinician engage in the decision-making process. Information and values are shared; both the physician's technical knowledge and experience and the patient's experience, culture, and preferences are used to come to a decision. This is also referred to as "concordance," which describes and encourages a partnership between patients and professionals when making decisions about health care and drug therapy.[11]

In terms of the pharmacist's relationship with patients, the pharmacist may be in a decision-making position when discussing self-medication, but in the case of prescribed medication, the pharmacist is more in a position of mediating the relationship between physician and patient. It has been noted that a large barrier to shared decision making is efficiently and effectively educating patients so that they can participate in decisions. It is also a challenge for physicians to ascertain patients' preferences and values.[9] Pharmacists are in an ideal position to assist the patient and physician to share information and common understanding. Patients can be educated such that they are able to discuss treatment options with the physician, and they can be helped to recognize their values and preferences and coached to divulge this to the physician. The result should be concordance between patient and his or her health professionals.

DEFINITION OF PATIENT COUNSELING IN PHARMACY

From this discussion it can be seen that counseling is essentially a helping process.[12] The "helper" role for pharmacists has been clearly identified by pharmacy organizations such as the Joint Commission on Pharmacy Practice, which declared in 1991 that "The mission of pharmacy practice is to help people make the best use of medications."[13]

In order to help patients, the pharmacist must also educate them about their illnesses and their medications. An overall definition of patient medication counseling may be stated: Patient medication counseling is pharmacists talking with patients about the medications they are intended to take in order to educate them about medication-related issues and to help them get the most benefit from their medications.

Thus, there are both helping and educational goals of patient counseling in pharmacy.

HELPING GOALS OF PATIENT COUNSELING IN PHARMACY

In order to help patients, the pharmacist must first establish a relationship with the patient and develop trust.[14] The pharmacist must also demonstrate concern and care for the patient in order for him to know that the information the pharmacist is providing and the questions the pharmacist is asking are in the patient's interest.[14]

What does the patient need help with? The essence of all counseling is to help a person cope effectively with an important problem or concern.[12] In the case of patient medication counseling, that problem involves the individual's health and the need to fit medication use into his or her daily life. For example, a patient may need help in planning how he or she can take an antibiotic every 6 hours when he or she is at work part of the day and asleep at night.

Patient counseling might also involve helping the patient cope with illness and with the changes it is likely to bring about in his or her lifestyle. For example, patients with illnesses such as diabetes and high blood pressure may require help in coping with changes in diet as well as changes in work habits and recreational activities.

In addition to dealing with immediate problems, counseling involves interventions to prevent the occurrence of later problems and to develop the individual's capacity to deal with such problems if they should arise.[15] Through patient medication counseling, problems can be anticipated and then prevented or at least minimized through discussion with the patient. Future problems might involve the patient's ability and intention to adhere to the medication directions. For example, a patient going to a party might decide to skip one of his prescribed high blood pressure pills so that he can enjoy a potentially interacting alcoholic beverage at the party. If such situations have been anticipated and discussed with the pharmacist, then the patient can make better decisions when the time comes. The pharmacist could point out the risks of missing a dose of the medication and suggest alternatives to the patient such as restricting himself to nonalcoholic beverages, such as mineral water with lemon, while taking the medication.

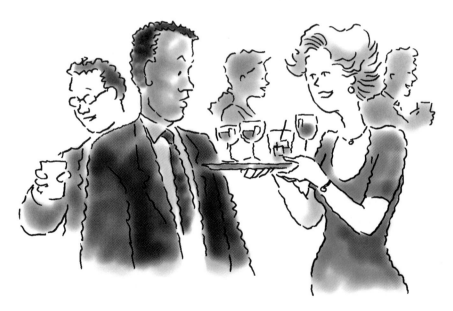

The pharmacist said "no alcohol," but surely one drink can't hurt.

Other future problems might involve the development of side effects or adverse effects. The occurrence of side effects such as constipation or discolored urine may alarm or disturb a patient sufficiently to cause him or her to discontinue the medication. If the patient is forewarned, however, he or she will recognize the symptom as a side effect and know how to handle it (e.g., use a stool softener for constipation), while continuing on the medication.

Similarly, if a patient is told about the signs of possible adverse effects, then such effects can be detected at an early stage, and the physician can be notified before more serious effects set in. In addition, patients who fear possible adverse effects will be reassured by knowing how rarely they occur and by understanding how they can be

TABLE 2-2	Helping Goals of Patient Counseling

1. To establish a relationship with the patient and to develop trust
2. To demonstrate concern and care for the patient
3. To help the patient manage and adapt to his or her medication
4. To help the patient manage and adapt to his or her illness
5. To prevent or minimize problems associated with side effects, adverse effects, or present and future nonadherance
6. To develop the patient's capacity to deal with such problems
7. To help the patient and other health professionals to work together toward shared decision making

detected at an early stage, or even modified. The unknown is often more frightening than the known. Knowing what to expect and what action to take allow the patient to exert some control over unavoidable events.

In the case of repeat medications, the goal of counseling is to detect any of the above problems and ensure that things are proceeding well.

Once present and future problems with medication use have been detected, the goal of counseling is to develop the patient's capacity to deal with such problems. Although some problems will involve the intervention of the physician and perhaps other health professionals (e.g., community visiting nurse), the patient is still an integral part of the problem solution.

Through counseling, the pharmacist can explore the patient's present and future needs. The pharmacist must discover what the patient needs to know; what skills he or she needs to develop; and what problems need to be dealt with. In addition, the pharmacist must determine which behaviors and attitudes need to be modified.

Finally, pharmacists can provide education and gather information from the patients about their needs and preferences in order to support the physician–patient relationship. For example, a patient may tell the pharmacist things that he or she does not want to discuss with the physician, or ask what the pharmacist thinks of the physician's treatment choices. The pharmacist can help both parties to come to a better understanding by encouraging patients to discuss issues with all health professionals and, with the patient's permission, talking with other health professionals on the patient's behalf.

A summary of the helping goals of patient counseling in pharmacy is found in Table 2-2.

The techniques involved in counseling the patient in order to attain these goals will be discussed in Chapters 5–8.

EDUCATIONAL GOALS OF PATIENT COUNSELING IN PHARMACY

To attain the counseling goals of helping the patient in various ways, the pharmacist must also take steps to educate the patient. Education involves enhancing skills and knowledge in order to bring about changes in related attitudes and behaviors.[5]

Pharmacists often think of education as providing verbal or written information. Simply providing information, however, does not guarantee that patients' skills and knowledge about their illnesses and medications will improve, or that the necessary changes in related behavior and attitudes will be affected.

The pharmacist's educational goal will be to provide information that meets the specific needs of each patient. Through discussion with a patient, the pharmacist must first determine how much the patient already knows about the medication in question, and whether he or she holds any misconceptions about the medication or the illness it is meant to treat. For example, a patient may believe that his or her high blood pressure is the result of bad nerves; that "hypertensive" medication is meant to relieve "tension"; and that the medication is needed only when he or she is feeling "hyper." On discovering that the patient holds such views, the pharmacist will know that he must convey clear information about the meaning of high blood pressure, the purpose of the medication, and the importance of taking the medication regularly.

The educational goals of patient counseling also involve investing patients with the skills and techniques they need to optimize their prescribed therapy. For example, a patient may need instruction in the proper use of an inhaler or assistance in devising a method for remembering and following a complicated dosage schedule.

The pharmacist must provide information and instruction in a way that makes them effective for *this* particular patient in *this* particular situation. For example, the information and instructional methods required by a young patient receiving an inhaler for the first time will be quite different from those needed by an elderly patient receiving a new prescription for diabetes treatment in addition to several repeat prescriptions treating arthritis and congestive heart failure. The approach taken in the educational process is an important aspect of dealing with the individual needs of the particular patient and the particular situation.

Finally, pharmacists have opportunities to educate other health professionals about drug-related issues. This may occur in a formal setting such as educating nurses in a nursing home or educating through hospital grand rounds; or the pharmacist may contact a physician or nurse to inform them of a drug-related problem and find the need to educate them about the problem (e.g., mechanism of an interaction) and alternative solutions.

These educational goals of patient counseling are summarized in Table 2-3.

TABLE 2-3   **Educational Goals of Patient Counseling**

1. To provide information appropriate to the particular individual and the particular problem
2. To provide skills and methods that the patient can use to optimize the usage and effects of the medication
3. To present information and instruction using educational methods that are appropriate to the particular individual and the particular situation
4. To educate other health professionals about drug-related issues

PHARMACISTS AS HELPERS AND EDUCATORS

Now that the goals of patient counseling have been discussed, the way that pharmacists attain these goals should be considered. As discussed above, the goals involve helping and educating the patient; it follows, then, that the pharmacist must approach the patient-counseling encounter as a helper and an educator.

The Helping Approach

Pharmacists have traditionally been involved in the preparation and dispensing of medication, at the direction of the physician. As such, they have been strongly allied with the medical profession and, hence, with the view that the health professional should be in control of the patient. But, with the shift in the model of pharmacy from a focus on the medication to a focus on the patient, there is a need for a shift in the pharmacist's approach as well. This shift can be described as moving from the health professional–centered "medical-model" approach to the patient-centered "helping-model" approach.

The medical model and the helping model contrast with respect to the relationship between the health professional and the patient, which differs in the two models in a number of areas: The role of each party in the relationship; the basis for trust; the approach to problem solving; and the allowance for the solving of future problems.[16]

In the medical model, the health professional is active and the patient is passive; in the helping model, both patient and health professional are active. In the medical model, the basis for trust is the presumed expertise and authority of the health professional, to which the patient automatically responds. In the helping model, trust is not automatic, but grows slowly, based on the personal relationship—trust develops mutually between the professional and the patient.

Although in both models a need to solve a problem is the reason for the relationship, their approaches to problem solving are considerably different. In the medical model, the health professional identifies the problem, analyzes information, arrives at a diagnosis, and gives direction to work on the solution. The patient is responsible only for answering questions and following directions. In the helping model, the professional assists the patient in exploring the problem and possible solutions. The patient is responsible for drawing conclusions, making decisions, and selecting a solution he or she can follow.

In the medical model, the patient becomes dependent on the professional. As a result, the patient must return to the health professional to deal with future problems in the previously learned way and to seek help if necessary. In the helping model, the patient develops self-confidence to manage his or her own problems.

The relationship between the health professional and the patient in the medical model is more akin to a parent–child relationship than to the equal, adult relationship that characterizes the helping model.

The comparison as summarized in Table 2-4 is very black and white, and is probably an oversimplification of what is indeed a complicated process.[16] In reality, a range of approaches exists, on a continuum from the health professional–centered medical-model

TABLE 2-4	The Helping Approach: Relationship between Health Professional and Patient

Medical Model	Helping Model
Patient is passive	Patient is actively involved
Basis for trust is expertise and authority of health professional	Trust is based on personal relationship developed over time
Health professional identifies problems and determines solutions	Health professional assists patient in exploring problem and possible solutions
Patient is dependent on health professional	Patient develops self-confidence to manage problems
Parent–child relationship	Equal relationship

Adapted from Anderson TP. An Alternative Frame of Reference for Rehabilitation: The Helping Process versus the Medical Model. In: Marinelli R, Dell Orto A., eds. The Psychological and Social Impact of Physical Disability. New York: Springer, 1977: 18–20, with permission from The American Congress of Rehabilitation Medicine and the American Academy of Physical Medicine and Rehabilitation.

approach to the patient-centered helping-model approach. Pharmacists must decide for themselves where on the continuum they feel most comfortable in their relationship with the patient, and also where the patient may feel most comfortable. To attain the counseling goals most effectively, however, the pharmacist must lean more heavily toward the helping-model approach.

The Educational Approach

When pharmacists approach the educational aspects of patient counseling, they often become "teachers," adapting a style that they recall from when they were taught as children. However, in the majority of cases, patient counseling involves dealing with adults. Although fundamentally adults and children learn in the same way, differences exist between learning process and in conditions surrounding learning when dealing with children (pedagogy) compared to adults (andragogy).[17]

There are four basic concepts that illuminate the conditions and processes of adult learning as summarized in Table 2-5: (a) self-concept; (b) experience; (c) readiness to learn; and (d) time perspective and orientation to learning.[17]

Self-concept

When educating children, the relationship between teacher and learner is a directing one, in which the learner is dependent and the teacher dominant. Adults tend to resent being treated as though they were children and perceive this as a lack of respect, being talked down to, or being judged.[17] As a result, they may not follow medication directions and may not admit to nonadherence or concerns about their conditions since they may fear being ridiculed or scolded.

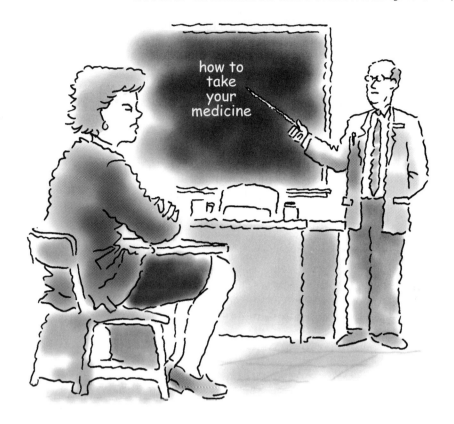

Adults don't like to be taught as if children.

TABLE 2-5	**The Educational Approach: Conditions and Process of Adult Learning**

1. Helping relationship, with reciprocity
2. Patient's experience is drawn upon as a resource in learning
3. Educational methods involve two-way communication techniques such as group techniques, discussions, simulation, role-playing, and skill-practice sessions
4. Educational tasks involve subjects of immediate concern and importance in the individual's daily life
5. Adults choose what they want to learn, and when
6. Learning is problem-centered, and involves identifying and solving the problem in the present

Based on information presented in Knowles MS. What is andragogy. In: The Modern Practice of Adult Education. Englewood Cliffs, NJ: Prentice Hall Regents, 1970; 40–62.

In adult education, the teacher and learner develop a helping relationship, characterized by reciprocity in the teaching–learning transaction.[17] The pharmacist must join with the patient to help solve problems relating to his or her illness and medication use.

Experience

Adults accumulate a vast range of experience over the course of their lifetime, which contributes to the way they view and interpret new experiences, and the way they approach the need for new information.[17]

In relation to illness and medication, patients may have certain beliefs arising out of previous experiences of their own or out of those of others that they have heard about. For example, a patient may have experienced an unpleasant side effect from a medication taken in the past, and therefore may be reluctant to use medication, even when it is prescribed for the treatment of a life-threatening condition.

When teaching adults, pharmacists can draw upon patients' experiences as a resource. Two-way communication techniques, such as group discussions, simulation, role-playing, and skill-practice sessions, will allow this.[17] The use of a variety of techniques, rather than simply presenting a lecture about medications, is likely to be most effective. Such techniques will be discussed in Chapters 5 and 6.

Readiness to Learn

The subjects that adults need to learn are usually of immediate concern and importance in their daily lives.[17] This is certainly the case in pharmacy, where for example, a patient may need to learn how to use an inhaler or how to cope with an illness while continuing to work and participate in other social functions.

Adults make themselves available for learning because of their perception of a particular need in a particular area (e.g., in the context of health, the need for assistance with breathing). Adults will choose what they need to know (e.g., how to use an inhaler) and when they want to learn about it (e.g., when they pick up the prescription or later when they have time to talk). Patients must perceive the need for the medication and for proper instruction in its use before they will be prepared to learn about, for example, inhaler use, and make themselves available for the necessary instruction. Rather than forging ahead with instructions, the pharmacist must act as a resource person to help patients discover their own learning needs.

Time Perspective and Orientation to Learning

Adult education involves issues of concern in the individual's life at present and is problem-centered.[17] Through discussion with the patient, the pharmacist can avoid providing extraneous information—the kind that does not apply to the particular patient or the particular situation. Instructing a patient to avoid operating hazardous machinery while using a medication, for example, is a useless exercise for both the pharmacist and patient if that patient is an 80-year-old woman who neither drives nor works in a factory. It is up to the pharmacist to discover from the patient the kind of information that will be useful for solving that patient's specific problems and then tailor the counseling to the particular patient. Aspects of "tailoring" in patient counseling will be discussed in Chapter 8.

SUMMARY

This chapter has defined patient counseling in pharmacy, the goals and the approach to counseling. Throughout it has been emphasized that the patient is at the center of the patient-counseling approach. Therefore, it is important for the pharmacist to try to understand patients' perspectives in relation to illness and medication use. This will be discussed in the following two chapters.

REFLECTIVE QUESTIONS

1. Demonstrating how to use a blood glucose monitor would be considered patient education. What could be added to the interaction with the patient to fit the definition of patient counseling?
2. According to the humanist school of thought, what elements need to be considered when counseling a patient on smoking cessation?
3. What aspects of the helping and educational processes would be applied in the following steps of pharmaceutical care: Collecting and interpreting patient information; listing and ranking drug-related problems; determining feasible alternatives; selecting and individualizing the most appropriate drug regimen; and designing a drug-monitoring plan?
4. What principles of adult education make parenting groups an ideal opportunity to talk to people about medication safety and poison control?

REFERENCES

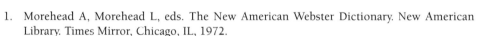

1. Morehead A, Morehead L, eds. The New American Webster Dictionary. New American Library. Times Mirror, Chicago, IL, 1972.
2. Funk CE. New Practical Standard Dictionary. Funk and Wagnalls, New York, 1950.
3. Corsini RJ. Introduction. In: Current Psychotherapies, 3rd Edition. FE Peacock Publishers, Inc., Itasca, IL, 1984, p. 1–13.
4. Lively BT. The community pharmacist and health education. Contemp Pharm Pract. 1982;5:14–20.
5. Knowles MS. What is Andragogy? In: The Modern Practice of Adult Education. Prentice Hall Regents, Englewood Cliffs, NJ, 1970, p. 40–62.
6. Wilson G. Behavior Therapy. In: Corsini R, eds., Current Psychotherapies, 3rd Edition. FE Peacock Publishers, Inc., Itasca, IL, 1984, p. 239–278.
7. Davis H, Fallowfield L. Counseling Theory. In: Davis H, Fallowfield L, eds., Counseling and Communication in Health Care. John Wiley & Sons, Chichester, England, 1991, p. 23–58.
8. Meach B, Rogers C. Person-centered Therapy. In: Corsini R, eds., Current Psychotherapies, 3rd Edition. FE Peacock Publishers, Inc., Itasca, IL, 1984, p. 142–195.
9. Coulter A. Partnerships with patients: The pros and cons of shared clinical decision making. J Health Serv Res Policy. 1997;2(2):112–121.
10. Stevenson F, Barry C, Britten N, et al. Doctor–patient communication about drugs: The evidence for shared decision making. Soc Sci Med. 2000;50:829–840.
11. Smith F, Francis S, Rowley E. Group interviews with people taking long-term medication: Comparing the perspectives of people with arthritis, respiratory disease and mental health problems. Int J Pharm Pract. 2000;8(6):88–96.

12. Eisenberg S, Delaney DJ. The Counseling Process, 2nd Edition. Rand McNally College Publishing, Chicago, IL, 1977, p. 12–31.
13. Anonymous. JCCP provisional draft mission statement for pharmacy practice. NARD Newsletter. 1991:4.
14. Leibowitz K. Improving your patient counseling skills. Am Pharm. 1993;33:465–469.
15. Krumboltz JD, Thoresen CE. Counseling Methods. Holt, Rinehart and Winston, New York, 1976, p. 1–25.
16. Anderson TP. An Alternative Frame of Reference for Rehabilitation: The Helping Process Versus the Medical Model. In: Marinelli R, Dell Orto AE, eds., The Psychological and Social Impact of Physical Disabilities. Springer-Verlag, New York, 1977, p. 18–20.
17. Ingalls JD. A Trainer's Guide to Andragogy. Data Education, Inc., Waltham, MA, 1976.

CHAPTER 3

Understanding Patients' Needs, Wishes, and Preferences

Objectives

After completing the chapter, the reader should be able to

1. explain how factors described in the Health Belief Model help to explain people's behaviors in relation to medication use.
2. describe patients' potential emotional reactions to illness and how they may affect their behavior.
3. describe how people feel about medication use and information about it.
4. discuss strategies pharmacists can use to improve patients' quality of life (QOL).

From the preceding discussion about the goals of counseling, it follows that, in each counseling situation, the pharmacist needs to determine the particular needs, wishes, and preferences of each individual patient's health. The specific details of what needs to be done to accomplish those goals for each individual patient need to be determined. Consider the following two patients:

Mrs. Jones is receiving a prescription for high blood pressure and says to the pharmacist, "I know Dr. Harris told me I need this, but I feel fine. My mother and father both lived into their 90s and never needed pills. Maybe I don't really need them."

The next patient, Mr. Hoffman, receives a prescription for the same medication as Mrs. Jones. He comments to the pharmacist, "I know my blood pressure is pretty high, and I should be taking these pills regularly, but I have a busy schedule and I find it difficult remembering to take them."

These two patients have different counseling needs. Mrs. Jones needs help in understanding her illness and the necessity to take medication daily, whereas Mr. Hoffman needs help in remembering and scheduling his medication.

Decisions about the patient's needs, preferences, and wishes must be made fairly quickly, sometimes without the aid of complete background information. The specific goals of counseling for the individual can be determined in part through discussion with the patient—by means of open questions and probing. These techniques will be discussed further in Chapter 7.

The pharmacist must also gain a sense of what a patient's feelings and concerns are in order to establish a relationship with the patient, to help direct the discussion, and to decide on an approach to the patient's situation. Pharmacists who have a general

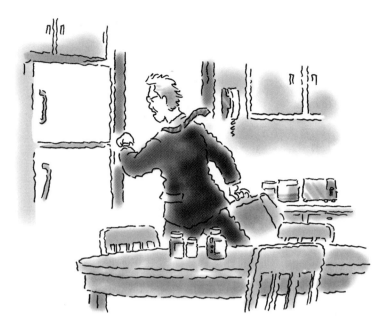

"I have a busy schedule and I find it difficult to remember to take my medication."

understanding of how people feel about being ill and about using medication will have a better idea of how to proceed with the individual counseling session.

ILLNESS AND SICKNESS: THE PATIENT'S PERSPECTIVE

The World Health Organization defines health as "a state of complete physical, mental, and social well being, and not just the absence of disease and infirmity."[1] Conversely, then, illness can be seen as more than just the presence of disease. The terms *illness* and *sickness* are used interchangeably by most people, but they actually suggest different perspectives.[2] *Sickness* refers to the limited scientific concept of a diagnosed medical condition, whereas *illness* refers to an individual's perception of any condition that causes that individual to be concerned and seek help. The study of illness behavior, or health-related behavior, considers issues surrounding the individual's perceptions of symptoms.[2]

Symptoms are perceived, evaluated, and acted on (or not acted on) differently by different people and in different social situations.[2] Individuals may differ in their attentiveness to pain and symptoms; in the way that they define pain and symptoms; and in the extent to which they seek help, make claims on others, and adjust their schedules to accommodate illness.

In understanding the individual's perception of illness, it is important to recognize that illness does not lend itself to rigid definition. The individual continually evaluates and re-evaluates the severity and meanings of symptoms in various situations.[3] Illness behavior involves an attempt to make sense of symptoms and to cope with them.[2] The evaluative and coping processes, and the decisions that result from them, may be limited by the individual's intelligence, as well as by his or her social and cultural understanding.[2,4]

The pharmacist who provides pharmaceutical care must think in terms of the patient's illness rather than the medically defined sickness condition. The patient's perception of illness in this sense can affect his or her attitude and behavior in relation to using medication. Consider that when a patient is receiving a prescription for an antibiotic, he or she is not just a case of "strep throat," but rather an individual who is experiencing discomfort swallowing, who has had to take the day off from work, and who wants some sympathy from family members. Likewise, when dispensing refill prescriptions, the pharmacist should consider that a patient's perceptions of illness may be changing; an original lack of concern about a sore throat may now have become worry over the implications of a longer-term condition, concern over being off work longer than expected, and possibly questions about the physician's and pharmacist's abilities to treat the condition.

HEALTH BELIEFS AND BEHAVIOR

Health-related behavior has been the subject of considerable research and theorizing. Theories pertaining to health-related behavior were developed primarily to understand the failure among patients to adhere to medical treatments and to follow preventive health measures, such as immunization and regular health examinations.[5] A variety of models have been constructed to help explain such behaviors.[2] One such model—the Health Belief Model—contains elements that are also found in many of the others, and therefore it will be used here as the basis of a discussion of the general concept of health-related behavior. Figure 3-1 illustrates this model.

The Health Belief Model suggests that the likelihood that an individual will take action in the interest of his or her health depends largely on that person's perception of the threat posed by a particular disease.[6] For example, patients who believe that high blood pressure may result in a heart attack are thought to be more likely than others to take their high blood pressure medication, watch their diet, exercise, and have regular physical checkups.

The perception of the threat of disease, however, depends on many factors, including so-called modifying factors, individual perceptions, and triggers to action.[6] Modifying factors can include a host of variables ranging from the demographic (age, gender, race, ethnicity, and so on) and the socio-psychologic (personality, social class, peer and reference-group pressure) to the structural (knowledge about the disease, prior contact with the disease, and so forth). For example, a sexually active girl who is cautious by nature, knows about birth-control methods, and has a friend who became pregnant may perceive that the chances of becoming pregnant are high. She is therefore very likely to use birth control.

Individual perceptions of the seriousness of a disease and of personal susceptibility to that disease may also affect a person's perception of its threat. For example, an individual may believe that high blood pressure is not a serious disease at all, and that it is unlikely to have a life-threatening effect.

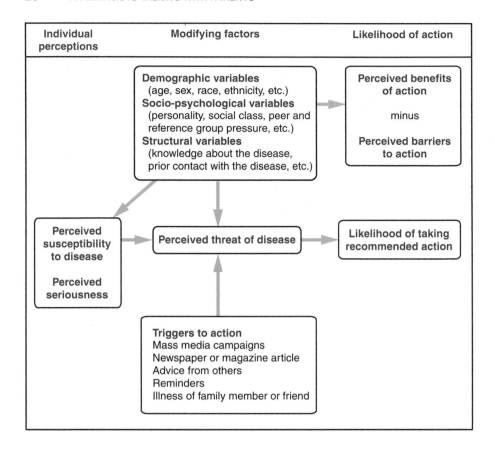

Figure 3-1   **The Health Belief Model (Adapted from Becker MH, Rosenstock IM. Compliance with Medical Advice. In: Steptoe A, Mathews A, eds., Health Care and Human Behaviour. Academic Press, London, 1984.)**

Individual perceptions are determined, to a degree, by modifying factors.[6] For example, an individual whose parents lived to a very old age and who believes that any serious illness should have some obvious symptoms may believe that his or her family is not very susceptible to heart disease and that his or her diagnosed high blood pressure is not very serious. Therefore, he or she may not consider the condition to be much of a threat and may consequently fail to take prescribed medication or follow advice about diet and regular checkups.

External factors can also affect an individual's perception of the threat of a disease and act as a trigger to action. Articles or campaigns in the media, advice from others, and similar illness among family members or friends may constitute triggers to action.[6] For example, reports in the media about the spread of an influenza virus, combined with reports of numerous deaths from the flu among the elderly population, might trigger the perception in elderly individuals that influenza poses a real threat to them, and lead them to get influenza vaccinations.

Even though the perceived threat of disease may be high, an individual may still fail to take action because of various factors that limit his or her ability to do so; in other words, because the perceived barriers to action outweigh the perceived benefits of action.[6] For example, an individual who has difficulty paying for high blood pressure medication may fail to take it regularly, even though he or she believes that it would be beneficial to do so.

In a review of 46 studies involving the Health Belief Model, Janz and Becker found that barriers to action represented the most important variable in explaining health-related behavior. This was followed, in descending order of importance, by perception of susceptibility, benefits of action, and perception of seriousness or severity of the condition.[7]

Interestingly, the findings of studies exploring preventive-health behavior are significantly different from those of studies that seek to explain nonadherence. This suggests that certain variables are more important in some situations than in others.[6] In addition, studies involving patients in various age groups, with differing medical conditions, find different factors to be important.[8] Perhaps the most important outcome of this research is the recognition that health-related behavior is extremely complicated and involves many variables—not just an individual's knowledge or personality.

For the pharmacist, this means that each counseling situation must be approached with an open mind with respect to the way the patient may be feeling about his or her illness and about medication use. Together, pharmacist and patient must explore the factors that are involved in the patient's individual situation, and determine which of them might be most important. For example, a patient whose job involves driving a truck will be concerned about the barriers to taking his prescribed medication regularly—he won't want to risk possible drowsiness on the job and may not have the opportunity to take regular doses. Another patient may think that there is not much point in taking his high blood pressure medication because he isn't very concerned about this condition and doesn't believe that the medication will do much good anyway—i.e., perception of threat is low.

PATIENTS' FEELINGS ABOUT ILLNESS

Another important aspect of illness that a pharmacist needs to consider when dealing with a patient is the individual's emotional reaction to illness. Although people seek help for symptoms for a variety of reasons, they are most often prompted by concern about the potential seriousness of their symptoms or by the disruption of their normal ability to function, or both. In some cases, the symptoms and the series of events leading up to seeking and receiving help can arouse strong feelings. If pharmacists are able to recognize and understand these emotions, they will be able to interact and help patients more effectively.

The range of emotions that may be experienced by individuals can include frustration, fear and anxiety, feelings of damage, anger, dependency, guilt, depression, and loss of self-esteem.[9,10] These feelings may occur in varying degrees in different people and in different situations, and may even be encountered in patients with seemingly minor conditions, such as hemorrhoids or acne.

Frustration

It isn't difficult to understand the frustration associated with being ill. Most people have a routine in their lives, which is disrupted, to various degrees, by being ill. Perhaps the least of the disruptions is taking the time to visit the physician, and then the pharmacy. Frustration results from having to delay usual activities, as well as from unfamiliar restrictions, such as the inability to perform simple actions—for example, walking a certain distance or even laughing without pain or discomfort. The patient may also feel frustrated by the loss of certain pleasures, such as eating a highly spiced gourmet meal or enjoying sexual activities.[9] The treatment for the condition may also cause frustration if it results in loss of pleasure, for example, not being allowed to drink alcohol because of its interaction with the medication.[9]

Such frustrations may manifest themselves in the patient's anger or impatience toward the pharmacist or in nonadherence, or both.[10] Although pharmacists cannot counteract the causes of these frustrations, they can encourage patients to find alternative pleasures and ways to minimize the inconvenience of delaying routine activities. They can also encourage patients, where appropriate, to resume as many of their normal activities as possible.[9]

Fear and Anxiety

Patients may experience feelings of fear as a result of real or imagined problems relating to their illness.[9,10] They may fear the physical outcome of their disease (e.g., pain, disfigurement, death, or long-term disability); the worsening of symptoms (e.g., more severe pain or permanent disability); the adverse effects of treatments; or the social consequences of the illness (e.g., the shock, disgust, or fear experienced by friends or family, embarrassment, and loss of employment).

Although fear is often apparent in the patient's physical appearance and manner (nervousness, pallor, and perspiration), it can be less obvious and more difficult to detect. The patient may report physical symptoms such as stomach upsets, diarrhea, headaches, raised blood pressure, and muscular tension. Fear can also manifest itself in the patient's behavior—in the nervous repetition of questions, the demand for attention, and the need for reassurance.

When the pharmacist perceives that fear is present, he or she can help the patient by making it clear he or she recognizes and accepts these feelings and by encouraging the patient to discuss them. The pharmacist may also be able to help alleviate certain fears by explaining symptoms and their possible outcomes, and by putting such fears into proper perspective. Reassurance can be given where appropriate, and aid in terms of referral to self-help groups or counseling may also be offered.[9]

Feeling of Damage

Another emotion sometimes aroused by illness is a feeling of damage.[9] This emotion may occur not only in illnesses where disfigurement or paralysis is evident, but in association with other illnesses as well. Patients may perceive themselves to be impaired or "different" in some way, simply because their bodies are no longer functioning in their normal capacities, or because they need to take medication. The patient's self-image and body image have been damaged.[9]

By recognizing this emotion and by allowing the patient the opportunity to discuss it, the pharmacist may be able to help the patient come to terms with the feeling and, possibly, to see ways of resolving it.

Anger, Dependency, and Guilt

A patient's experience of illness is affected by his or her background of emotional reactions to previous illnesses, and by patterns of behaving and coping developed during his or her lifetime.[9] Emotions such as anger, dependence, and guilt are expressed during illness primarily as a result of previous life experiences.[9]

Feelings of anger by the patient may or may not be verbalized. If such feelings are verbalized, they may be disruptive and upsetting to all; if they are not, they may still result in destructive behavior by the patient.[9] The pharmacist must recognize that anger shown by the patient, for example, while waiting for a prescription, may simply be the result of frustration as discussed above. This would best be dealt with by the pharmacist discussing the cause of anger with the patient.

As a result of their life experiences, patients sometimes become very dependent during illness, or alternatively refuse to become dependent at all.[9] Although dependence is necessary to a degree during severe illness, patients should be encouraged to become self-dependent.

For various personal reasons, patients may also feel guilt regarding their illness, or an inability to function normally.[9] Patients who experience guilt may appear passive and tolerant, communicate minimally, and appear withdrawn. Again, the pharmacist will need to discover if the patient's passivity is a result of guilt, and let the patient know that he or she recognizes, accepts, and understands such feelings.

Depression and Loss of Self-esteem

When the emotions discussed above are allowed to continue without relief, they may progress to feelings of depression and loss of self-esteem.[9] Depression is recognizable by withdrawal and unwillingness to talk, eat, or engage in activity as well as difficulty sleeping and loss of enjoyment of previously enjoyable activities. Pharmacists should deal with depression by being aware of it and by directing the patient to professional psychological help.[9]

Self-esteem is a combination of one's values, attitudes, and assumptions about oneself.[9] Prolonged or severe illness and the resulting dependency on others can result in loss of self-esteem. This is more difficult for the pharmacist to recognize, but may be apparent in the patient's acceptance of illness and an attitude of defeat. Again, the pharmacist should be alert to identifying this feeling and should recommend additional help. There are also some ways that pharmacists can help improve a patient's self-esteem. For example, pharmacists can allow patients to have some feeling of control over their illness or treatment (e.g., involving them in treatment choices, showing them how to monitor symptoms, allowing them to decide whether they want a tablet or liquid, twice or four times daily dosage). The pharmacist can further improve the patient's self-esteem by showing concern about, and interest in, the patient.

Feelings Connected with Death and Dying

The most extreme and difficult situation that the pharmacist must deal with is one involving a dying patient and his or her family. Health professionals often try to avoid such situations, because they don't know how to react to the patient. In addition, the situation may arouse the pharmacist's own fears associated with death as well as frustration at not being able to prevent the patient's death and suffering.[11]

In a pioneering study, Elisabeth Kübler-Ross observed dying patients and identified five stages that the terminally ill patient may go through.[12] Not all patients progress through each stage in the same order, and some may remain in one stage or even repeat stages. The five stages, as described in Table 3-1, are denial, anger, bargaining, depression, and acceptance.

TABLE 3-1	Stages of Dying and How the Pharmacist Can Help	
Stage	**Patient Behavior**	**How the Pharmacist Can Help**
Denial "No, not me"	A self-protective reaction mechanism in response to the initial shock Patient may dismiss or question the diagnosis even after it has been confirmed by a second opinion	Understand, listen May need to repeat information since patient may not absorb it all Do not try to convince
Anger "Why me?"	Anger toward people and objects May blame, question, and challenge, envying those who are well Feeling of helplessness Often complains continually and drives others away, thus becoming lonely	Try not to get angry in return Don't just take the anger but try to find out why the patient is angry Let patient vent feelings Listen Empathize, recognize that the patient is not angry with you
Bargaining "Yes, me—but..."	Tries to accept the situation Tries to bargain with God and people for more time	Listen Help patient focus on what is possible, rather than on the impossible
Depression "Yes, me"	Realizes the truth and now grieves and mourns May be very silent; may cry	Allow patient to express sorrow Allow privacy, but listen if patient wants to talk
Acceptance "I'm ready"	No longer angry or depressed Not bitter resignation, but a need to deal with unfinished business May separate himself or herself from others and wish to be with only one loved person by his or her side	Allow for privacy

Adapted from Jang R. Emotional Reaction to Illness and Treatment. In: Communication Skills in Patient Counseling on OTC Drugs. Health Sciences Consortium, Chapel Hill, NC, 1980; Kübler-Ross E. What is it like to be dying? Am J Nurs. 1971;71(1):54–60; Okolo N, McReynolds J. Counseling the terminally ill. Am Pharm. 1987;27(9):37–40.

Denial is a common first reaction for patients to go through on discovering they have a terminal illness. This is a kind of self-protective mechanism during which the patient copes with the situation by questioning the diagnosis even after a second opinion, or simply dismisses the prognosis. Although the patient is trying to assimilate information about his or her illness, the patient may need information to be repeated by the pharmacist. The pharmacist should not attempt to convince the patient of the truth of the situation, and should be prepared to be understanding of the patient's point of view and simply listen.

When coping with terminal illness, patients may become angry, and express anger toward various people and objects. They may blame, question, challenge, and continually complain, often driving people away so that they become lonely. The pharmacist should try not to take the anger personally. He or she should listen, allow the patient to vent his or her feelings, and try to empathize.

Patients often try to accept their situation by bargaining with caregivers and with God for more time. Again the pharmacist should be prepared to listen, but may also help by trying to focus on the possible rather than the impossible.

Because of the hopelessness of the illness and treatment, imminent separation from loved ones, and loss of contact with the outside world, terminally ill patients often become depressed. The patient is grieving and may become silent or often cry. The pharmacist should provide privacy, but be prepared to listen and encourage sharing of feelings if the patient wishes.

Some patients reach an acceptance of their situation, during which they seem ready to die. They may appear devoid of feelings, but are not bitter. They may wish to be alone with loved ones only. The pharmacist should honor this wish for privacy, and offer help where appropriate in dealing with unfinished business.

Pharmacists can help their patients and their patients' families by recognizing these stages and dealing with them accordingly. Suggestions for communicating with critically ill patients will be discussed further in Chapter 8.

PATIENTS' FEELINGS ABOUT MEDICATION AND COUNSELING

From the medical perspective discussed in the previous chapter, patients take medication because it has been prescribed and because they have been advised by a medical authority to do so. From the helping perspective, however, we recognize that patients take medication for a variety of personal reasons. In order to help patients get the most benefit from their medication, the pharmacist must learn to view medication use from the patient's perspective.

Patients with different disease conditions may have different beliefs about medications and different patient groups may also have different needs and desires for information and counseling.[13–17]

Reasons for Taking Medication

Patients may have a variety of personal reasons for taking medication.[13] In a study of anticonvulsant users, the reason most commonly given was practical. Patients saw medication use as a fact of life, necessary if seizures were to be controlled, and social and personal disruptions avoided. The second was psychologic—to reduce worry. The third reason was the desire to ensure "normality," in the sense of leading a "normal life" without seizures. In addition, for these individuals, using medication was not only a part of everyday life, but became a sign of illness, symbolizing, to themselves and others, that they were different and, perhaps, inferior.

Patients are constantly making independent decisions about whether to take their medication and about the manner in which they will do so.[14] When patients are given information and advice from health professionals, they make decisions to modify their health behaviors by considering new information in light of previously held information, experiences, beliefs, and biases.[14]

Bias affects the way patients acquire and process information during the decision-making process. For example, patients don't always gather information from all sides before making a decision, and some patients decide that the information they have gathered does not necessarily apply in their particular case.

In addition, patients have difficulty processing large amounts of "probabilistic information," such as the chances of side effects occurring or the consequences that could arise if their condition were to continue unchecked.

Most importantly, it has been found that patients' decision-making processes are not always logical. Pharmacists need to understand this decision-making process and be nonjudgmental about the illogical ways in which people make decisions.

Beliefs about Counseling and Information

Pharmacists generally believe that patients primarily want information about how to take their medication and how to store it, and that too much information deters adherence.[18,19] But studies show that patients most desire information about side effects and drug interactions; and that providing information does not harm, and in fact correlates with improved adherence.[16,18–21]

Patients want basic information about the medical condition being treated, and specific information about side effects, duration of treatment, and range of available treatment options.[19] However, patients may vary in their preferences for information and involvement in the treatment process.[22] Morris et al. classified patients in terms of how they viewed information as physician reliant, pharmacist reliant, questioners, and the uninformed (those that received little information and believed that one need not ask questions if one trusts the doctor).[23]

Patients want information at different times in their treatment. Zehnder et al. found that one-third of patients studied wanted comprehensive drug information only after they asked, one quarter wanted the most important aspects provided each time; one third wanted comprehensive information only the first time they received a drug, and one tenth wanted comprehensive drug information each time.[16] There was also a slight variation between the type of information desired for prescription and nonprescription drugs.

The patients' need for cognition has the strongest effect on their expectation for counseling from pharmacists.[24] Older patients were found to perceive less need for cognition, but their previous experience with counseling and self-perceived need for knowledge increased the expectation for counseling.[24]

It has been suggested that pharmacist–patient interaction is reliant on the patients' desire for information, so that if they do not see the need for information, do not know that the pharmacist can provide it, or if they are too embarrassed, intimidated, or shy, they will not ask for information.[24] As a result the pharmacist will provide less information, spend less time counseling, or may even be unable to counsel.[24]

Not all patients ask questions.[25] For patient-centered health care, patients need to be empowered to participate. Factors influencing question-asking in the pharmacy include explicit invitation to participate, encouragement, expectations for information, ability to articulate the question, and actually getting answers.[26]

Patients also desire a qualitative dimension to the patient–pharmacist interaction.[27] Patients want to feel at ease in the pharmacy, to have privacy, and to feel included. They want to understand the information, feel confident in the quality of counseling, and to feel genuine concern from the pharmacy staff.[27]

Feelings About Risk

Patients generally want information about side effects, but how risk is presented and understood makes this a challenge. Studies of how to present side-effect information reveal that when given a verbal description of risk, e.g., very common or very rare, people tend to overestimate the likelihood of the adverse effect compared to numerical risk information, e.g., 1 in 100,000.[28]

Patients can, however, get information overload, decreasing their ability to assimilate information provided.[29] It is helpful to present risk in a balanced and simple way, comparing risk of medication with everyday risks, e.g., risk of road accident.[29] Patients expect pharmacists and physicians to share the responsibility of risk counseling about the appropriate choice of medication; and they expect pharmacists to provide information on how to manage and avoid risk.[24]

CONSIDERING HEALTH-RELATED QUALITY OF LIFE

When we consider how patients feel about being ill and taking medication, we should also take into consideration the effects of illness and medication on the patient's quality of life (QOL). This concept takes into account a person's physical, emotional, mental, and intellectual capacity; his or her ability to function at work, in social situations, and within the family; perception of his or her abilities; and satisfaction with those abilities.[30]

Health care policy makers, pharmaceutical companies, third-party payers, and the Food and Drug Administration now recognize QOL issues when evaluating pharmaceuticals.[30] In terms of pharmaceutical care, pharmacists must consider the patient's QOL when they identify and prioritize medication-related problems, determine treatment goals, and develop monitoring protocols. For example, when pharmacists consider outcomes of treatment, they should realize that measures such as sedimentation rate or blood pressure mean little to the patient, but that physical discomfort, the ability to walk briskly up the stairs, and financial impact have real-world significance. They can realize that a patient taking antihypertensive medication may perceive that his or her QOL has actually been reduced because of unpleasant side effects, reduced feeling of well-being, increased medical expenses, and restricted activities. This may result in

TABLE 3-2 Pharmacist's Contribution to Patients' Quality of Life
1. Discuss with the patient whether the therapy is likely to interfere with important aspects of his or her lifestyle
2. Explain to the patient what he or she can and cannot expect from therapy and help the patient weigh the benefits against costs
3. Offer suggestions on how to minimize the impact of negative effects of therapy on the patient's QOL
4. Be prepared for medication-induced patient complaints
5. Communicate medication-related QOL complaints to the physician and suggest alternatives
6. Include lifestyle characteristics such as hobbies and occupation on the patient's medication profile

Source: Smith M, Juergens J, Jack W. Medication and the Quality of Life. Am. Pharm. 1991; NS31(4):27–33.

nonadherence, reduced confidence in physician and pharmacist, as well as worsening of the medical condition because of a negative outlook. The physician, however, may see blood pressure reduced and consider therapy to be a success.[30]

Although pharmacists don't have access to detailed information about patients' lives when counseling, some of it can be illuminated through discussion. Pharmacists can at least anticipate QOL effects and help the patient and physician take them into consideration in selecting and evaluating therapy. Some suggestions of how the pharmacist can contribute are listed in Table 3-2.

SUMMARY

This chapter has touched on the very complicated area of health and illness theory. These findings about patients' feelings and beliefs regarding illness and taking medication seem to suggest at least one thing very clearly: That simply telling patients to take their medication, or simply providing information about the medication, will not necessarily result in patient adherence—the subject of the next chapter.

REFLECTIVE QUESTIONS

1. What aspect(s) of the Health Belief Model can be used to explain why teenagers often do not see smoking as a threat to their health?
2. How might a patient diagnosed with diabetes display feelings of dependency?
3. What can a pharmacist do to help the patient in the previous question?
4. You have noticed that a patient with worsening chronic obstructive pulmonary disease is much less talkative than usual when picking up refill medications at the pharmacy. He is also less responsive to your attempts to make conversation. What possible emotional reaction to his illness could be responsible for these changes?

5. An elderly patient with arthritis does not ask questions during counseling. What might be the cause of this?
6. How might you use QOL considerations in helping a patient choose between treating migraine headaches as needed with a product such as sumatriptan or going on a preventative medication like amitriptyline?

REFERENCES

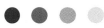

1. Chappell N, Strain L, Blandford A. Health Status and Aging. In: Aging and Health Care: A Social Perspective. Holt, Rinehart and Winston, Toronto, 1986.
2. Mechanic D. Illness Behavior. In: Medical Sociology, 2nd Edition. Free Press, New York, 1978.
3. Alonzo A. Everyday illness behavior: A situational approach to health status deviations. Soc Sci Med. 1979;13A:397–404.
4. Rakowski W. Health psychology and late life: The differentiation of health and illness for the study of health-related behaviors. Res Aging. 1984;6(4):593–620.
5. Cummings KM, Becker MH, Maile MC. Bringing the models together: An empirical approach to combining variables used to explain health actions. J Behav Med. 1980;3(2):123–145.
6. Becker MH, Rosenstock IM. Compliance with Medical Advice. In: Steptoe A, Mathews A, eds., Health Care and Human Behaviour. Academic Press, London, 1984.
7. Janz N, Becker MH. The health belief model: A decade later. Health Educ Q. 1984;11(1):1–47.
8. Owens N. Patient noncompliance: Subset analysis. Drug Topics. 1992;Supp 136(13):11–15.
9. Bernstein L, Bernstein RS. Emotions in Illness and Treatment. In: Interviewing: A Guide for Health Professionals, 4th Edition. Appleton-Century-Crofts, New York, 1985.
10. Jang R. Emotional Reactions to Illness and Treatment. In: Communication Skills in Patient Counseling on OTC Drugs. Health Sciences Consortium, Chapel Hill, NC, 1980.
11. Okolo N, McReynolds J. Counseling the terminally ill. Am Pharm. 1987;27(9):37–40.
12. Kübler-Ross E. What is it like to be dying? Am J Nurs. 1971;71(1):54–60.
13. Conrad P. The meaning of medication: Another look at compliance. Soc Sci Med. 1985;20(1):19–37.
14. Dolinsky D. How do the elderly make decisions about taking medications? J Soc Admin Pharm. 1989;6(3):127–137.
15. Horne R, Weinman J. Patients' beliefs about prescribed medicines and their role in adherence to treatment in chronic physical illness. J Psychosom Res. 1999;47(6):555–567.
16. Zehnder S, Bruppacher R, Hersberger K. Drug information sources used by patients. J Soc Admin Pharm. 2003;20(5):156–160.
17. Mackowiak J, Manasse H. Expectation vs. demand for pharmacy service. J Pharm Market and Manage. 1988;2:57–72.
18. Airaksinen M, Vainio K, Koistinen J, et al. Do the public and pharmacists share opinions about drug information. Int J Pharm. 1994;8(4):994–996.
19. Nair K, Dolovich L, Cassels A, et al. What patients want to know about their medications. Can Fam Physician. 2002;48(1):104–110.
20. Haynes R, Wang E, Da Mota Gomes M. A critical review of interventions to improve compliance with prescribed medications. Patient Educ Couns. 1987;10:155–166.
21. Myers E, Calvert E. Information, compliance and side effects: A study of patients on antidepressant medication. Br J Clin Pharmacol. 1984;17:21–25.
22. McCann S, Weinman J. Empowering the patient in the consultation: A pilot study. Patient Educ Couns. 1996;27:227–234.

23. Morris L, Grossman R, Barksdoll G, et al. A segmentational analysis of prescription drug information seeking. Med Care. 1987;25:953–964.

24. Schommer J. Patients' expectations and knowledge of patient counseling services that are available from pharmacists. Am J Pharm Educ. 1997;61(1):402–406.

25. Taylor J, Gilbertson A, Semchuk W, et al. Effect of verbal encouragement on patient question-asking behaviour during medication counselling. Int J Pharm Pract. 2001;9:253–259.

26. Roter D. Patient participation in patient-provider interaction: The effects of patient question asking on the quality of interaction, satisfaction and compliance. Health Educ Monographs. 1977;5:281–315.

27. Norris P, Rowsell B. Interactional issues in the provision of counselling to pharmacy customers. Int J Pharm Pract. 2003;11:135–142.

28. Berry D, Raynor D, Knapp P, et al. Patients' understanding of risk associated with medication use. Drug Safety. 2003;26(1):1–11.

29. Edwards A, Elwyn G, Mulley A. Explaining risks: Turning numerical data into meaningful pictures. Br Med J. 2002;324(6):827–830.

30. Smith M, Juergens J, Jack W. Medication and the quality of life. Am Pharm. 1991;NS31(4):27–33.

Helping Patients with Adherence and Decision Making

CHAPTER 4

Objectives

After completing the chapter, the reader should be able to

1. list the potential outcomes of medication nonadherence.
2. describe the current thinking on patient-centered decision-making and nonadherent behavior.
3. describe how various health beliefs, communication, and psychological factors are related to adherence.
4. describe barriers to adherence.
5. tailor patient counseling to identify, assess, and prevent potential causes of nonadherence.
6. utilize strategies to prevent and resolve nonadherence consistent with its underlying causes.

While preparing a refill prescription for a beta-blocker for an elderly patient, a pharmacist notes from the patient record that the previous quantity of medication would have lasted only 30 days, and it has now been 40 days since the prescription was dispensed. She plans to discuss this with the patient, since she knows about the possible serious implications of suddenly stopping beta-blockers, and of the long-term results of uncontrolled high blood pressure. As a concerned pharmacist, she is well aware of the issue of compliance/adherence.

DEFINING THE ISSUES

Compliance has been defined as "the extent to which a person's behavior (in terms of taking medications, following diets, or executing lifestyle changes) coincides with medical or health advice."[1] Medication nonadherence has been defined as the number of doses not taken or taken incorrectly that jeopardizes the patient's therapeutic outcome.[2] As noted in Chapter 1, failure to adhere to medication is a significant problem. Nonadherence has been designated by the National Council on Patient Information and Education as "America's other drug problem."[3] In a 1992 survey conducted by Schering Laboratories, 19% of patients admitted to not following prescription directions exactly and 8.7% to not filling initial prescriptions.[4] However, self-reports of adherence can be expected to underestimate the problem. Depending on the group being studied, the type of medication, and various other factors, studies find nonadherence rates with drug therapy range from 13% to 93% with an average rate of 40%.[3] Nonadherence is a continuous rather than a dichotomous measure so that patients are not clearly either adherent or nonadherent but more likely to range from 0% to 100% adherent. About 50% to 60% of patients may be considered compliant, taking 80% or more of prescribed doses at the correct times; 30% to 40% of patients are "partial compliers" and take 20% to 79% of prescribed doses; and 5% to 10% of patients are resistant to treatment and take less than 20% of prescribed doses.[5,6]

The outcome of nonadherence should be of utmost concern to pharmacists who wish to provide pharmaceutical care. Pharmaceutical care requires the identification, resolution, and prevention of drug-related problems, three of which pertain to nonadherence: (a) taking or receiving too little of the correct drug, (b) taking or receiving too much of the correct drug, (c) not taking or receiving the drug prescribed.[7] The concept of pharmaceutical care further requires the pharmacist to take responsibility for the outcome of medication use. Nonadherence results in a number of undesirable outcomes including prolonging or worsening of the medical condition; hospital and nursing home admissions; and in the extreme case, death.[7] In addition, the incalculable effects of nonadherence complicate the evaluation and approval of new pharmaceutical agents at the clinical investigations stage where optimum dosing is determined; and at the postapproval stage where unanticipated problems with dosing and side effects are monitored.[8] Finally, there is an enormous cost to society and the health care system, not only costs of treating the harmful results of nonadherence, but also costs of wasted medication and lost work days.[6]

In light of pharmacists' recognized responsibility to affect outcomes of treatment, it becomes important for pharmacists to understand the factors that contribute to nonadherence and to employ techniques and approaches to overcome it.

ADHERENCE IN TERMS OF PATIENT DECISION MAKING AND BEHAVIOR

What makes a patient miss taking his or her medication? Does the patient make a conscious decision or is it a mistake? As a starting point to understanding this it might be useful to consider the terms used: Compliance, self-regulation, adherence, persistence, and concordance. The word *compliance* itself suggests the paternalistic medical-model approach: The patient must follow the physician's orders and "comply" with his or her directions.[1,9,10] In fact, the dictionary definition of compliance is "yielding to the wishes of others."[11] This way of thinking implies that there is no place for the patient in decision making about drug use.

Also implicit in the concept of compliance is the notion that following the recommended advice is always correct and in the patient's best interest. There is an assumption that the condition being treated has been properly diagnosed; that the treatment is appropriate and effective, and does more good than harm; and that the prescribed regimen is understandable and achievable (i.e., directions are simple, dosing is convenient, and cost and side effects are acceptable).[12] Patients, however, often do recover without having rigidly adhered to their physician's directions, and, conversely, prescribed treatments are not always effective—some "compliant" patients do not recover and some even get worse. In addition, drugs are on occasion prescribed unnecessarily or simply in an attempt to placate the patient.[13] In fact, reduction or discontinuance of medication may be warranted in cases where unpleasant side effects and possibly dangerous adverse effects occur, often referred to as *intelligent noncompliance*.[8] Such facts certainly challenge the premise on which the notion of compliance is based.[9,13]

Rather than considering the issue in terms of *noncompliance*, we should see it from the perspective of *self-regulation* or, at least, *nonadherence*.[1,9,10] From this patient-centered perspective, patients are seen to be active agents in their treatment. The most popular term used in American health literature today is *adherence*, with the term *persistence* referring to long-term adherence.[14]

It has also been suggested that we view nonadherence as a behavioral disorder with various causes and risk factors that can be identified; it can be assessed and monitored and interventions can be applied to prevent and treat nonadherence; and since it has a variable course, patients need to be reassessed periodically.[15] Considering nonadherence as a behavioral disorder also leads us to consider theories of behavior change since adherence to medication often requires a change in behavior.

CAUSES OF MEDICATION NONADHERENCE

A number of theoretical models have been proposed to help us understand the phenomenon of nonadherence, and studies have considered many different factors as contributors to nonadherence.[16–20] The main contributing factors to nonadherence identified include various patient factors and beliefs, the nature of communication between the patient and health professionals, and various behavioral factors.[10] In addition, there are various barriers to adherence that make it difficult for a patient to comply, even if they would otherwise have the inclination. Understanding these factors can help us develop approaches to preventing and treating nonadherence.

Patient Factors Affecting Nonadherence

A number of factors included in the Health Belief Model discussed in the previous chapter may contribute to nonadherence. Other theories such as the Theory of Reasoned Action suggest that patients will modify their behavior based on logical thought into the risks of the disease and benefits of the treatment, with various internal and external factors modifying these thoughts.[19,20] A number of the factors suggested in these models and theories have been found to be significantly related to adherence.

The individual's perception of the seriousness of his or her condition has been found to be associated with nonadherence.[9] In a study of patients taking a short-term antibiotic regimen, compliers perceived their condition to be worse than did noncompliers.[21] An individual may not believe that his or her condition is sufficiently serious to warrant attention or may even deny that a problem exists. This often occurs in the case of psychiatric disorders, where the illness may compromise the patient's perceptions of threat.[3] The immediate threat of problems if medication is not taken appears to be significant. Patients taking anticonvulsants were found to be more likely to be adherent than those on antihypertensives.[22]

Patients apparently do a kind of cost-benefit analysis. A study of beliefs and adherence in patients from four chronic illness groups (asthma, renal, cardiac, and oncology) revealed that although 89% believed their medication was necessary, over one third had concerns about their medication based on beliefs about the dangers of dependence or long-term effects. Higher reported adherence rates were associated with higher necessity scores and lower concern scores.[23] Type of condition was a factor so that having heart disease was related to adherence, whereas having asthma was related to nonadherence.

Perception of the condition may also relate to personal values of treatment—for example, isotretinoin, used for cosmetic reasons for acne treatment, was found to be more likely to be complied with than antihypertensive drugs.[22]

The individual's perception of the efficacy of a prescribed treatment has also been found to be a relevant factor in adherence.[9] Patients may believe that no medication can alleviate their particular condition, or they may misunderstand the manner in which a medication is intended to help and therefore interpret it to be ineffective. For example, a medication such as amitriptyline may not exhibit an effect for several weeks, during which time the patient, seeing little or no change, may come to believe that the drug is ineffective. Adherence to lipid-lowering drugs has been found to be correlated with perceptions of efficacy in preventing cardiovascular events.[24]

Another factor influencing adherence is the effect of family and friends (social support). In one study, although 43% of patients on antihypertensive therapy reported feeling better, only 1% of companions reported improvement, and 99% reported worsening of the patient's condition.[12] These companions may serve to deter medication-taking behavior.[12] Alternatively, the availability of a social support network to encourage medication use can improve adherence.

Communication Factors

Various factors involved in the communication between the patient and health professional have been considered for their effects on adherence.[19] It has been suggested that if a message from a health professional is sent, received, comprehended, retained, and believed by a patient then the result will be adherence. Various factors affecting the communication process may affect adherence such as reinforcing information, cuing, and verbal and written communication.[19] Communication skills will be discussed in Chapter 7.

Nonadherence has been associated with minimal medical supervision, whereas higher adherence rates have been found to occur when patients are given explicit and appropriate instructions, more and clearer information, and more and better feedback.[10]

The content of the communication is of course important. Many have believed that discussing side effects would increase nonadherence due to fear. Although fear of side effects can contribute to nonadherence, being informed can reduce it. In a survey about the risks of drugs, 90% of patients reported that precaution and warning information would encourage them to take the drug exactly as prescribed.[25] However, patients must not be scared into taking medication, with dire warnings about what would happen if they do not adhere, as this may worsen adherence.[26] Rather, communication should help patients make personal decisions about treatments and find ways to integrate medication taking into his or her daily routine.[27]

The effectiveness of the patient–health professional interaction appears to reside less in the improvement of the patient's knowledge than in the way that patient education is approached. To be most effective, the interaction has to involve strategies that modify the patient's health beliefs and attitudes.[13]

The emotional content has also proven to be relevant in matters of adherence—essentially, the lower the patient's satisfaction with the interaction, the greater the likelihood of nonadherence.[18] Studies of patient–physician interactions suggest that nonadherence is higher when patients find their physicians unfriendly or when their expectations of their physicians are not met.[10] Patients' perception of physician time spent explaining cholesterol and chronic heart disease (CHD) affected adherence to lipid-lowering medication.[24] In another study, nonadherers were judged to be less assertive, and less friendly during consultation with their physician than compliers.[21] In a study involving pharmacists, patients were more likely to follow nonprescription drug advice when the pharmacist was introverted rather than extroverted in personality.[28] The researchers suggested that patients might have perceived extroverted pharmacists as overbearing, unreliable, or untrustworthy.

Further evidence of the importance of satisfaction with pharmacist and physician was found in a 1992 survey of patients. A high percentage of patients who failed to take the proper dosage, did not take medication at proper times, or did not take the medication for the full duration found fault with the medication in some way. However, the perception that the medication failed was found to be partially related to dissatisfaction with the health professional interaction, since patients who reported being dissatisfied with the pharmacist's instructions and with the doctor's counsel were more likely to report that their medication failed.[4]

Simply interacting with the patient can make a difference in the case of the pharmacist–patient situation. Nonadherence was reduced by 25% when the pharmacist, rather than the clerk, handed the medicine to the patient.[4] Concern for the patient by the health care professional and involvement by the patient in decisions regarding therapy also improve adherence.[3]

These findings suggest that if adherence is to be improved, the encounter must provide the patient with significantly more than simply factual information, but must also include involvement of the patient in discussion. Consultations that acknowledge patients' autonomy and tailor treatment to accommodate patients' values and personal circumstances are more likely to result in adherence and better treatment outcomes.[29]

Behavioral Factors

Various behavioral factors have been found to affect adherence. As noted above, nonadherence can be considered a behavioral disorder; therefore, behavioral learning theories have been suggested to help find ways to explain and modify nonadherence.[19]

Patients' decision-making and cognitive abilities may affect their adherence with medication: Patients formulate action plans, appraise the plans, and find ways to cope. They use their cognitive skills and emotional experiences to solve problems regarding their medication use, resulting in adherent or nonadherent behavior.[19]

Studies exploring factors involved in medication use point to the importance of the decision-making aspects of nonadherence, as well as to experiential learning. For example, nonadherence may be the result of an individual's decision to test the efficacy of the drug. In interviews of patients with epilepsy, Conrad found that patients often altered or discontinued their medication to test if it was having any effect, and to determine whether they still had epilepsy.[10]

Experience may also be a positive aspect, in that experience taking medication on a regular basis may improve adherence. In one study, adherence improved as the number of concurrent medications increased.[22] The authors hypothesized that patients were forced to develop a dosage-administration strategy that ensured adherence.

An individual may also be nonadherent in an attempt to assert control—over the doctor–patient relationship or over the medical condition itself, especially if it is one that appears to be beyond control, such as epilepsy.[10] As discussed in Chapter 3, suffering from an illness, taking medication, and relying on health professionals can be perceived by the individual as increased dependence. Patients may attempt to regain that independence by means of altering their medication regimens.[10]

The patient's knowledge about the disease or the medication has not been shown to be directly related to adherence.[13] Knowledge is of limited value without the understanding or desire to apply it. Studies show that a patient's knowledge only improves adherence when it is imparted in a manner that modifies the patient's health beliefs and attitudes.[13]

Various individual characteristics have been proposed to affect adherence. However, in most studies conducted to date, no consistent relationship has been found to exist between adherence and demographic factors such as social class, age, gender, education, or marital status and there is no evidence to date to suggest that a nonadherent type of individual exists.[9,18,21]

Barriers to Adherence

Recognizing the various factors that contribute to nonadherence, it is clear that there are barriers to adherence which must be overcome to improve or prevent nonadherence.

One issue is the complexity of medication regimen and difficulties in following the prescribed regimen.[9] The more complex the regimen, the less adherent patients are likely to be. Many studies have found that as the number of required doses increases adherence decreases: Once daily being most complied with, twice or three times daily dosing being equally poor compared to once daily, and four times daily being least adhered to.[21,22] Difficulties in remembering to take medication several times daily or in fitting medication use into a daily routine have been suggested as reasons for this reduction in the likelihood of adherence.[21]

Therapy of a longer duration is also less likely to be adhered to. This may result from the patient's difficulties in remembering and in scheduling doses. Decreasing adherence over time may also involve decreasing concern with the condition, or attempts to test the need for continued medication.[10]

The presence of adverse effects or side effects has also been found to reduce adherence, due to discomfort or fear of more serious effects, or both.[4,30] This may be particularly true if the patient has not been warned about the possibility of side effects or has not been given suggestions about how to minimize such effects. As noted above, precaution and warning information about a prescription reportedly encourages patients to take the drug exactly as prescribed.[25] Apparently, it is not simply the occurrence of adverse effects that interferes with adherence, but rather difficulty with particular adverse effects that the patient cannot tolerate or manage.[3]

When patients are unable to understand the reasons for medication use or the directions for use because of literacy, cognitive ability, or language barriers, then it is likely that they may be unable to take medication as directed. Patients with mental disorders such as depression and anxiety have been found to have lower adherence to lipid-lowering medications.[14] However, low intelligence or poor memory have not been found to be consistently related to nonadherence.[18]

If patients have difficulty accessing their health professional or pharmacy, through disability or lack of services, they may find it difficult to receive medication in a timely manner, and therefore may not take medication at all, or take it irregularly. A study of patients on statins found that those on Medicaid were significantly less likely to have high persistence (greater than 80% of doses) than those with higher annual incomes.[31]

A patient may also be unable to take a medication because he or she physically cannot administer the medication, i.e., open the container, correctly hold a puffer.

To summarize, studies have found that multiple factors and barriers are related to patient nonadherence, often working together within the same situation. In particular, the patient's perceptions and involvement in therapy decisions are important.[21] A summary of the factors that have been found to contribute to nonadherence is shown in Table 4-1.

TABLE 4-1	Causes of Medication Nonadherence
Patient factors	Perceived lack of seriousness of the disease and outcomes of nontreatment
	Perceived ineffectiveness of the treatment
	Negative views of family and friends or lack of social support
Communication	Low degree of medical supervision
	Lack of instruction that is explicit, appropriate, clear, adequate in quantity, and including feedback
	Lack of balanced information on risks and side effects
	Lack of strategies by health professional to modify attitudes and beliefs
	Low patient satisfaction in the interaction with the health professional
	Little or no interaction with health professional
	Health professional is perceived as unfriendly, lacking concern
	Health professional does not allow involvement of patient in decisions
Behavioral	Desire to test the efficacy of the drug
	Desire to assert control over the doctor–patient relationship, or even over a condition that appears to be beyond control
	Lacking or negative experience with medication
	Lack of knowledge of disease
Barriers to adherence	Complex regimen
	Length of duration of therapy
	Presence of adverse or side effects
	Poor literacy, cognitive ability, language barriers
	Physical/financial barriers to care

PATIENT DECISION MAKING AND EMPOWERMENT

Considering nonadherence as a behavioral issue leads us to consider how patients make decisions about taking their medications and about changing their behavior from non-adherent to adherent.

Stages of Change Theory

The Transtheoretical Model of Change, also known as *stages of change*, developed by Prochaska et al., has been used to develop effective interventions to promote change in many health behaviors including smoking cessation, weight control, mammography screening, and medical compliance.[32,33] The model describes how people make decisions to change behavior in stages of emotion, cognitions, and behaviors that facilitate change. It draws on the Health Belief Model and other behavioral models to explain how people weigh the pros and cons of a certain behavior and progress through experiential then behavioral processes that stimulate and reinforce change. The stages of change are described in Table 4-2 including precontemplation, contemplation, preparation, action, maintenance, and relapse prevention.[32]

TABLE 4-2 Stages of Change	
Precontemplation	Not considering change
	Feeling of no control
	In denial or feels immune—does not believe advice applies to them
	Believes consequences are not serious
	May have tried unsuccessfully to change before but given up
Contemplation	Ambivalent about change
	Feel sense of loss to give up enjoyed behavior
	Assessing barriers as well as benefits of change
Preparation	Prepare to make specific change
	Experiment with small changes
	Determination to change gradually increases
Action	Actually changing behavior more consistently
Maintenance and relapse prevention	Must change behavior over long period
	May have slips in behavior
	May return through previous stages to return to action stage before change is established
	Relapse may be demoralizing
	Relapse is normal part of change

Based on information presented in Prochaska JO, Velicer WF. The transtheoretical model of health behavior change. Am J Health Promot. 1997;12:38–48.

In order to encourage adherence to medication, pharmacists should help the patient move through the stages of change. Methods to do this will be discussed in the next section.

Making Decisions and Reaching Concordance

Considerations of how patients come to health decisions like whether to take medication have led to research into issues such as decision making, the relationship between patients and health professionals, and communication about risk. As discussed in previous chapters, the current trend is for shared decision making so that the patient and health professional build a consensus about the preferred treatment, share information, and agree on the treatment.[29] The result is concordance, whereby patients are working in partnership with their health professionals.

A key element is education of the patient about treatments and the communication of risk. How risk is presented can affect patients' decisions. Decision aids have been developed to assist this process, typically including such elements as information about the clinical problem, information about options and outcomes, outcome probabilities, examples of other patients, and guidance in the steps of decision making.[34] Decisions are not always made on a rational basis; patients may need more than facts to make decisions. A caring health professional who can support the patient through this process is equally important.[34]

Equipped with this understanding of the factors that contribute to nonadherence and patient behavior change, we can now consider ways in which the pharmacist can help to reduce nonadherence. Pharmaceutical care requires that pharmacists engage in a systematic and comprehensive process whereby they identify a patient's actual and potential drug-related problem; resolve the patient's actual drug-related problems; and prevent the patient's potential drug-related problems from becoming actual problems.[7] Approaches to improving adherence among patients will now be discussed as they relate to prevention, identification, and resolution of nonadherence.

PREVENTION OF POTENTIAL NONADHERENCE

What can pharmacists do to encourage and assist their patients to be adherent? All patients should be viewed as potentially nonadherent.[3] As such, each situation must be considered individually in terms of the risks of nonadherence for this individual patient in this particular situation.

In developing a plan to prevent nonadherence, the pharmacist must consider the reasons for adherence and barriers to adherence. Attention should be focused on three aspects of patient counseling: (a) communication with the patient, (b) provision of information, and (c) strategies to prevent nonadherence.

Communication with the Patient

As discussed above, in order to prevent nonadherence, there must be communication with the patient. The pharmacist must engage the patient in discussion to establish a relationship with the patient. Further communication must occur to allow the pharmacist to proceed through the pharmaceutical care process to gather appropriate information, determine methods to prevent nonadherence, and carry them out.[7]

The following aspects of communication with the patient can help prevent nonadherence: Patient satisfaction, tone, nature, content, frequency, and method. Communication tips to prevent adherence are summarized in Table 4-3. These and other aspects of communication with patients and the use of various counseling aids will be discussed in further detail in Chapters 6 and 7.

Provision of Information

Through appropriate communication with the patient, the pharmacist is able to determine what type of information would best prevent nonadherence, and how best to present that information.

As has already been pointed out, simply providing information about medication use is of limited effectiveness. Although adequate information and clear instructions for use are obviously essential, they are not sufficient to encourage adherence.[9,13] A review of studies evaluating strategies for improving adherence found that providing information was shown to be effective in only slightly more than half of the studies.[16]

Providing information may, however, have some effect on attitudes and beliefs, and this may in turn have an effect on adherence.[16] In addition, the attention received by the patient in the course of instruction on medication use may contribute to improving adherence.

There are a number of factors concerning the provision of information that are important in preventing nonadherence.

1. *Persuasiveness*: It appears that the effectiveness of information provision depends on the persuasiveness of the health professional's communication and on the extent of his or her attempts to motivate the patient.[9,10] Therefore, the method of information provision and communication techniques of the pharmacist are critical.

2. *Information Regarding Use*: Of course, in order to adhere to medication use, a patient must always be provided with correct, appropriate, and complete instructions including how much medication to use, when to take it, how long to continue use including refill information, and what to do if a dose is missed.

3. *Information Regarding Illness and How and When Medication Will Help*: In addition, the patient needs information about his or her condition and the ways in which the medication is expected to help the condition. For example, a patient prescribed an antibiotic and H_2-receptor antagonist for a *Helicobacter pylori*–induced ulcer needs to understand that an ulcer is a lesion in the stomach resulting in part from a microbial infection, and that the medication will help to treat the infection, and along with the H_2-blocker will allow the ulcer to heal. This will hopefully prevent the patient from using the medication intermittently "as needed" rather than completing the course of treatment.

    The patient should also be made aware of the amount of time it may take before pain and discomfort are reduced—in other words, when some effect of the medication is likely to be felt. This will help prevent any misperceptions on the patient's part about the seriousness of the condition or the effectiveness of the medication.

TABLE 4-3	**Communication Tips to Prevent Nonadherence**
Patient satisfaction with communication	Engage the patient in conversation regarding his or her medication[3,14]
Tone of communication	Should not be coercive, frightening, threatening, or demeaning[3]
	Should not insist that the patient comply, but rather should offer the patient help with gaining the most benefit from his or her medication
	Convince the patient that adherence would be in his or her own best interest
	Must not frighten the patient regarding possible adverse effects, or threaten him or her regarding the dangers of nonadherence
Nature of communication	Discussion as well as presentation of information
	Involve patient as much as possible in the interaction and in decisions regarding medication use (e.g., when to take and dosage form preferred)
Content of communication	Inquire into the patient's perceptions of medication use to determine the kinds of misperceptions that may be at play and the types of information and behavioral strategies that might be most beneficial for that patient
	Try to discover some of the costs and benefits as perceived by the patient, and to address them before they occur
	Directly ask the patient if he or she perceives any difficulties with taking the medication
	Address misperceptions or beliefs through further discussion, provision of information, and specific strategies
Frequency of communication	Encourage future communication
	Suggest that the patient call to discuss any problems or concerns that arise in the future
	Follow the patient's progress and continue to interact with him or her after the initial prescription has been dispensed since the patient's decision making about his or her illness and medication use is a continuous process
	During refill prescription counseling explore any changing beliefs and perceptions about the illness or medications
Method of communication	Combination of verbal and written communication is most likely to improve adherence and is preferred by patients[3,19]
	Avoid the use of jargon
	Match the patient's language and education levels

4. *Information about Side Effects*: Since the occurrence of side effects or fear of side effects occurring have been found to contribute to nonadherence, patients should be told about the signs of any common side effects that may occur. The provision of information about side effects and adverse effects reduces nonadherence by reducing fear and by allowing for a more appropriate handling of problems.[35,36] This positive effect may also arise out of the patient's greater sense of control over the effects of the medication. As mentioned above, patients report that such information would encourage them to be adherent.[10]

    Patients should also be told what they can do to prevent or minimize side effects. Signs of adverse effects should also be explained. The pharmacist should emphasize that these effects are very rare, but that it is nonetheless important to be able to recognize them as soon as they occur in order to allow for their early detection and management.

    As noted above, although some pharmacists hesitate to discuss side effects and adverse effects with patients for fear that this may cause suggestible patients to later imagine that they are indeed experiencing the described effects, studies have shown that patients who receive such information generally have no greater experience of side effects than those who do not.[37,38]

    It has also been found that patients find it difficult to comprehend the magnitude of risk and generally overestimate it, particularly if it is stated in words such as rare, unlikely, common, and so forth. Studies have illustrated that patients, university students, and even doctors overestimated the numerical meaning of these words. Whereas "rare" has been designated in Europe as 0.01% to 0.1%, patients grossly overestimated risk to a mean of 8%.[39] Although numerical statement of risk is also problematic, there may be better ways to provide this information. This will be discussed further in Chapters 5 and 6.

5. *Special Techniques*: Information regarding techniques to apply the medication, if necessary, and ways to remember medication use should also be provided to reduce the chance of nonadherence due to difficulties following the regimen.

6. *Quantity and Level*: Information should not be too comprehensive or detailed for a patient to absorb or understand according to his or her education level, disabilities, or emotional state, since this may actually compromise rather than enhance adherence.[3] The specific types of information that can benefit patients, and the best ways to present such information, will be discussed in greater detail in Chapters 5, 6, and 7.

Strategies for Preventing Nonadherence

Since nonadherence is considered a behavior that is affected by beliefs, experience, and so forth, a variety of behavioral strategies are recommended to prevent nonadherence.[3,9,13,15,40] Such strategies may include the following:

1. Working with the physician to simplify medication schedules by reducing the number of drugs, reducing the number of daily dosage intervals, and adjusting the dosage regimen to better accommodate the patient's daily routine.
2. Supplying medication reminders and organizers, such as pill containers with alarms or organized compartments, and individualized drug-taking check-off charts.
3. Reminding patients by telephone or mail about their prescription refills.

4. Enlisting the support of the patient's spouse or other family members to remind and encourage the patient to take the prescribed medication.

These methods not only help to prevent incidents of nonadherence that arise out of practical difficulties in taking medication, but they also attempt to change individuals' attitudes or beliefs.

IDENTIFICATION OF NONADHERENCE

Although the pharmacist may have applied all the above techniques and strategies when a patient first received medication, most studies report that almost all adherence strategies decline over time.[3] When a patient comes to the pharmacy to pick up a refill prescription, the pharmacist has an opportunity to identify nonadherence. Identification of nonadherence requires the pharmacist to gather information to detect whether nonadherence is occurring; to assess the nonadherence, its frequency, and the situations that precipitate it; and to determine the factors that are contributing to nonadherence. This information will assist the pharmacist in developing strategies to deal with the situation.

Detecting Nonadherence

Direct and indirect methods of detecting nonadherence can be used.[15] Although direct methods such as serum levels or other clinical indicators may be a more precise check on adherence, they require the cooperation of the patient for blood and urine sampling and are therefore impractical in most cases.[15]

Indirect methods involve pill counts, refill records, and measurement of health outcomes. Refill records have been found to result in about 10% higher apparent adherence than direct serum assay.[19]

When reviewing the patient record, the pharmacist should keep in mind that nonadherence may not be the only explanation for an apparent late or early refill. Other reasons could be that the patient received verbal instructions from the physician to alter the dosage or had the prescription filled at a different pharmacy in the interim. Alternatively, nonadherence may not be apparent from the patient record. Patients sometimes continue to reorder medication on a regular basis, while stockpiling medication, possibly because they want their doctor to believe they are being adherent, or because in some cases the medication is being paid for by a third party and the patients feel they should "save it up" for a time when they may no longer receive such benefits.

In addition, pill taking is often intermittent and random rather than systematic, and patients often omit or delay doses or miss a day or more at a time, but may make up for it just before a physician visit (known as the *white coat effect* or *toothbrush effect*).[3,18] This irregular dosing may not be readily apparent from the patient's chart.[12] The pharmacist must therefore interview the patient to determine if nonadherence is occurring, either as indicated on the patient record or in the absence of such evidence.

A meta-analysis showed that simply asking patients about adherence can be fairly accurate; patient interviews have been found to identify 80% of nonadherent patients as verified by pill counts.[14,41] This should be done with an open mind and with careful attention to the tone of the inquiry (i.e., it should not sound like an inquisition). Use of open-ended questions to encourage the patient to provide as much information as possible and gentle probing to determine when the medication is usually taken will help determine the extent of nonadherence without alienating the patient. Some suggested open-ended statements are shown in Table 4-4. Communication and interview techniques will be discussed further in Chapters 5 and 7.

Apart from refill counseling, nonadherence may come to the pharmacist's attention during a medication management consultation with a patient. Techniques for the

TABLE 4-4	Probes to Detect and Assess Nonadherence
Probes to detect nonadherence	"Many people have difficulty taking all the medications we prescribe. During the past week, how many tablets (capsules) have you missed?"
	"Are there any days over the previous 2 weeks that you have run out of any medicine or missed any doses?"
	"Are there any future events that may interfere with taking your medication?" "How do you plan to cope?"
Assessing patient factors	"What results do you expect to receive from this medication?"
	"What concerns do you have about your illness or its treatment?"
	"Are you satisfied with your current treatment plan?"
Assessing medication factors and barriers	"How do you take this medication?"
	"Do you use any memory aids to help you remember to take your medication?"
	"What might prevent you from following the recommended treatment plan?"
	"How do you remind yourself to take medication on schedule?"
	"Please describe for me how you remember to take your medicine."
	"How do you remember to take your medicine on the weekend—when you eat out, when you visit, when you travel, and so forth?"
	"What do you think you could do to solve the problem of missing doses?"
Assessing support	"Does anyone help you take your medications?"
Assessing patient–physician–pharmacist factors	"Do you feel comfortable asking your physician about your medications?" "What about asking the pharmacist?"
	"Where do you get information about your medication and condition?"

Based on information presented in Jacobson TA. The forgotten cardiac risk factor: Noncompliance with lipid-lowering therapy. Medscape Cardiol. 2004;8(2). Available at: www.medscape.com/viewarticle/496144 (accessed January 4, 2005); and Nichols-English G, Poirier S. Optimizing adherence to pharmaceutical care plans. J Am Pharm Assoc. 2000;40(4):475–485.

detection of nonadherence during a medication management consultation will be discussed further in Chapter 5.

Nonadherence may also come to the pharmacist's attention through a comment or inquiry by the physician or patient regarding poor response to medication or the occurrence of side effects. These outcomes may be a result of improper use, for example, heart rhythm abnormalities resulting from intermittent use of beta-blockers.

In addition, pharmacists can detect nonadherence through sponsoring or becoming involved in medication review, or "brown bag," programs such as that promoted by The National Council on Patient Information and Education.[6] Such programs encourage patients to bring all their prescription and nonprescription medications to an announced place where pharmacists and other health care professionals review them. Pharmacists involved in these programs are ideally situated to discuss regular medication use with patients and to detect nonadherence.

On a more formal level, a medication review clinic may be conducted, where patients are seen regularly for the purpose of assessing drug-related problems, including adherence, through self-assessment by patients and through interviews by pharmacists.[42,43]

Assessing Nonadherence

Once the pharmacist has found that nonadherence is indeed occurring, he or she can proceed to assess the situation. This assessment will help the pharmacist to evaluate if indeed this is a serious problem to be reported to the physician (since it may be causing a poor response that may be misinterpreted by the physician) or rather it is a minor or temporary problem that can be corrected by the pharmacist and patient alone. It also helps the pharmacist in the pharmaceutical care process to list and rank the problems.

The pharmacist must probe to find out the details of frequency, duration, and degree of nonadherence and the situations that surround it. Nonadherence may be occurring only occasionally, as in the case of the patient who skips a dose when going to a party because he or she doesn't want to mix alcohol with medication. Alternatively, it may be very frequent, as in the case of the patient who uses medication only for symptomatic relief rather than on a continual basis as prescribed for the prevention of symptoms. It may occur regularly at a certain time of day; for example, afternoon doses might be skipped on workdays only.

Sensitivity in questioning the patient is important. General questions about any difficulties that the patient may be experiencing with the medication are likely to be most productive, inviting the patient to divulge problem situations (Table 4-4). More specific questions can then follow to determine the relevant details. Suggested dialogues and further aspects of such probing will be discussed in Chapters 5 and 7, and Appendix B.

Determining Factors Contributing to Nonadherence

After ascertaining the details of nonadherence, the pharmacist must investigate the contributing factors to that nonadherence before attempting to resolve it. Pharmacists often make erroneous assumptions about the reasons for nonadherence, particularly in assuming that patients simply forget to take their medication. In the previous section many possible reasons for nonadherence were suggested, and patients may exhibit one or a combination of these.

In the course of discussion, the pharmacist should explore the possible factors involved in nonadherence, from health beliefs to patient–physician communication and behavioral factors and barriers. A systematic way to approach evaluation is to focus on the patient, then the medication, spouse/family/peers, and the patient–health professional relationship.[44] Recommended questions and probes to do this are shown in Table 4-4.

1. *The Patient*: Factors such as the patient's knowledge, attitudes, values, and perceptions about their illnesses or therapies need to be investigated.[43,44] The pharmacist must determine whether the patient has become apathetic or frustrated about the treatment and whether the patient has lost confidence in the ability of the medication to treat his or her symptoms. If the patient has lost confidence, the pharmacist must determine why. It is also important to assess what stage of change in terms of nonadherent behavior the patient is in. It has been suggested that making a simple statement advising the patient to take his or her medication, e.g., "I recommend that you take this medication regularly as prescribed" would elicit a response from the patient that may suggest what stage he or she is in—from not planning to comply (precontemplation) to regular use (maintenance).

2. *The Medication*: The skills of the patient and difficulty following a regimen need to be investigated, as well as the lack of availability of resources and services that could help the patient with adherence.[43,44] In particular, the pharmacist should focus attention on the medication regimen. Does it need to be simplified, in particular with regard to decreasing the number of daily doses? How can it be organized to coordinate better with the patient's daily routines? In addition, the pharmacist must determine whether side effects have emerged that might be discouraging the patient from using the medication. Is the patient reluctant to continue use because side effects are causing discomfort, because they are inconvenient, or because they cause fear?

3. *Spouse/Family/Peers*: Attitudes and behaviors of peers, family, and employers should be considered.[43,44] The pharmacist should pay attention to aspects of the patient's social life. Are family members or, possibly, friends involved in supporting adherence? If not, can they become more actively involved? Is the patient receiving any help with the medication?

4. *The Patient–Health Professional Relationship*: The pharmacist must explore the patient's relationship with his or her physician, as well as with the pharmacist him- or herself.[43,44] Has the patient become dissatisfied with some aspect of these relationships? Perhaps there is a personality conflict with one of the health professionals, or the patient feels a lack of confidence in the health professional's knowledge regarding his or her condition. On a more subtle level, the patient may simply feel powerless with regard to his or her own treatment.

RESOLUTION OF NONADHERENCE

Once nonadherence has been detected by the pharmacist, it is now his or her responsibility to resolve this problem. The pharmacist should proceed to identify the desired outcomes of his or her intervention, develop a plan, select strategies that motivate the patient, select various techniques and tools, then follow-up to ensure that desired outcomes result.

Identifying the Desired Outcomes of a Plan to Resolve Nonadherence

Depending on the factors that the pharmacist has determined to be contributing to the patient's nonadherence, the desired outcome of the pharmacist's action may be any one or all of the following:[7]

1. The patient should receive the appropriate medication (e.g., requiring a medication change to improve the effectiveness, prevent side effects, or offer simpler dosing).
2. The patient should receive the appropriate dose of a drug at the appropriate time and interval (e.g., a change in the dosage to a long-acting medication to simplify dosing, or a change in the patient's beliefs and behavior regarding medication).
3. Side effects the patient is experiencing should be removed (e.g., suggest taking medication with food to reduce stomach irritation).

The pharmacist also needs to specify how he or she will determine that the outcomes of actions to resolve nonadherence have been accomplished. The following parameters should be noted: The change in the patient that can be identified, e.g., a laboratory finding; progress in terms of degree of improvement expected; and time frame, e.g., the patient will be able to walk to the bus stop after continuing on anti-inflammatory therapy regularly for 3 weeks.[7]

The pharmaceutical care model also specifies that the plan should be documented.[7]

Developing a Plan to Resolve Nonadherence

Once the outcomes have been decided, the pharmacist must develop a plan to accomplish them. The plan should include: Assessing needs; specifying goals and objectives; delineating content, strategies and resources; and evaluating the program.[43]

One important aspect of the plan to resolve nonadherence is the need for communication with the physician and other health care workers. Any needed alterations in regimens and dosage forms to improve adherence must be negotiated with the prescribing physician. There is also a need for the pharmacist to advise the physician of regularly occurring nonadherence by a patient, since such behavior could be causing distortion in the physician's evaluation of the efficacy of the prescribed treatment. In addition, the physician and other health professionals, such as nurses and social workers, may be able to help formulate the plan aimed at resolving nonadherence. Disclosure to the physician should be discussed with the patient, in consideration of patient confidentiality. The pharmacist's interactions with other health professionals will be discussed further in Chapter 7.

When developing a plan for resolution of nonadherence, attention must again be drawn to the different types of patient–health provider relationships. In shared decision making, the aim of treatment should *not* be to *make the patient comply*, but rather to *join with the patient* to overcome perceived problems relating to medication use. The pharmacist must convey to the patient an attitude that says, "I'm here to help you get the most benefit from your medication."

Armed with the information gathered during the process of identification of nonadherence, the pharmacist, together with the patient and other health professionals, can proceed to select various strategies. These involve some of the strategies discussed above with respect to preventing nonadherence, as well as the educational approaches discussed in Chapter 2. The plan should include techniques to motivate the patient, as well as various interventions specific to overcoming that particular patient's problems with medication use. A summary of techniques to resolve nonadherence is shown in Table 4-5.

TABLE 4-5	**Methods for Resolving Nonadherence**
Changing behavior	Determine patient's stage of change by direct recommendation that patient adhere to medication
Precontemplation	Discuss pros and cons of treatment and encourage patient to think about this
	Let patient know you are available to help
Contemplation	Help patient articulate the pros and cons from their point of view
	Provide further information
	Bolster confidence to take next step
Preparation	Provide tools and skills to help take action
	Praise and encourage
Action	Regularly reassess
	Praise and encourage
Maintenance/relapse	Monitor
	Deal with relapse in positive way
Motivational methods	Use motivational interviewing techniques to overcome ambivalence and help patient to feel change is important and within his or her ability and control
	Discuss benefits and risks/pros and cons of medication use
	Raise patient's awareness of body cues indictating need for medication
	Explain how patient can self-evaluate
	Help patient develop coping mechanisms
Tools and techniques	Adherence aids
	Enlisting support of the spouse or other family members or patient support groups
	Increase supervision
	Social-service intervention
	Switching to an alternative dosing schedule or dosage form
	Verbal or formal contracts
	Controlled therapy
	Self-monitoring programs

Changing Behavior

In terms of the stages of change, a nonadherent patient may be in precontemplation, contemplation, or preparation stages. The pharmacist should engage the patient in discussion to increase his or her readiness for counseling, and move the patient toward the action stage.[33,45] The discussion would include a direct and simple recommendation that the patient take prescribed medication as directed. If the patient responds that he or she doesn't intend to change the nonadherent behavior, then the patient is in the precontemplation stage. By discussing the pros and cons of the treatment, the pharmacist can help the patient move from precontemplation to contemplation. The pharmacist can also encourage the patient to think about this and let the patient know that help is available when he or she is ready to change.

If the patient begins to discuss pros and cons, then he or she is in the contemplation stage. The pharmacist can help the patient articulate the pros and cons, provide further information about the pros and cons of treatment, and bolster patient confidence to take the next step, i.e., preparation.

In the preparation stage the patient has made the decision and could benefit from tools and skill to help take action, for example, memory aids, dosing schedules, techniques to reduce adverse effects or to administer medication easily. The patient will also benefit from praise and encouragement that he or she has the ability to adhere and that it is the best thing for them.

Once the patient is in the action stage where they are already adhering to medication regimens, the pharmacist still needs to be involved, helping to maintain the behavior and deal with the threat of relapse as needed. This involves regular reassessment of adherence, when the patient gets refills of medication or at intervals by telephone.

Finally, when the patient is in the maintenance stage, he or she is regularly adherent but needs to remain so. The pharmacist can monitor the patient to prevent relapse or deal with it in a positive way if it does happen.[33]

Motivating the Patient

Patients—particularly those who are nonadherent—are often unwilling recipients of counseling. Patients may not expect to be counseled and may not have actually asked for help. Nonadherent patients may also feel embarrassed or guilty about their nonadherence and may therefore be reluctant to discuss the subject.

During counseling the nonadherent patient, the pharmacist must motivate the patient. Motivational interviewing is a behavior change technique to motivate change by exploring and resolving ambivalence.[46] It is suggested that a nonadherent patient is in an ambivalent state in which he or she wants to change but at the same time does not want to change. When patients are motivated, they feel that change is important, that they are able to change, and that they are in control of their ability to change. This must come from within the patient rather than from an outside source.

Motivation involves getting the patient's cooperation as a partner in attaining optimal therapy. Motivational interviewing uses empathy and reflective listening (these skills are discussed in Chapter 7) along with key questions that are patient-centered but also directive.[33] First, rapport and a trusting relationship must be established, then the patient's feelings and concerns can be elicited, drawing the patient to explore his or her own perspectives, personal values, and goals to come to his or her own argument for change. The patient's confidence in his or her ability to change must be raised and the patient will eventually take responsibility for change, feeling empowered.[46]

Resistance results from the patient trying to resolve the discomfort of ambivalence. Rather than arguing with the patient, resistance may be approached by the pharmacist asking the patient directly—but in a nonconfrontational manner—about reasons for nonadherence, countering the patient's reasons with questions about how the patient feels and the actions the patient thinks can help him or her change.

Depending on the factors contributing to nonadherence in a patient and the stage of change, the pharmacist can motivate and help the patient move toward the action stage using a variety of motivational methods.[3,47,48] These motivational methods have been found to be particularly effective for long-term medication use.[47] A combination of the appropriate motivational methods is generally more successful than one method alone.[3,19] The following motivational methods are summarized in Table 4-5:

1. *Discuss the Pros and Cons of the Medication*: The pharmacist should try to answer the patient's unspoken question, "What's in it for me?" This addresses health beliefs and misperceptions of susceptibility of the disease as well as misperceptions of the value of the medication that often affect adherence. This must be balanced with discussions of the risks in a way that does not scare the patient, but rather presents a realistic view that helps the patient see that when weighed against each other, the pros outweigh the cons.

2. *Raise Awareness of Body Cues*: Raising the patient's awareness of the body cues that signal the need for the medication helps the patient to see the benefits of medication use. For example, a patient with high blood pressure might be shown how to take his or her own blood pressure and how to identify the initial high-level reading that registers before medication use.

3. *Explain Ways to Self-evaluate*: Similarly, cues can be devised to help the patient to evaluate the outcome of therapy. For example, the pharmacist may encourage the patient to continue taking his or her own blood pressure on a regular basis, thus proving to himself or herself that the medication effectively keeps blood pressure down.

4. *Help Develop Coping Mechanisms*: The pharmacist can also help the patient develop coping mechanisms to deal with circumstances that make it difficult to adhere to medication use. For example, if a patient is concerned about co-workers' reactions to his or her use of an anticonvulsant, the pharmacist might discuss the feared reactions and help the patient devise ways to broach the issue with his or her co-workers or to take the medication without others knowing (e.g., by means of alternative dosing).

Techniques and Tools to Resolve Nonadherence

In addition to motivating nonadherent patients to adhere to medication regimens, pharmacists should provide patients with tools and techniques to overcome barriers to adherence and change behavior.[2,4,14] Interventions used should be tailored to the patient's needs, and multiple strategies should be employed for maximum effectiveness.[31] The following tools and techniques are summarized in Table 4-5:

1. *Adherence Aids*: A variety of aids have been developed for pharmacists to offer to patients. These include: Special medication containers to remind patients when to administer doses; medication caps with timepieces and alarms; pill-reminder packages; compliance packaging that provides the patient with one treatment cycle in a ready-to-use package; calendars or drug-reminder charts to check off doses taken; and telephone or mail reminders for refills.[3,6] These types of devices will be discussed further in Chapter 6.

2. *Enlisting Support*: Another technique the pharmacist can use to resolve nonadherence involves enlisting the support of the spouse, other family members, or members of the patient's support network to encourage and remind the patient to take medication. The pharmacist should investigate the views and perceptions of family members carefully, since they may have negative views of the treatment or condition and actually may be a cause of the nonadherence.[12] The pharmacist can try to gain the support of these individuals and suggest ways they can help with patient adherence, such as reminders to take medication, reassurance over the effectiveness of treatment, and the need to treat the condition.

   Another form of support is the use of patient support groups. Particularly in the case of long-term treatment and conditions requiring significant lifestyle changes, support groups and ongoing counseling can help the patient to self-regulate and to deal with issues that interfere with adherence as they occur.

3. *Increasing Supervision*: Shortening the intervals for refills may help improve adherence by allowing the pharmacist to review medication use and to discuss this with the patient. This allows the pharmacist to detect problems that contribute to nonadherence over time such as the development of side effects; changes in social support; changes in attitudes and beliefs; changes in personal schedules; and so forth. Regular visits to the physician and personalized attention by the pharmacist and physician have been found to improve adherence.[12] In addition, follow-up counseling by telephone or in person can allow the pharmacist to discuss these issues with the patient.

4. *Social Service Intervention*: Social service intervention by means of a visiting nurse, a public health nurse, a social worker, or a home care worker may be recommended in certain cases to monitor and encourage the patient. This is particularly helpful where the patient has little or no social support, or where disabilities or cognitive deficits may be contributing to nonadherence.

5. *Alternative Dosing*: The pharmacist may need to recommend that the physician switch the patient to an alternative dosing schedule or dosage form (e.g., long-acting medications and transdermal drug delivery system). Since most studies find more frequent and complicated dosing significantly increase nonadherence rates, this is a simple remedy that should be considered in many cases. However, long-acting medications may not be appropriate in all patients or conditions, particularly where toxic levels may accumulate, or where variations in dosing may be needed.

6. *Contracts*: Drawing up a "contract" between the patient and the health professional that spells out behavioral expectations, incentives, and rewards for adherence has

been used successfully in some situations.[3] Through this technique, the patient is assisted by having the specific behavior outlined, by being involved in the decision-making process, by making a formal commitment, and by receiving rewards or incentives for achieving therapeutic goals.[3] Although such a formal process is not needed for most individuals, it may be suggested in situations where other methods have been tried and failed. Alternatively, a less formal, verbal contract can be entered into with a nonadherent patient whereby the pharmacist asks the patient to try to adhere to his or her therapy for a particular period.

7. *Controlled Therapy*: Controlled-therapy programs can also help nonadherent patients, particularly when long-term therapy is involved or when the patient has been dependent on caregivers administering medication previously. Such programs are sometimes organized as part of a hospital discharge program, whereby patients begin taking responsibility for administering their own medications before discharge. This allows time for difficulties with the medication or regimen to be detected and resolved before discharge. It also trains patients to organize their medications and to remember to take them.

8. *Self-monitoring Programs*: Patients may be assisted in self-monitoring programs that assist patients to monitor and adjust medications as needed, e.g., use of a blood glucose monitor. This has also been successful in pain management, where patients can actually administer doses of analgesics at their own rates (subject to some limits). This tends to reduce the underuse or overuse of such medications and results in improved relief of symptoms.

Follow-up to Nonadherence Intervention

Once the pharmacist has selected various techniques to resolve nonadherence, he or she should arrange and conduct follow-up consultations with the patient. Having arranged with the patient when follow-up would occur, the pharmacist can either telephone the patient or speak with him or her in the pharmacy to determine if adherence is improved and if the planned outcomes are occurring.

Special Programs

Although adherence is largely an individual matter, groups of individuals with similar characteristics, such as age or type of condition, have similar adherence problems and therefore can be targeted with special programs to deal with nonadherence.[15] For example, parents of children with acute otitis media were found to have high motivation to treat the condition initially because of accuracy of the diagnosis and their children's symptoms of pain and discomfort. However, after 5 to 6 days of a 10-day antibiotic regimen, adherence decreased to only 20% to 30% because the motivation has been significantly reduced as the symptoms abated. Adherence programs for this group should therefore be aimed at increasing motivation to treat during the latter term of the treatment.[49]

The chronically ill older patient presents another high-need situation regarding adherence intervention because of the complexities of multiple diseases; risk of cognitive impairment; multiple drug use; and increased risk of drug reactions.[15,49,50] Specific education programs developed for the elderly should be aimed at increased supervision of medication use as well as greater discussion with the patient to explore health perceptions and cognitive ability.[49]

Other groups of patients who have been found to benefit from special programs include schizophrenic and other psychiatric patients, sight-impaired and hearing-impaired patients, low-literacy patients, and ethnic minorities.[15,33,38,43,51] The specific needs of these patients and counseling issues will be discussed further in Chapter 6.

THE NEED FOR CAREFUL PROBING WHEN DEALING WITH A NONADHERENT PATIENT

An important part of refill counseling involves the identification and resolution of nonadherence. In order to do this effectively, the pharmacist must use careful probing. Let's look at Counseling Situation 4.1.

COUNSELING SITUATION 4.1: Dealing with a Nonadherent Patient

Mrs. Preston is a middle-aged woman who is picking up a refill prescription for hydrochlorothiazide, 50 mg. When the pharmacist checks the patient profile, she notes that the interval since the last refill was appropriate. She proceeds to counsel the patient as follows:

Pharmacist: Hello, Mrs. Preston, your prescription is ready. It looks like things are going OK for you. Have you been feeling all right?

Patient: Yes, pretty good, but a little tired.

Pharmacist: That sounds like low potassium. You were told to drink orange juice or eat a banana every day. You are doing that aren't you?

Patient: *(feeling too foolish to admit forgetting about that)* Oh, well, sometimes.

Pharmacist: Well, try to remember in the future. I guess we'll see you in another 3 months when these run out.

Patient: OK.

This pharmacist did not plan to investigate nonadherence with the patient because the patient profile did not indicate a problem. She made a poor attempt to assess the effectiveness of the medication and to rule out any medication-related problems. When a problem did come to light she did not pursue appropriate questioning to explore the problem further or attempt to resolve it in an effective manner. Now let's look at Counseling Situation 4.2.

COUNSELING SITUATION **4.2:** The Use of Careful Probing

Pharmacist: Hello, Mrs. Preston, how are you today?

Patient: Oh, pretty good, but a little tired.

Pharmacist: Oh, I know the feeling. Why don't you come and have a seat over here where we can spend a few minutes discussing your medication to make sure you're getting the most benefit from it.

Patient: Thanks, that would be good.

Pharmacist: You're getting a refill of your hydrochlorothiazide. I see you've been taking it for a while now. How is it working for you?

Patient: Well, I guess it's working OK. It sure makes me lose water like it's supposed to. I even have to get up in the night to go to the bathroom. It's wearing me out.

Pharmacist: Yes, you mentioned that you've been tired. That can't be very pleasant having your sleep disturbed.

Patient: I get so tired. Sometimes I stop taking it for a few days just so I can get some rest. I know I have to keep taking it to keep my blood pressure down, so I only stop for a few days, then I start again.

Pharmacist: I see. How often would you say you stop taking them like that?

Patient: Oh, maybe every few weeks. Then my ankles get so swelled up that I take a few extra to make up for it.

Pharmacist: That doesn't sound so good. So, the problems are that you feel tired and that you have to get up during the night to go the bathroom.

Patient: Yes.

Pharmacist: Let's see what we can do about that. Can you tell me when you usually take your pills?

Patient: Well, I usually take them in the morning.

Pharmacist: Most people forget to take their pills sometimes. How often do you find you forget?

Patient: Well, several times a week I forget to take them in the morning, then I take them when I remember, usually after supper.

Pharmacist: It's important to take this medication regularly. When you stop taking them, the fluid builds up as you've found, and when you start the pills again, you have to go to the bathroom more than usual. Also, taking them late in the day increases the chance of having to get up during the night to go to the bathroom. Try taking them every day, first thing in the morning. I'll give you a calendar and a pill-reminder package to help you keep on track.

Patient: Oh, I get it now. I really need to take them regularly. Those reminders sound like a good idea to help me remember too.

Pharmacist: Now, about your tiredness. It may be a result of having to get up during the night, or it could be caused by low potassium resulting from the

COUNSELING SITUATION **4.2:** (Continued)

hydrochlorothiazide. I mentioned a while ago that with these pills you need to have a banana or a glass of orange juice every day for extra potassium. I know it's hard to remember everything. I wonder if you've been getting enough of those foods?

Patient: Oh, I forgot about that. I haven't been doing that at all.

Pharmacist: Well, that may be the problem then. I suggest that you see your doctor. I'll call to tell her about how you've been feeling, and I'll tell her that you haven't been taking the orange juice or bananas. She'll probably want to check your potassium. If it's low, she may prescribe some potassium pills to make it up.

Patient: OK. I'll make an appointment today.

Pharmacist: Do you have any questions?

Patient: No, I think I understand now that I should take the pills every day, and that if I take them in the morning, I should be OK by bedtime. And I'd better start eating those foods with potassium.

Pharmacist: Good. I'll call you in a few days to see how you're doing and to find out what the doctor suggested.

Patient: OK. I'll talk to you then. Goodbye.

Pharmacist: *(returns to the dispensary to telephone the physician, then documents the intervention and discussion on the patient's profile)*

This time, the pharmacist conducted a complete refill counseling session. She asked appropriate probing questions to identify nonadherence, including the details of nonadherence and factors contributing to the nonadherence. She made sure not to judge the patient's forgetfulness or lack of understanding about her medication, and made it easy for the patient to fully disclose her nonadherence. Along with the patient, the pharmacist discovered how best to resolve the nonadherence, then obtained the patient's implicit agreement to discuss it with her physician. Finally, the pharmacist arranged to follow up with the patient to monitor the success of the resolution of nonadherence, then documented her intervention. Counseling for refill prescriptions will be further discussed in Chapter 5.

SUMMARY

The discussion of nonadherence in this chapter has emphasized the need for the pharmacist to deal with the patient in a helping manner. The importance of keeping an open mind and of remaining nonjudgmental when dealing with nonadherent patients has also been stressed. It has been pointed out that the content and quality of communication between the patient and the pharmacist is crucial in preventing, identifying, and resolving nonadherence problems. In addition, the pharmacist should communicate in an appropriate and timely manner with physicians and other health care workers in dealing with nonadherence by their patients. A variety of methods and tools have been discussed as they pertain to adherence counseling, and the scenario has illustrated these points.

The following three chapters will discuss more specifically the content of communication with the patient, patient–education methods, and communication skills for patient counseling.

REFLECTIVE QUESTIONS

1. Describe how the helping model and shared decision making might prevent some of the communication-related causes of nonadherence.
2. List three reasons why discussing medication side effects and adverse effects may prevent problems with nonadherence.
3. List four methods pharmacists can use to identify nonadherence.
4. Adele K. is a 57-year-old woman with hypercholesterolemia who has discontinued the use of her cholesterol-lowering medication. What factors may have contributed to this?
5. On probing you discover that Adele K. discontinued her medication due to its high cost and the fact that she did not notice any improvement in how she felt. What strategies might you use to encourage her to restart her medication?
6. Use the parameters of patient, progress, and time frame to prepare a sample plan for evaluating whether your suggestions to resolve Adele K.'s nonadherence have been effective.

REFERENCES

1. Sackett D, Snow J. The Magnitude of Compliance and Noncompliance. In: Haynes R, Taylor D, Sackett D, eds., Compliance in Health Care. The Johns Hopkins University Press, Baltimore, MD, 1979, p. 11–22.
2. Smith DS. Patient Compliance: An Educational Mandate. Norwich Eaton Pharmaceuticals, Inc. and Consumer Health Information Corp., McLean, VA, 1989.
3. Bond W, Hussar D. Detection methods and strategies for improving medication compliance. Am J Hosp Pharm. 1991;48(9):1978–1988.
4. Anonymous. Schering Report XIV. Kentucky Pharm. 1992;6:176–178.
5. Insull W. The problem of compliance to cholesterol altering therapy. J Intern Med. 1997;241:317–325.
6. Clepper I. Noncompliance: The invisible epidemic. Drug Topics. 1992;136(16):44–50, 56–65.
7. Strand LM, Cipolle RJ, Morley PC. Pharmaceutical Care: An Introduction. Current Concepts. The Upjohn Co., Kalamazoo, MI, 1992, p. 15.
8. Lasagna L. Noncompliance data and clinical outcomes: Impact on health care. Drug Topics. 1992;Suppl 136(13):33–35.
9. Becker MH, Rosenstock IM. Compliance with Medical Advice. In: Steptoe A, Mathews A, eds., Health Care and Human Behavior. Academic Press, London, 1984.
10. Conrad P. The meaning of medication: Another look at compliance. Soc Sci Med. 1985;20(1):29–37.
11. Morehead EA, Morehead L, eds. The New American Webster Dictionary. New American Library. Times Mirror, Chicago, IL, 1972.

12. Rudd P. Partial compliance in the treatment of hypertension: Issues and strategies. Drug Topics. 1992;Suppl 136(13):16–21.
13. Christensen D. Understanding patient drug-taking compliance. J Soc Admin Pharm. 1985;3(2):70–77.
14. Jacobson TA. The forgotten cardiac risk factor: Noncompliance with lipid-lowering therapy. Medscape Cardiology. 2004;8(2). Available at: www.medscape.com/viewarticle/496144 (accessed January 4, 2005).
15. Nichols-English G, Poirier S. Optimizing adherence to pharmaceutical care plans. J Am Pharm Assoc. 2000;40(4):475–485.
16. McKenney J. The Clinical Pharmacy and Compliance. In: Haynes R, Taylor D, Sackett D, eds., Compliance in Health Care. The Johns Hopkins University Press, Baltimore, MD, 1979, p. 260–277.
17. Di Matteo M, DiNicola D. The Compliance Problem: An Introduction. In: Achieving Patient Compliance. Pergamon Press, New York, 1982, p. 18–27.
18. Ley P. Memory for Medical Information. In: Communicating with Patients: Improving Communication, Satisfaction and Compliance. Croom Helm, New York, 1988, p. 27–52.
19. Fisher R. Patient education and compliance: A pharmacist's perspective. Patient Educ Couns. 1992;19:261–271.
20. Ried LD, Christensen DB. A psychological perspective in the explanation of patients' drug taking behavior. Soc Sci Med. 1988;27(3):277–285.
21. Cockburn J, Gibberd R, Reid A, et al. Determinants of noncompliance with short term antibiotic regimens. Br Med J. 1987;295:814–818.
22. Hamilton R, Briceland L. Use of prescription-refill records to assess patient compliance. Am J Hosp Pharm. 1992;49(7):1691–1696.
23. Horne R, Weinman J. Patients' beliefs about prescribed medicines and their role in adherence to treatment in chronic physical illness. J Psychosom Res. 1999;47(6):555–567.
24. Kiortsis DN, Giral P, Bruckert E, et al. Factors associated with low compliance with lipid-lowering drugs in hyperlipidemic patients. J Clin Pharm Ther. 2000;25:445–451.
25. Slovic P, Kraus N, Lappe H, et al. Risk perception of prescription drugs: Report on a survey in Canada. Pharm Pract. 1992;8(1):30–37.
26. Rudd P. Maximizing compliance with antihypertensive therapy. Drug Therap. 1992;22:25–32.
27. Mullen PO, Green LW, Pessinger GS. Clinical trials of patient education for chronic conditions: A comparative meta-analysis of intervention types. Prev Med. 1985;14:753–757.
28. Nichol M, McCombs J, Johnson K, et al. The effects of consultation on over-the-counter medication purchasing decisions. Med Care. 1992;30(11):989–1003.
29. Coulter A. Partnerships with patients: The pros and cons of shared clinical decision-making. J Health Serv Res Policy. 1997;2(2):112–121.
30. Morris LA. A survey of patients' receipt of prescription drug information. Med Care. 1982;20(6):596–605.
31. Avorn J, Monette J, Lacour A, et al. Persistence of use of lipid-lowering medications: A cross-national study. JAMA. 1998;279:1458–1462.
32. Prochaska JO, Velicer WF. The transtheoretical model of health behavior change. Am J Health Promot. 1997;12:38–48.
33. Zimmerman G, Olsen C, Bosworth C. A stages of change approach to helping patients change behavior. Am Fam Physician. 2000;61:1409–1416. Available at: www.aafp.org/afp/20000301/1409.html (accessed November 2, 2004).
34. O'Connor A, Rostom A, Fiset V, et al. Decision aids for patients facing health treatment or screening decisions: Systematic review. Br Med J. 1993;319:731–734.
35. Regner MJ, Hermann F, Ried LD. Effectiveness of a printed leaflet for enabling patients to use digoxin side effect information. Drug Intell Clin Pharm. 1987;21(2):200–204.
36. Seltzer A, Roncari I, Garfinkel P et al. Effect of patient education on medication compliance. Can J Psychol. 1980;25(12):638–645.

37. McBean BJ, Blackburn JL. An evaluation of four methods of pharmacist-conducted patient education. Can Pharm J. 1982;115(5):167–172.

38. Morris LA, Mazis M, Gordon E, et al. A survey of the effects of oral contraceptive patient information. JAMA. 1977;238(23):2504–2508.

39. Berry D, Holden W, Bersellini E. Interpretation of recommended risk terms: Differences between doctors and lay people. Int J Psychoanal Psychother. 2004;12:117–124.

40. Simpkins C, Wenzloff N. Evaluation of a computer reminder system in the enhancement of patient medication refill compliance. Drug Intell Clin Pharm. 1986;20(10):799–802.

41. Stewart M. The validity of an inteview to assess a patient's drug taking. Am J Prev Med. 1987;3(2):95–100.

42. Nagle BA, German TC, Coons SJ, et al. Developing a compliance screening program to monitor and minimize noncompliance in the elderly. Abstract of Meeting Presentation. ASHP Midyear Clinical Meeting 26 P-456D, 1991.

43. Opdycke RA, Ascione F, Shimp L, et al. A systematic approach to educating elderly patients about their medications. Patient Educ Couns. 1992;19:43–60.

44. Stoudemire A, Thompson T. Medication noncompliance: Systematic approaches to evaluation and intervention. Gen Hosp Psychiatry. 1983;5(12):233–239.

45. Eisenberg S, Delaney DJ. Working with Reluctant Clients. In: The Counseling Process, 2nd Edition. Rand McNally College Publishing, Chicago, IL, 1977.

46. Lau Carino J, Gulanick M. Using motivational interviewing to reduce diabetes risk. Prog Cardiovasc Nurs. 2004;19(4):149–154. Available at: www.medscape.com/viewarticle/496829 (accessed January 13, 2005).

47. Leventhal H, Safer MA, Panagis DM. The impact of communication on the self-regulation of health beliefs, decisions, and behavior. Health Educ Q. 1983;10(1):3–29.

48. Given C, Given B, Coyle B. The effect of patient characteristics and beliefs on responses to behavioral intervention for control of chronic disease. Patient Educ Couns. 1984;6(3):137–140.

49. Owens N. Patient noncompliance: Subset analysis. Drug Topics. 1992;Suppl 136(13):11–15.

50. Moore SR. Cognitive variants in the elderly: Integral part of medication counseling. Drug Intell Clin Pharm. 1983;17(11):840–842.

51. Schoepp G. For kids only. Drug Merch. 1990;71(1):26–31.

The Counseling Session

Objectives

After completing the chapter, the reader should be able to

1. list and describe five phases of the patient-counseling session.
2. list the types of information that should be gathered and provided for a new prescription.
3. describe how the following situations might differ from a patient-counseling session for a new prescription: Refill prescriptions, monitoring follow-up, and self-care consultations.
4. explain the purpose and content of a medication management consultation.
5. be prepared to conduct a counseling session and a medication management consultation.

Having considered the goals of counseling, and patients' needs and concerns with respect to medication use, let us now turn to the specifics of the counseling session. In studies of pharmacist-counseling activities, the counseling session has generally been found to consist of a sequence of instructions with little input from the patient other than token responses such as "okay" or "mhmm."[1] However, the patient–pharmacist encounter should consist of an exchange of information, feelings, beliefs, values, and ideas between the patient and the pharmacist—much like any other conversation between two people. It should not consist of a one-sided lecture by the pharmacist.

The manner adopted in asking questions and the wording used to present information may be critical to the outcome of the counseling session. Most importantly, there should be two-way communication, with multiple opportunities for discussion and for the patient to ask questions. This shows genuine concern for the patient and allows the pharmacist to monitor the patient's cognitive processing.[2,3] Suggested dialogues to use during counseling are provided in Appendix A, and the communication skills involved are discussed in Chapter 7.

It may be useful at this point to refer back to Chapter 2 and review the purpose of counseling, remembering that there are both counseling and educational goals. The pharmacist's main purpose is to educate patients about medication-related issues and to help them get the most benefit from their medications. This involves more than providing information, and should include enhancing patients' skills, knowledge, attitudes, and behavior with respect to their illnesses and their medications.

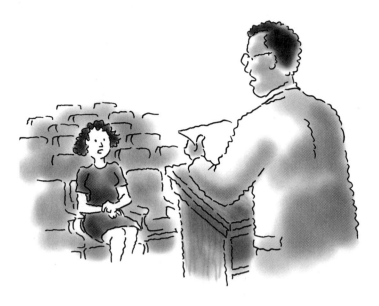

It is helpful to follow a set format for counseling, in order to help the pharmacist be as efficient and effective as possible, keeping focused on the task and covering all necessary areas. It is also most effective for patients with respect to memory and understanding, when a standard schema is adhered to.[4]

The specific details of the discussion during the counseling session will depend on the nature of the encounter and the reason the counseling is taking place. It may involve a new patient or a returning patient. It may concern a new medication or a refill, a prescription or a nonprescription medication. Some counseling sessions are not focused on a medication, but rather on gathering information such as a medication management consultation, follow-up medication monitoring, or a response by the pharmacist to an inquiry by the patient regarding a specific condition, symptom, or medication. Each of these requires modification of the counseling content.

Since all patients are individuals with varying needs, the content of counseling should be tailored to meet those needs. Some patients may be overwhelmed by too much information, resulting in feelings of frustration or information overload, and therefore the counseling may be conducted over several sessions or supplemented with printed information.[2] Other patients may need specific types of information about their condition or about treatment choices. Tailoring counseling to the needs of various patients will be discussed further in Chapter 8.

PREPARING FOR THE COUNSELING SESSION

If possible, the pharmacist should prepare for the counseling session. In the case of prescription counseling for a returning patient, the pharmacist has an opportunity to prepare for the counseling session during the dispensing process. Through review of the patient's medication record, the pharmacist may identify real or potential problems such as nonadherence (over- or underuse), drug interactions, allergies to prescribed drugs, or interference with existing conditions. In addition, the pharmacist should note any information that may affect counseling or medication use such as disabilities (e.g., impaired hearing or eyesight) or language barriers.

In the case of a new patient to the pharmacy, this information needs to be gathered through a medication management consultation, which is discussed in detail later in this chapter.

If real or potential problems are identified at this point, appropriate prevention or resolution of problems may be considered and appropriate action may be necessary prior to meeting with the patient. This may involve discussion with the physician, consultation of references, and/or consideration of nonadherence resolution methods described earlier. Further problem identification and resolution will be carried out during the patient-counseling session.

Preparation for the patient-counseling session may also involve a review by the pharmacist of information concerning the medication and the condition being treated. In addition, any available patient education materials regarding the condition being treated and the medication should be selected for the patient.

A further consideration the pharmacist should make before entering into discussion with the patient is the need for privacy. All counseling should be conducted with a relative degree of privacy in order to maintain confidentiality of patient information. It will encourage the patient to disclose appropriate personal information, as well as allow the pharmacist to interact with the patient in an atmosphere free from distractions. If the medication involves a condition that might be embarrassing for the patient, instructions that may be complicated, or issues that need to be addressed that may be time-consuming, counseling will be more suitable—and more productive—if it takes place in a private area away from the main dispensing area. If this is not possible, it may be better to suggest to the patient that the counseling be carried out over the telephone. The issue of pharmacy design to ensure privacy will be discussed in Chapter 9.

THE FIVE PHASES OF THE COUNSELING SESSION

The counseling session should proceed in a logical manner. It has been found that patients understand and remember information better when information is grouped into categories and tasks.[4] As illustrated in the diagram in Figure 5-1, the counseling session may be divided into five phases: (1) the opening discussion; (2) discussion to gather information and identify needs; (3) discussion to resolve problems and develop a pharmaceutical care plan; (4) discussion to provide information and educate; (5) the closing discussion.

This is only a suggested protocol, and the patient may alter the flow at any point by asking a specific question requiring immediate discussion. If the question does not relate specifically to the medication counseling, however, the pharmacist might choose to postpone the discussion until after the counseling is completed. In any event, the question should not be ignored. It may also be necessary to break the counseling into several sessions as noted above.

1. Opening discussion
• Introduction • Explain purpose of counseling

2. Discussion to gather information and identify needs

New patient
• Gather patient information
• Conduct medication management consult

Returning patient
• Confirm patient information
• Confirm medication use information

New Rx
• Knowledge about purpose, medication, regimen and condition, and treatment goal
• Potential problems

Refill Rx/Follow-up monitoring
• Adherence problems
• Details of medication use
• Evidence of side effects
• Effectiveness of treatment
• Potential problems

Self-care
• Description and duration of symptoms
• Has physician been consulted?
• What treatment has been used previously?

3. Discussion to develop care plan and resolve problems
• Discuss real or potential problems
• Agree on alternatives
• Implement plan
• Discuss outcomes and monitoring

4. Discussion to provide information and educate

New prescription
• Provide information on condition and medication
• Adherence and self-monitoring
• Refill and follow-up monitoring

Nonprescription drug

Medication recommended
• Provide information on condition and medication
• Future treatment
• Reassurance
• Self-monitoring
• Side effects and precautions
• Non-drug treatment
• Pharmacist follow-up

No medication recommended
• Refer to physician
• Suggest non-drug treatment
• Provide information needed
• Reassurance
• Pharmacist follow-up

Refill Rx/Follow-up monitoring
• Clarify drug or condition information
• Self-monitoring information
• Refer to physician prn
• Resolve side effects
• Reassure

5. Closing discussion
• Recap • Get feedback • Encourage questions • Confirm monitoring follow-up

Figure 5-1 **The Five Phases of the Counseling Session**

    The pharmacist must also decide where to place the emphasis in the counseling protocol to maximize its effectiveness and efficiency. This involves "tailoring" the counseling to the specific patient, medication, condition, and situation as noted above.

    Counseling Situation 5.1 illustrates the difficulties of conducting an effective and efficient patient-counseling session without adopting the suggested phases of counseling.

COUNSELING SITUATION 5.1: Counseling Without a Protocol

Mrs. Hampton is a middle-aged woman. It is her first time in this particular pharmacy, and she has not previously been counseled by a pharmacist. She gives the pharmacist a new prescription for minocycline. The pharmacist notices that Mrs. Hampton's name is not familiar.

Pharmacist: Hello, Mrs. Hampton. Have you had prescriptions filled here before? *Closed*

Patient: No, I usually go to the pharmacy close to my office.

Pharmacist: You'll have to fill out this patient history form then. What's your *No sm talk* address, phone number, and drug-plan information?

Patient: (*indignantly*) If this is going to be a problem, I can go back to the other pharmacy.

Pharmacist: (*quickly*) No, no. We can fill the prescription for you here. Just *Increase / disagreed?* fill this form out while you're waiting. I just need your name, address, and drug-plan information to get started.

Patient: (*reluctantly*) OK.

. . .10 minutes pass.

Pharmacist: Mrs. Hampton. Your prescription is ready now.

Patient: (*returns to the pharmacy counter and hands over the patient history form*) Here's your form. I don't know why you need all this information. My doctor has it all.

Pharmacist: It's just for our records. Now, let me see. (*glances at the patient* *Patronized* history form) You seem to have filled this out correctly.

Patient: (*getting more aggravated by the minute, not realizing that the antacid she takes occasionally for stomach upset and the calcium supplement she takes are considered nonprescription medications*) I don't see the point in all this information, just let me have my prescription.

Pharmacist: (*not wanting to aggravate the patient any further*) Well, I guess that's OK then. I'll just take a minute to go over your new medication with you. It's a type of antibiotic called minocycline.

Patient: Look, I've taken antibiotics before. (*She thinks she will need to take it four times a day for a few weeks as previously for an infection.*) Now, can I go?

Pharmacist: Yes. Well, here's some more information on this sheet. (*attempts to review it with the patient*)

Patient: (*snatches the sheet from the pharmacist's hands*) Fine, I'll read it at home.

Pharmacist: OK. Well, if you have any questions after you read this feel free to call.

Patient: Sure. (*She walks away thinking, "What a waste of time! Next time I'll just go back to the other pharmacy. They never hassle me like this." When she gets home she takes the prescription out of the bag and throws the bag with the information sheet inside into the garbage, forgetting that it is there and proceeds to take four capsules daily without reading the label.*)

This pharmacist had very good intentions to learn about the patient's medication use before proceeding to counsel this new patient. But something went wrong! The patient wasn't at all receptive. In fact, she viewed the discussion as an aggravation. As a result, the pharmacist was not able to develop sufficient rapport with the patient to allow complete assessment of the medication use, or even to conduct appropriate counseling for a new prescription. If the pharmacist had properly conducted the five phases of counseling, starting with an opening discussion, gathering necessary information appropriately, he or she would have been able to identify drug-related problems, resolve the problems, and educate the patient as needed. The pharmacist would have discovered the potential overuse and drug interactions and would have been able to proceed to counsel the patient about appropriate use.

The following sections will describe each of the five phases of counseling in detail. Figure 5-1 summarizes the information to be gathered, with slight variations depending on whether it is for a new or returning patient, new or refill prescription, follow-up monitoring, or a nonprescription drug, which will be discussed in more detail later in this chapter.

The Opening Discussion

Patients report that they want to feel at ease, participate in the counseling, have confidence in the quality of counseling, and feel genuine concern by the pharmacist.[3] The purpose of the opening discussion is to do this. It will build rapport with the patient, developing a helping relationship and a sense of trust in the pharmacist.

During the next phase of the counseling session, the pharmacist will need to ask a number of personal questions to gather information and to make appropriate decisions regarding the nature of the patient's real or potential problems and methods to resolve them. Such questions may affect the patient's self-image (*face*) and may not be expected from a pharmacist (although patients expect them from the physician).[3] The pharmacist can reduce this threat to face through the opening phase of counseling by being polite, explaining the need for the questions, and attempting to set a caring and conversational tone.

If the patient and pharmacist have not previously met, the pharmacist should introduce himself or herself, stating his or her name and position clearly. The patient's identity should also be verified to ensure that the correct patient is receiving the prescription and to confirm that the person picking up the prescription is indeed the patient. The patient's name should then be used during the counseling session to help personalize the encounter.

If the person is not actually the patient being discussed, the pharmacist must determine whether the information can be reliably transmitted to the patient. If at all possible, it is advisable to arrange to speak with the patient in person or by telephone at least to confirm that all information and instructions have been relayed and understood, and to explore any problems or concerns that the patient may have. Pharmacy regulations in some jurisdictions require that an "offer" to counsel the patient be made "in person" whenever possible, or through access to toll-free telephone service.[1]

As a further attempt to set the patient at ease and create a friendly atmosphere, the pharmacist should try to engage the patient in casual conversation. For example, the pharmacist might comment on the weather or inquire after the patient's family. Although this "warm-up conversation" should be brief, it should not appear rushed.

Following the introduction and warm-up conversation, the purpose of the counseling should be made clear to the patient. The pharmacist should explain what will follow, why, and how long it will take. This will prepare the patient for the potentially personal nature of the discussion and may motivate the patient to participate. The purpose should be presented in terms of the benefit to the patient—with the main purpose always being for the patient to get the most benefit from the medication.

If the patient indicates that he or she does not have time to discuss the medication immediately (even after being told of the importance of the information to the outcome of the therapy), then it may be necessary to arrange for the conversation to take place, either in person or by telephone, at an alternate time. It can be very difficult to counsel an unwilling patient, and beyond a certain point, any attempt to do so is likely to prove a waste of time and effort. In this case, the pharmacist should be sure to document that the offer to counsel was made and that the patient refused. If possible, written information should be provided, along with the pharmacist's card and encouragement to call later with any questions or concerns. Keep in mind the following guidelines:

1. *Opening Discussion for a New Prescription*: The need to introduce counseling is especially important if the patient has never been counseled by a pharmacist before. In such circumstances, patients are sometimes disconcerted by the pharmacist's attention, unprepared to discuss personal information, and possibly unwilling to spend the necessary time talking with the pharmacist. For a new patient with a new medication the amount of information to be gathered and provided in the next two phases of counseling can be quite time-consuming. Patients can become overwhelmed and so it is important to explain this to the patient, and perhaps make arrangements to conduct some of the counseling at a more convenient time.

2. *Opening Discussion for a Refill Prescription or Follow-up Drug Monitoring*: Some patients and pharmacists may expect that since the patient was counseled when the medication was first received, there is no need for further discussion. However, it is important to follow-up with patients to assess the effectiveness of medication and monitor the patient's medication use to identify actual or potential drug-related problems, particularly nonadherence or side effects. Evaluation of the patient's current status and outcome of medication use is an important role in pharmaceutical care.[5]

Ideally, a pharmaceutical care plan is prepared at the time of a new medication being dispensed, with a monitoring plan set in place. With the first refill of medication, or at another agreed-upon interval, the pharmacist can start to follow the patient's progress and may determine the degree of success of treatment and the plan implemented during counseling.[5] This important part of pharmaceutical care requires the pharmacist to take responsibility for ensuring that outcomes of drug therapy are positive.[5]

In the opening phase of counseling, it is necessary to explain this to the patient, reminding him or her of any previously arranged follow-up monitoring. As there is usually less need to provide information, there may be more time for the pharmacist to take the opportunity to get to know the patient through the warm-up conversation.

Discussion to Gather Information and Identify Needs

In this phase of the counseling session, the pharmacist's aim is to gather any information from the patient with a view to identifying real or potential problems with the medication, as well as to identify the patient's information needs.

Information Gathering with a New Patient

If the patient is new to the pharmacy, the pharmacist will need to gather basic patient information. This should include the following information: Name, address, telephone number, age, and gender.[6] In addition, information should be recorded regarding the patient's history where significant, including disease state or states, known allergies and drug reactions, and a comprehensive list of medications and relevant devices. The pharmacist's comments relevant to the individual's drug therapy should also be noted.[6]

Gathering patient history through a medication management consultation will be discussed in further detail later in this chapter. It may be practical to gather as much as possible of the above information and brief details pertinent to the medication being dispensed during the medication-counseling session, and to schedule a complete medication management consultation for a time more convenient for the pharmacist and patient.

Information Gathering with a Returning Patient

For a returning patient, certain information should already be available from a previously conducted medication management consultation and from the patient record or chart. In this case, the pharmacist simply has to inquire to confirm that there are no changes such as new conditions or medications received elsewhere, either prescription or nonprescription.

Information Gathering for a New Prescription

If the encounter involves a new prescription, the following information should be obtained from the patient, in addition to the patient information and medication-history information discussed above:

1. *Previous Use*: The pharmacist must first determine whether the patient has ever taken the medication before. Even for a returning patient for whom the medication does not appear on the patient record, the patient may have received the medication from another pharmacy, directly from the physician, or during a hospital visit. If the patient has taken the medication previously, the remainder of the counseling will be geared to a refill, rather than a new prescription.

2. *Knowledge about Medication Purpose and Condition*: If the prescription is indeed new, the pharmacist must determine the condition being treated and the patient's understanding and perception of this. The pharmacist should ask what the physician has told the patient about the purpose of the medication. This will allow the pharmacist to gauge the level of the patient's understanding about his or her condition and the purpose of the medication, and will allow the patient the opportunity to express concerns or problems regarding his or her condition. The pharmacist will then be able to assess the patient's information needs in this

regard, and to identify potential misunderstanding or lack of motivation that may lead to nonadherence.

This discussion also provides the pharmacist with an indication of the patient's language level. The pharmacist should then adopt this language during the following discussion as much as possible (e.g., if the patient refers to his or her epileptic seizures as *blackouts*, the pharmacist should use the same term). If knowledge of the language of the country or a language the pharmacist can speak is a concern, then this must be addressed (Chapter 8 for further discussion).

Through the discussion the pharmacist will also gain information to evaluate whether the prescribed medication is an appropriate choice. Although the patient's view of the purpose of the medication may or may not be accurate, the discussion will bring out any gross errors. If possible, the pharmacist should supplement this information with the actual medical diagnosis or treatment goal from the physician.

3. *Knowledge of Medication Regimen*: The pharmacist must then determine the patient's understanding of how the medication is to be used. The pharmacist should ask the patient what the physician has said about medication use and whether the patient anticipates any difficulties taking the medication as prescribed. This will allow the pharmacist to assess the patient's information needs and may save time if the patient demonstrates that he or she already understands the information clearly. Again, this will give the patient the opportunity to raise anticipated concerns or potential difficulties with the regimen, and will allow the pharmacist to identify potential nonadherence or dosing problems.

4. *Treatment Goal*: The patient may also be asked what he or she would like to accomplish by taking this medication. This will further elucidate any perceptions regarding medication use that would lead to nonadherence.

5. *Potential Problems*: At this point, the pharmacist can start to identify potential problems. Inquiring about how the patient feels about taking the medication and whether there are any difficulties that they foresee with taking the medication may alert the pharmacist to further issues to investigate.

(6) Reservation or fears

Information Gathering for a Refill Prescription or Follow-up Medication Monitoring

If the encounter involves a refill prescription or a follow-up medication-monitoring interview, the following information should be gathered, in addition to the patient information and medication use information discussed above, where necessary:

1. *Details of Medication Use*: The pharmacist should determine how the patient is using the medication and whether the patient has experienced any difficulty thus far in taking the medication (e.g., overuse or underuse). If a review of the patient record has indicated nonadherence, questioning should concern the actual frequency of medication use and the possible reasons for nonadherence. As stressed in the previous chapter, this should be a gentle probing, not an inquisition. Factors contributing to nonadherence should be explored as discussed in the previous chapter (e.g., difficulties with dosing regimen, misunderstanding about use, and perceptions about need).

2. *Effectiveness of Medication*: The pharmacist should also attempt to assess whether the medication is effective. The pharmacist should ask if the medication is helping and if it is accomplishing what was expected. In addition to the patient's perceptions, the pharmacist should ask specific questions about symptoms that would indicate medication effectiveness in a clinical sense (e.g., blood pressure levels). The patient may not be the most accurate source of this information so that, where possible, this should be supplemented with actual clinical data from the physician, patient chart, or measurements taken in the pharmacy (e.g., blood pressure).

    This discussion also allows the pharmacist to identify any misgivings or concerns that the patient might have (e.g., the patient may report reduced blood pressure readings, but that he or she doesn't notice any difference in how he or she feels, and therefore sees little point in continuing with medication use).

3. *Presence of Adverse Effects*: The pharmacist should determine if any adverse effects are occurring. Such questioning should always be prefaced by a general statement about the rarity of adverse effects and the necessity of checking for signs to allow for prompt treatment should they occur. It should also be balanced with mention of the benefit of medication. The patient should be asked if he or she has felt any different than usual while on this medication. Probing regarding specific adverse effects can follow. Note that in this discussion, symptoms should be described rather than providing the medical names of conditions (e.g., *unexplained fever* rather than *blood dyscrasias*). It is important to gather information regarding the duration and severity of side effects in order to allow the pharmacist and physician to decide if a change in medication is warranted or if the side effects are manageable. The patient's perceptions and quality of life are important here since he or she may be unwilling to tolerate a side effect that is considered clinically manageable (e.g., constipation).

Discussion to Develop a Care Plan and Resolve Problems

Having gathered complete information, the pharmacist is now in a position to resolve actual or potential problems identified and develop a pharmaceutical care plan.[5] In some situations, the pharmacist may have the luxury of time to break at this point to document and assess the information gathered in order to develop a detailed pharmaceutical care plan. In other cases, this must be done on the spot, with a short pause for the pharmacist to complete documentation of data gathered and to collect thoughts. It is generally recommended that documented notes should follow the SOAP format (subjective, objective, assessment, plan) used in medicine for the problem-oriented medical record system.

Developing a Care Plan for a New Prescription

Developing a pharmaceutical care plan will require thought on the pharmacist's part, as well as discussion with the patient. If real or potential problems have been identified, then the pharmacist should inform the patient that there are some important things to discuss. The patient and pharmacist should then negotiate the order of importance.[5]

Next, desired pharmacotherapeutic outcomes for each real or potential problem should be established.[5] This should be done through discussion with the patient, and should include ways the patient could identify these outcomes.[5] For example, for a patient experiencing constipation as a result of medication use, the pharmacist may discuss the situation with the patient and determine that the patient would like the constipation alleviated so that his or her normal once-daily bowel movement would return, and that this would occur by the end of 2 weeks.

If discussion with the patient results in a conclusion that the patient's therapy should be altered, then the pharmacist must identify alternatives.[5] These alternatives should be discussed with the patient, and, if a change in a prescribed drug is involved, then with the physician. For example, the patient experiencing constipation as a result of medication use may require a change to a medication that does not cause constipation, or the addition of an extra medication to alleviate constipation.

As a result of these deliberations, the pharmacist should then determine the best pharmacotherapeutic solution and individualize the therapeutic regimen.[5] The patient should again be involved in a discussion regarding the choice of drug, dose, formulation, and regimen. For example, for the patient with constipation, the choice of laxative should be discussed with the patient to be sure that it meets his or her wishes as far as dosage form, time to effect, and frequency of need.

Any changes in therapy should then be initiated and documented by the pharmacist.[5]

Finally, the pharmacist should discuss a follow-up monitoring plan with the patient.[5] This may involve a telephone call to the patient, who would keep track of symptoms; the patient returning to the physician at set intervals; or the patient returning to the pharmacy at set intervals, when the prescription is refilled or at more frequent intervals. At this point, any information or education needs should be apparent.

Developing a Care Plan for a Refill Prescription or Follow-up Medication Monitoring

Strategy for adherence

This phase of counseling for a refill prescription or during a medication-monitoring interview involves documenting any changes to the treatment plan and documentation regarding success of the plan to date as evidenced by the discussion with the patient.

This phase of counseling is difficult to implement when patients do not always frequent the same pharmacy. The pharmacist can help implement monitoring by explaining to the patient during new prescription counseling that this service will occur if he or she continues to patronize this pharmacy exclusively.

Discussion to Provide Information and Educate

Now that any real or potential problems have been identified, and a plan has been developed to deal with problems where necessary, informational and educational needs should be satisfied.

The pharmacist will most likely need to provide the patient with information about the medication he or she is receiving and, if necessary, about the condition for which he or she is being treated. As discussed in Chapter 4, this may prevent any potential adherence problems (provided it is presented in an appropriate way). Along with verbal information, additional information sources, such as print information and audiovisual materials, may be given to the patient for future reference either at this stage of the counseling session or later during the closing phase of the session. Patient information materials will be discussed in Chapter 6.

In the past, there has been some controversy about how much information a patient should be given about his or her medication and condition, and which health professional should provide it. As mentioned in Chapter 1, pharmacists have legal and professional obligations to provide sufficient information; in some jurisdictions legislation and regulations clearly specify the details to be provided. There are sometimes concerns about infringing on the physician's responsibility. However, even if the physician has provided information, it is helpful for the pharmacist to review this, as patients often do not retain all the information provided in an often-rushed physician consultation, and may need clarification or have further questions.

The pharmacist must often decide the extent of detail that is appropriate on the basis of several considerations. One consideration is that of the patient's rights and preferences. Members of the public have become increasingly aware of their rights to know about their drug treatments, alternative treatments, and possible risks of treatment.[7] Studies of patients find that they want to know about their medications and specifically about risks and adverse effects.[8,9]

Another consideration is the pharmacist's perception of the patient's ability to understand the information based on the patient's level of education, language barriers, and so on.

The pharmacist must weigh these considerations for each individual patient and situation, but the needs of the patient identified during the information gathering and care plan development phases of counseling should be the ultimate guide to the selection of information. Information that the patient indicated knowledge of during the previous phase of counseling can be omitted and specific questions the patient raised about his or her therapy or condition should be addressed here.

Providing Information for Refill Prescription or Follow-up Monitoring

If problems such as nonadherence, side effects, or adverse effects were not detected during the information-gathering phase, the patient may not need to be given any new information. In this case, the pharmacist might simply reinforce previous information provided to the patient about precautions that should be observed while on the medication. The need for continued use of the medication should be affirmed and encouraged, and the availability of refills and further follow-up should be confirmed.

Resolution of identified adherence problems may involve providing information about the patient's medical condition; information about the way the medication is intended to work; reassurance about the efficacy of the medication; suggestions for altering the regimen to improve adherence; education about how to self-monitor progress; suggestions for further discussion with the physician; or motivational strategies discussed in the previous chapter.

If side effects or adverse effects were detected, the patient may need information about actions to reduce side effects (e.g., take with food); reassurance that the effects are mild or that they are likely to decrease with continued medication use; methods to continue monitoring side effects and actions to take if they become more severe; or recommendation to consult a physician for further assessment.

Providing Information for a New Prescription

For a new prescription, the patient needs to be educated about all aspects of the medication. Since this is often a good deal of information, it is important to provide it in a succinct and organized manner. It has been found that a commonly preferred schema by patients is general information about the medication (name, purpose), how to take (dose and schedule), and outcomes (warnings, mild side effects, severe side effects).[4] The specific types of information that may be necessary to provide for a new prescription include the following:

1. _The Name and Description of the Drug_: Although the name of the drug appears on the label of the prescription, generic and trade names may be somewhat confusing for the patient, and the relationship between the two should be clarified. The dosage form of the drug should be made clear, e.g., liquid medicine to be taken by mouth.

2. _The Purpose:_ The purpose of the medication and, briefly, how it is intended to work should be stated in the simplest terms. If necessary, more detail may be provided regarding the condition being treated.

3. _How and When to Take_: The patient should be shown the label on the prescription package, and the instructions should be read from it. Further explanation may be necessary in some cases, for example, that "every 4 hours" means "around the clock."   *missed*
   clock."   *closes*
   If the medication must be ingested or applied in a particular way, the patient should be instructed concerning the proper procedure, then encouraged to practice it. If the instructions are complicated or require skill development, as in the case of inhaler use, the patient should be asked to repeat the instructions back to the pharmacist (placebo inhalers are available from manufacturers for demonstration purposes). In addition, any special directions or precautions regarding preparation or use should be provided (e.g., use in a ventilated area; may stain clothes).

4. _Adherence Suggestions and Self-monitoring_: The patient should be asked if he or she foresees any difficulty in using the medication as instructed, and if so, suggestions for overcoming them should be made, as discussed in the previous chapter. Potential nonadherence problems should also be anticipated as a result of previous information gathered, and suggestions should be made to prevent nonadherence such as techniques to remember medication use, suggestions of how to involve family or friends, and so forth. Information should also be provided about what to do if a dose is missed, particularly if a missed dose would be critical (e.g., with oral contraceptives).
   Self-monitoring symptoms is important in preventing nonadherence. The patient needs to know how to evaluate the effectiveness of the medication and the basis on which to decide whether, or when, to discontinue medication use (e.g., what blood pressure should be and what to do if it registers above or below a given range). This may involve suggesting the patient learn to take his or her own blood pressure readings or keep a diary of symptom severity and improvement.

5. _Side Effects and Adverse Effects_: As noted above, the depth to which information on this subject is provided will depend on the patient and the situation. Patients generally want more information than pharmacists expect, but too much information can result in feelings of frustration or information overload.[1]
   The pharmacist should preface the discussion with a statement about the rarity of such effects, and balance this statement with the benefits of the medication. As discussed in Chapter 3, when patients are properly prepared, they are

likely to feel more in control of the situation and are less apprehensive about their medication use.

Only the symptoms of adverse effects should be described, and complicated names of conditions (e.g., blood dyscrasia) should be avoided. It is very important that the patient be told how to handle the symptoms, whether by employing actions that will minimize them (such as taking the medication with food or plenty of water) or by contacting the prescribing physician immediately.

The patient should be told which symptoms are minor and of little concern and which symptoms necessitate contact with the physician. The patient should always be reassured that these effects are not likely to occur, but that, if they do, early detection and treatment are essential.

There is controversy about how best to word discussions of the degree of risk of treatments. Pharmacists often use very vague terms such as *sometimes, possibly*, or *might occur*.[1] In Europe, guidelines have been published which suggest verbal descriptors ranging from *very rare* (less than 0.01% frequency) to *very common* (greater than 10% frequency).[10] However, studies have found that patients tend to overestimate the likelihood of side effects occurring when these verbal descriptors are used.[10]

Patients may prefer to be given numerical frequency descriptors (10%, 1%, less than 1%) and have been found to make more accurate predictions of their personal likelihood of experiencing adverse effects when they are used.[1] These percentages can also be translated into integers, such as "a chance of 1 in 10," to help make it more understandable.[11] It has also been found helpful to make comparisons to familiar risks, for example, "less than the risk of having a car accident."[11] Pictorial representations, for example, showing a crowd of 100 people with affected people in a different color, or bar graphs and pie charts may be preferred for some patients, particularly the less literate.[11]

6. *Precautions, Contraindications, and Interactions*: The patient should always be advised about any precautions associated with the medication that apply specifically to the patient—for example, for a pregnant woman that the medication could harm a fetus or be transmitted to an infant through the mother's breast milk. Those that do not apply to the patient should not be mentioned.

   The pharmacist should also make the patient aware of possible interactions with certain nonprescription medications and alcohol. If a number of possible interactions exist, it might be more useful to instruct the patient to consult with the pharmacist or prescribing physician before using any nonprescription medications, and to inform any future physicians or pharmacists of current medication use. The topic of alcohol use should be addressed in a nonjudgmental manner, explaining the reason for mention. Suggested wording for such discussions is provided in Appendix A.

   Contraindications to medication use should also be addressed in case the patient develops the conditions in the future. For example, if a patient were to decide to try to become pregnant, a potentially teratogenic drug should be discontinued.

7. *Storage Instructions:* Any special storage instructions, such as the need to refrigerate the medication, should be stated, even if the relevant information appears on an auxiliary label affixed to the package.

8. *Refill Information and Follow-up Monitoring Plan*: The patient should be informed if the physician has indicated that the prescription may be refilled. If no such instructions have been supplied with the prescription, the patient should be asked whether the physician gave any verbal instructions regarding follow-up. If the physician has not discussed these matters with the patient, then the patient should be advised to consult with the physician.

   Further monitoring and follow-up by the pharmacist should be discussed here if it was not discussed in the previous section during discussion of the care plan. How often and through what means (telephone, pharmacist home visit, pharmacy appointment) can be negotiated with the patient and may also depend on the condition, the drug, and the patient. For example, a patient who appears confused about using medication or unsure about adhering should be followed-up at shorter intervals and more frequently than a patient who appears confident and adherent.

Closing Discussion

In closing the patient-counseling session, it is important to allow the patient an opportunity to consider the information he or she has received and to ask any further questions. If the patient appears to be confused or if a language problem is suspected, it may be useful to ask the patient to repeat the most important information, such as directions for use. People are often unsure of themselves and fear that they may appear stupid if they ask questions. The pharmacist needs to reassure patients that they should feel free to ask anything at all or to discuss any concerns, whether now or later.

The closing discussion should also be used to reiterate and emphasize the most important points of the counseling, since the last message heard is usually the one that is remembered best.

Additional information sources such as written information, if available, may be provided to the patient at this point as an alternative to during the information-giving phase of the session.

. Just to make sure I didn't leave anything out, please tell me how you are going to take the med...

SELF-CARE COUNSELING

As noted above, the purpose of the specific counseling session may call for a modification to the content of counseling. Although self-care counseling should still follow the recommended five phases shown in Figure 5-1, there will be an emphasis on the information-gathering phase in order to assess the appropriateness of medication use. Before discussing the protocol for self-care counseling, it is useful to review the issues of self-care and self-treatment, the need for self-care counseling, and the pharmacist's role in self-care counseling.

Self-care and Self-treatment

Self-care has been defined as "a process whereby a lay person can function effectively on his or her own behalf in health promotion and decision making, in disease prevention, detection, and treatment at the level of the primary health resource in the health care system."[12] Although self-care activities can range from breast self-examination to performing home pregnancy tests, or simply regular exercise, a frequent activity is self-treatment with medication.[13]

Self-treatment is very common: consumers self-treat four times more health problems than doctors and 60% to 95% of all illnesses are initially treated with self-care.[14] Nonprescription drug use is very common, with 77% of Americans reporting use in the past 6 months.[14] Nonprescription drugs are used either on a regular basis for chronic conditions such as stomach ulcers, or intermittently, for acute conditions such as colds. Most commonly they are taken for pain (78%); cough, cold, flu, or sore throat (52%); allergy or sinus problems (45%); heartburn, indigestion, and other stomach problems (37%); constipation, diarrhea, and gas (21%); minor infections (12%); and skin problems (10%).[15]

There is a growing trend toward self-care, and consumers often view self-medication as a right.[16] Part of the trend toward self-care has been the greater availability of effective nonprescription drugs. In the United States, the Food and Drug Administration (FDA) began conducting a comprehensive review of over-the-counter drug products in 1972, resulting in a gradual switch of many prescription drugs to nonprescription drug status.[16,17] From 1976 to 2001, 73 ingredients, dosages, or indications were switched from prescription to nonprescription drug status; more than 700 nonprescription products contained ingredients and dosages that were only available by prescription 30 years before.[14] Self-treatment by the patient has advantages for both the individual and the health care system. To relieve minor symptoms and ailments, patients can more conveniently and more readily treat themselves than if they seek professional help. Self-treatment also relieves medical services of a heavy burden, resulting in lower costs to individuals as well as state and federal governments. In America, drugs account for 60% of medications purchased, but only 3% of total US health care expenditures, making it a cost-effective form of health care.[13,18] By using nonprescription drugs to treat minor ailments, American consumers apparently save $20 billion in health care costs each year through savings on prescription costs, physician visits, loss of wages, and productivity.[19]

Other factors contributing to the self-care movement include improved education among patients, increased health awareness and availability of health information, escalating health care costs, an aging population with more health problems, advances in the technology of diagnostic aids and monitoring devices, and an increasingly hurried lifestyle.[13]

Need for Self-care Counseling by Pharmacists

Nonprescription drugs are considered to be relatively safe for use without professional supervision as long as labeled directions are followed.[20] This is not necessarily the case, however, since a wide range of potential problems can arise, including interactions with other prescribed or nonprescribed medicines or alcohol; interference with existing chronic conditions; interference with the course of pregnancy or fetal development; excessive dosing or chronic use leading to physical damage and habituation or addiction; delay in receiving a correct diagnosis and treatment for more serious disease; and adverse effects or allergic reactions.[21]

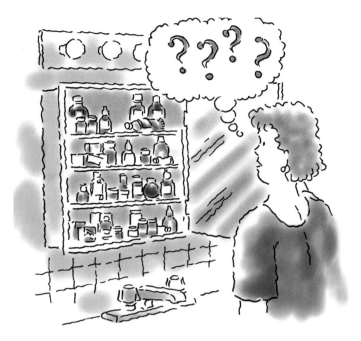

In a 2001 national survey in the United States, 48% of Americans said they take more than the recommended dose of a nonprescription medicine at times, and 36% said they would combine nonprescription medicines to treat multiple symptoms.[15,22]

Many problems have been detected through studies of hospital admissions or patient surveys.[23–25] Children and the elderly are particularly of concern. Only 40% of caregivers were found to be able to select a correct dose of acetaminophen for their child.[26] One-third of all nonprescription medicines sold in the United States are consumed by adults aged 65 and older. Many elderly people use nonsteroidal anti-inflammatory drugs (NSAIDs) resulting in serious adverse effects. A study of patients with arthritis found that they experienced gastrointestinal (GI) complications from NSAIDs resulting in 107,000 hospitalizations and at least 16,500 deaths annually.[27]

It is therefore evident that consumers need help in making decisions regarding self-treatment. Pharmacists are in an ideal position to provide the advice needed to ensure safe and effective self-treatment, because they are often the patient's first point of contact with the health care system.[28]

Pharmacist's Role in Self-care Counseling

According to a 2003 US national survey, only 43% of people consult a pharmacist when buying a nonprescription drug.[22] Pharmacists should not wait for patients to make requests, but should be proactive and offer their services to patients selecting a nonprescription drug. Patients often do not ask the pharmacist for advice about non-prescription drugs because they believe that they know all that is necessary or because they are unaware of potential problems.

Pharmaceutical care should not be relegated exclusively to prescription drug products.[13] The four outcomes that are sought by pharmacists in providing pharmaceutical care (curing disease, reducing or eliminating symptoms, arresting or slowing a disease process, or prevention of disease or its symptoms) can often be achieved with the use of nonprescription drugs, either at the request of the consumer or by the pharmacist's recommendation.[13]

When counseling a patient about self-treatment, the pharmacist should proceed through the patient care process.[5] By reviewing the patient's symptoms and considering various other factors, the pharmacist can differentiate between symptoms indicative of a serious condition that requires formal medical referral and symptoms that indicate self-limiting conditions amenable to symptomatic treatment. The pharmacist can decide when to refer, when to suggest no treatment, and when to suggest self-medication. Thus, pharmacists perform a triage or screening role—the sorting out and classification of patients presenting in the pharmacy with various conditions, to determine priority of need, and proper place and type of treatment.

If a self-treatable condition is identified, then goals of treatment can be agreed on and a care plan can be developed which may include nondrug as well as nonprescription drug treatment. If a nonprescription product is indicated, then the pharmacist can recommend an appropriate product and dosage regimen and counsel the patient accordingly. Most patients (80% in a recent US survey) purchase a nonprescription product when recommended to do so by a pharmacist, or do not purchase when advised against it (82%).[15]

Following the recommendation, expected outcomes should be discussed and follow-up arranged to further assess patient's needs.

Up until the mid-1960s, pharmacists in the United States had little direction with regards to nonprescription drug counseling. Activities were often limited to directing the customer to the item on the shelf, answering only specific questions, suggesting that the patient ask a doctor, or selling the newest or most expensive product. In 1965, the American Pharmaceutical Association (APhA) recognized the need of pharmacists for comprehensive information and guidelines regarding nonprescription drug counseling, leading to the first *Handbook of Nonprescription Drugs* in September 1967.[29]

The *Handbook of Nonprescription Drugs* provides treatment algorithms specific to a range of medical conditions that may be self-treatable. In particular, discussion of patient assessment questions and answers, patient counseling, patient education materials, treatment alternatives including nondrug treatments, and evaluation of treatment outcomes, help the pharmacist provide pharmaceutical care for patients seeking self-care for a wide variety of conditions.[30]

The APhA has also developed drug treatment protocols for self-treatable conditions to aid pharmacists in making drug therapy decisions.[31]

As described above for prescription drug counseling, it is helpful for the pharmacist to follow a set protocol consisting of five phases as shown in Figure 5-1. For nonprescription drug counseling, each of these phases differs slightly in the content from prescription counseling as described in the following sections.

Self-care Counseling Opening Discussion

As in prescription drug counseling, the purpose of the opening phase is to establish a helping relationship with patients and to help them feel comfortable discussing their symptoms and health concerns. The nonprescription counseling encounter may begin in a number of ways—with the patient approaching the pharmacist to ask for a recommendation with regard to a particular condition; with the patient asking for a particular product; or with the pharmacist approaching the patient to offer help in selecting a product.

Although patients' requests for help are often handled by a pharmacy technician or clerk, any such questions should be referred to the pharmacist. The atmosphere of the pharmacy and the availability of the pharmacist are important to encourage patients to come forward with requests regarding self-care. Since patients often do not expect to be counseled about a nonprescription medication, it is important to introduce the purpose of the questioning that will follow in the next phase. The pharmacist should explain to the patient the need for further questioning in a way that does not judge or belittle (e.g., "I'll need to ask you a few questions to find out the best medication for your situation," rather than, "I'd better ask you some questions to make sure you're buying the right thing").

As with prescription counseling, it is necessary to consider the personal and potentially embarrassing nature of the discussion and to provide at least a degree of privacy. Ways to improve the pharmacy atmosphere and availability of the pharmacist will be discussed in Chapter 9.

Discussion to Gather Information and Identify Needs

Since part of the aim of nonprescription drug counseling is to screen for appropriate self-treatment, the information-gathering phase is more extensive here than it is in prescription drug counseling.

The following information should be gathered:

1. _Identity of the Patient_: In many cases, the client may be purchasing a nonprescription medication for another person. If the client is familiar with the patient's medical history and symptoms, it may be possible to proceed with counseling. If not, however, it may be necessary to contact the patient, either by telephone or in person to gather this information.

2. _Description of the Patient_: The approximate age of the patient should be determined, because special considerations are likely to be involved with the very young or the very old. Elderly people and infants under 2 years of age often present with symptoms differently or react to medications differently than do other members of the population. Women of childbearing age should always be asked if they are pregnant or breast feeding before medication is recommended.

3. _Medical History_: Conditions such as high blood pressure, diabetes, heart disease, or liver or kidney disease are often contraindications to nonprescription drug use. Similarly, the patient may be allergic to certain ingredients in nonprescription drugs. Indeed, the symptoms that the patient intends to self-treat may be associated in some way with such conditions. The pharmacist must assess these possible relationships and any contraindications that might be present. If a patient profile or

medication record is available in the pharmacy, the pharmacist should refer to it at this point.

4. _Other Medication Used_: Many medications may potentially interact with nonprescription drugs. Also, certain symptoms presented for self-treatment—such as rashes, difficulty breathing or urinating, or upset stomach—may be side effects or adverse effects of medication. This can also be identified on the patient record but should be discussed to confirm that the information is up to date.

5. _Previous Diagnosis and/or Treatment of the Symptoms_: This information will help the pharmacist determine the recommendations that are most suitable. Patients sometimes want confirmation of their physician's diagnosis, or they disagree with it and want to self-treat even when advised against it. They may also have tried certain remedies in the past with varying degrees of success.

6. _Symptom Evaluation_: Thorough questioning is necessary to determine the nature of the patient's symptoms. Patients often omit information or describe symptoms in unclear or misleading ways. Careful probing and clarification of terms such as _an upset stomach_ or _a cold in the kidneys_ is required. References such as the APhA's _Handbook of Nonprescription Drugs_ can be consulted to assist the pharmacist in deciding on the types of questions that should be asked specific to the patient's complaint or the type of medication requested.[30] The aim of questioning is to elucidate the necessary details of the symptoms in order to screen for the appropriateness of self-treatment.

In general, the following information about the symptoms should be obtained[16,32]:

● _Location_: Where is the symptom located?

● _Quality_: What does it feel like?

● _Severity_: How severe is it?

● _Modifying Factors_: What seems to aggravate or alleviate it? Is there any particular time it occurs (e.g., on arising or after eating)?

● _Timing_: How long or how often has it been present? Has it changed over time?

● _Associated Symptoms_: Are there other, related symptoms?

● _Previous Treatment_: What has been done so far or in the past to treat this symptom? Has a physician been consulted now or in the past? If so, what happened?

In addition to gathering this information from the patient, the pharmacist should observe the patient's physical appearance. Obvious physical signs (e.g., skin pallor or rash) as well as facial expressions (e.g., grimacing with pain) and attitude (e.g., lethargy and agitation) may be apparent.[14,32]

Discussion to Develop a Care Plan and Resolve Problems

As in prescription counseling, the pharmacist must next develop a care plan that may include a variety of recommendations. The pharmacist must first decide if the symptoms the patient has described indicate the need for treatment. If the symptoms appear to be mild, the patient may simply need reassurance and possibly some suggestions for nondrug treatment. If the symptoms appear to be of a type, severity, and/or duration that indicate a non-self-treatable condition, the pharmacist must recommend that the patient seek the advice of a physician. Where appropriate, an interim measure may also be suggested (i.e., a nondrug treatment or temporary use of a nonprescription drug until the physician is contacted).

It is sometimes difficult for the pharmacist to make the decision to refer the patient to a physician. Six general criteria can be used to identify those patients for whom physician referral is most appropriate:[16,28,32]

1. *Age of the Patient*: In young children, particularly those younger than 6 months of age, conditions can change rapidly and consequences of apparently minor symptoms may be severe. Also, it is usually not possible to question the patient, and caregivers may not be observing important indicators to report. In the elderly, symptoms are often complicated by several health conditions and medications. In addition, some symptoms may be misleading, (e.g., earache is a possible symptom of angina, since pain can be referred to the neck and ear area as well as down the left arm). The elderly and very young may also react differently than the general population to certain drugs because of differences in the way they metabolize some drugs, and therefore, such patients may require adjusted dosages.

2. *Nature and Severity of Symptoms*: Symptoms such as chest pain; high fever; black, tarry stools; and colored sputum indicate severe problems that should not be self-treated. Symptoms such as pain that are reportedly too severe to be endured by the patient should also not be self-treated.

3. *Duration of Symptoms*: Symptoms that may initially appear appropriate for self-treatment cease to be so if they continue for a prolonged time, for example, diarrhea, pain of any kind, or fever. The duration that signals a need for medical attention varies with the symptoms and with other factors, such as the age of the patient. For example, an infant should not have diarrhea for more than 24 hours, whereas an adult may tolerate it for several days without alarm. If symptoms repeatedly return they should also be further investigated.

4. *Other Existing Conditions and Medication Use*: Patients with existing chronic conditions or those taking particular types of medication may be at greater risk of complications from minor conditions than others, and therefore should probably seek advice from their physicians for accurate assessment of their symptoms. For example, a patient with diabetes may easily develop gangrene from a blister on his or her foot; a patient taking immunosuppressive drugs can quickly develop pneumonia from a cold. In addition, some symptoms actually may be signs of side effects or of complications of the primary condition.

    Although pharmacists can certainly anticipate problems that might occur, they often do not have complete patient data to make accurate predictions, and therefore a physician may need to be consulted. For example, for a patient with high blood pressure, an oral sympathomimetic agent would be contraindicated, but a nasal spray may be safe; unless the pharmacist had access to more detailed information about the patient's blood pressure control, he or she would be unable to make a treatment decision.

5. *Pregnancy*: There is a lack of definitive information about the teratogenic effects of drugs, and therefore many nonprescription drugs pose a potential danger to the pregnant woman and her unborn child. In addition, there is concern that symptoms may be indicative of problems with the pregnancy, and that any treatments may stimulate

contractions. Although the mother's discomfort must be balanced with concern for the developing fetus, this is best done together with the patient's physician. The pharmacist should also be alert for symptoms in a female patient that may be indicative of pregnancy, such as nausea. The pharmacist should question the patient regarding this possibility before proceeding to make a treatment recommendation.

6. *Pharmacist's Concern*: If for whatever reason the pharmacist feels unsure about the patient's medical condition or need for treatment, then he or she should err on the side of caution and refer the patient for further medical assessment.[32]

A reference guide, such as the APhA's *Handbook of Nonprescription Drugs*,[30] may be consulted to assist pharmacists in making these decisions.

Discussion to Provide Information and Educate

If the symptoms indicate a self-treatable condition, as defined above, the treatment plan may include the recommendation of a nonprescription drug. If so, the following information should be provided regarding the nonprescription drug:

1. *Name of the Drug:* This should include the list of drugs included in the product since many products include similar ingredients for different purpose, for example, acetaminophen may be in a cold remedy as well as an arthritis remedy.

2. *Purpose of the Medication*: This should be stated in terms of the outcomes expected, for example, "This is a decongestant to help reduce stuffy nose."

3. *Directions for Use:* Although they are provided on the package label, the directions for use should be pointed out to the patient, and doses should be suggested in accordance with the age of the patient. If the product requires special instructions, such as insertion of eye- or eardrops, the pharmacist should explain and demonstrate where appropriate.

4. *Side Effects:* As in new prescription counseling, the pharmacist should preface the discussion of side effects with a mention of their rarity balanced with the benefits. The symptoms associated with possible side effects should be described, and the patient should be advised about how to avoid or deal with them (e.g., take with food to avoid stomach upset; stop taking it if a rash develops).

5. *Precautions*: Warnings should be provided against the use of interacting medications, and where appropriate, the pharmacist should warn the patient about use of the medication during pregnancy or breast feeding, or use with alcohol.

6. *Time Frame for Effectiveness*: The patient should be advised of the time frame within which the treatment should take effect, for example, a few days for a bulk laxative or immediately for a glycerin suppository. A patient equipped with this information will be less likely to discontinue treatment before it has had time to take effect or, conversely, to persist with a treatment that is ineffective.

Regardless of whether or not a nonprescription drug is recommended, the care plan should include the following information about the condition and symptoms:

1. *Advice Regarding Symptoms:* Since self-treated symptoms should be self-limiting and mild, a suggested time limit should be given for specified outcomes beyond which the patient should consult a physician. As with prescription counseling,

these outcomes should be discussed with the patient and measurable indicators should be agreed on to determine if the treatment is appropriate and effective. The time limit will vary for each type of symptom. For example, for diarrhea, medical advice should be sought after a few days, but for cold symptoms, advice should be sought only after a few weeks.

In addition, the patient should be told that certain changes in the original symptoms could indicate a more serious underlying condition that should be reported to the physician (e.g., changes such as the appearance of blood in diarrhea).

Patients should also be warned that continual or repeated use of a nonprescription medication may alleviate symptoms, but may mask more serious conditions. If symptoms such as abdominal pain, headaches, or indigestion recur frequently, they may be indicative of serious conditions.

2. *Advice Regarding the Condition*: Information may also be provided about the condition itself and about measures the patient can take to prevent further contagion or recurrence.

3. *Nondrug Treatment*: Where appropriate, the pharmacist should include in the treatment plan advice regarding other self-care treatments, such as use of a humidifier and increased fluid intake to reduce congestion.

4. *Follow-up:* The pharmacist should also encourage a follow-up consultation to ensure that the patient's symptoms are diminishing and that the medication is effective and is being used appropriately. At that time, the pharmacist can ensure that appropriate outcomes are occurring and can make further recommendations.

Closing Discussion

As in prescription drug counseling, the nonprescription drug-counseling encounter should end with a summary of important points and an attempt to get feedback from the patient to make sure that there are no misunderstandings. The patient should be encouraged to ask questions, whether at that time or later. If print information about the condition or medication is available, it may be given to the patient.

If the pharmacist has a patient record for that patient, he or she may make a record of the nonprescription drug purchase. Informing the patient that a record will be made may increase the patient's trust in both the pharmacist's counseling and the pharmacy's record-keeping services.

Monitoring and follow-up discussed during the information-giving phase should be confirmed and a time may be arranged for this.

A self-care documenting form has been proposed to allow the pharmacist to record the encounter for his or her own records, a copy of which can be given to the patient for a written reminder of the pharmacist's recommendations. Although it may take time to complete the form, it provides continuity of care for subsequent encounters with the patient, improved management of potential liability, and promotion of a perception in the patient's mind that a valuable health service is being provided.[13] Because the patient's medication use is part of any decisions made by the pharmacist, the medication list (a printout from the patient's computer record or a medication management form filled out at the time) should be attached to the documentation. An example of a Nonprescription Counseling Recording Form is provided in Appendix B.

THE MEDICATION MANAGEMENT CONSULTATION

Conducting a medication management consultation with a new patient is an important activity in both the hospital and the community-pharmacy settings. Community pharmacists often complain that it is difficult to counsel patients, because they don't know the patients' medical history or details of the conditions being treated.

Pharmacists in a hospital or clinic setting usually have the benefit of the patient's medical chart for reference. The chart will provide information regarding the condition or symptoms for which the medication has been prescribed, other existing conditions, and any medications the patient is currently using or has used in the past. With the development of real-time computer links and centrally located patient data sources, community pharmacists sometimes have access to patient data such as medications dispensed at any pharmacy, but more detailed medical information such as medical conditions and laboratory results is often inaccessible.

Complete information regarding actual medication use is not likely to appear on any type of record. The information in the patient chart was most likely gathered by a physician or a nurse, both of whom would not have been concerned with medication use. In addition, such records are often completed by several providers, who differ in the amount and type of information they record and in the terms they use, and therefore may be incomplete and confusing.[33]

In order to gather complete information regarding medication use, the pharmacist needs to interact with the patient and gain some understanding of his or her existing or potential concerns about, and problems with, medication use. The pharmacist is best able to gather this information, as studies have demonstrated that pharmacists generally gain more detailed information than physicians or nurses gathering a medication history.[34,35] Therefore, whether or not medical records are available for reference, it is important for the pharmacist to conduct a medication management consultation with the patient.

If the patient's medical record is not available, the pharmacist may need to supplement patient-provided information by contacting the physician. Patients have been found to be fairly knowledgeable and accurate in reporting health and functional status and medication use. There are, however, some areas that they often do not fully understand or about which they may not have been informed, for example, the types of laboratory test or even some major hospital procedures they have undergone or their results.[33]

Although pharmacists usually gather a certain amount of information from patients such as personal information, chronic conditions, and allergies, they often do not conduct complete medication management consultations because of time constraints. Conducting a complete consultation of this sort is admittedly a time-consuming process. To save time, the patient can be asked to complete a written questionnaire to start gathering information. A sample of this sort of questionnaire is provided in Appendix B.

Ideally, the pharmacist will be able to conduct a medication review consultation over several sessions with time away from the patient to research if necessary and to formulate care plan recommendations, consulting with the physician as needed, then meeting with the patient to discuss this. Discussion with the patient will allow determination of desired treatment outcomes and negotiation of recommended actions resulting in the best pharmacotherapeutic solution and individualized therapeutic regimen.

Since the medication management consultation may identify many issues, it may be necessary to arrange further consultations with the patient to resolve all the issues over time. For example, a time may be set up to educate the patient about his or her condition, to help develop skills in using a medication, or monitoring outcomes.

Goals of the Medication Management Consultation

Although many pharmacists do not make the time to conduct medication management consultations, they are a very useful and important part of pharmaceutical care. It is advisable to do this with new patients to the pharmacy as well as intermittently with ongoing patients. It may also be done when the pharmacist feels that there are a number of drug-related problems occurring or the physician, the patient, or the caregiver requests a complete review of medication use. Some pharmacists, working in conjunction with a physician, identify groups of patients for whom regular medication management consultations are most beneficial, such as those on more than a given number or types of drugs, with certain conditions (e.g., diabetes), or certain age groups (e.g., elderly over 75).

The main purpose of the medication management consultation is to assist the pharmacist in identifying real and potential problems with current and newly prescribed medications. It also provides a basis for the ongoing assessment of the patient's medication use. Specific information about the conditions being treated and the medications used in the past and present will help the pharmacist evaluate the appropriateness of the types and dosages of current and newly prescribed drugs. In addition, it will assist the pharmacist in evaluating the effectiveness of past and current treatments.

Information gathered in the medication management consultation will also help the pharmacist detect other real and potential problems associated with current or new medications such as drug–drug interactions, drug–disease interactions, side effects, adverse effects, allergies, or nonadherence. Further questioning of the patient can expose the factors contributing to these problems, such as misunderstandings or double doctoring, and possible solutions to these problems.

This information and information about the patient's occupation, language level, and perhaps attitudes and biases may also contribute to understanding and solving drug-related problems. Such information also allows the pharmacist to assess the patient's needs for future counseling and education. It may also provide valuable information about social support networks, cultural issues, and attitudes toward health and medication use.

The interaction with the patient that the medication management consultation affords will help create a helping relationship between the pharmacist and patient, which is an important part of the pharmaceutical care process.[5]

The information gathered in the medication management consultation will also assist the pharmacist in conducting an informed discussion with the patient's physician if the need arises.

Finally, conducting a medication management consultation allows the pharmacist to promote a "value-added" service offered by the pharmacy. Patients should be made

TABLE 5-1   Goals of the Medication Management Consultation
1. To provide a basis for ongoing assessment of medication use
2. To evaluate the appropriateness of the drugs selected and the dosing prescribed
3. To evaluate the effectiveness of past, current, and newly prescribed medications
4. To assist the pharmacist in identifying other potential and actual problems associated with current or newly prescribed medications such as drug–drug interactions, drug–disease interactions, side effects, adverse effects, allergies, and nonadherence
5. To identify factors contributing to these problems and their possible solutions
6. To allow the pharmacist to assess the patient's needs for future counseling and education
7. To provide valuable information about social support networks, cultural issues, and attitudes toward health and medication use
8. To assist the pharmacist in conducting informed discussions with the physician
9. To help create a helping relationship between the pharmacist and patient
10. To provide an "extra" service offered by the pharmacy to gain customer loyalty

aware that this consultation is of benefit to them and to their optimal health care, and that it is an added service provided by this particular pharmacy. This may encourage the patient to become a loyal customer, feeling that he or she is now "registered" at this pharmacy that offers "extra" services. They may also be willing to pay for this service.

A summary of the goals of the medication management consultation is found in Table 5-1.

Conducting the Consultation

Figure 5-2 illustrates the suggested format for a complete medication management consultation. Careful probing is necessary to gather complete data, while preventing an atmosphere of inquisition from developing and allowing plenty of time for the patient to respond to questions.[34] Communication skills involved with questioning and probing will be discussed in Chapter 7, and a suggested dialogue is presented in Appendix A.

The suggested protocol is recommended because it structures questioning in a logical sequence that helps the patient recall events and assists the pharmacist in assessing the information gathered. By staying on track, the pharmacist will be less likely to miss necessary information. The patient, however, may want to make comments or ask questions, and this input should not be ignored by the pharmacist. The patient's concerns may either be discussed briefly at the time (if they pertain to the information being gathered) or politely deferred until the end of the interview.

The pharmacist should resist making recommendations or giving advice until after all the information is gathered and a complete assessment has been made of the data.

Since personal data will be discussed during the interview, it is necessary to conduct the interview in a private setting—a separate cubicle or office.[34] If neither is available, the interview may be conducted over the telephone or in the patient's home.

Opening discussion
• Introduction • Explain purpose • Ensure confidentiality

Inquiry of personal information
• Age, occupation, etc. • Use of health care professionals and attitudes
• Social support and cultural issues

Discussion of medical conditions and medications used

Condition no. 1
• Name or symptom of condition • How long?

Current medications for condition no. 1
Medication A

• Name of medication
• Who prescribed it?
• How is it taken? (specifics)
• Does it help?
• If nonadherence detected, what are its causes?
• Side effects and adverse effects

Repeat questions about each medication

Past medications for condition no. 1
• Names of medications • Reasons for discontinuing use

Repeat questions about current and past medications for each condition

Nonprescription drug, herbals, alternative remedies used

• Name
• Usage—why, when, how used, how long?
• Side effects and adverse effects
• Effectiveness

Discussion of alcohol and tobacco use

Discussion of drug sensitivity

Discussion to develop care plan and resolve problems

• Discuss real or potential problems
• Agree on alternatives
• Discuss outcomes and monitoring
• Arrange for further consultations to educate
• Discuss with physician as needed and document

Closing discussion

Figure 5-2   Medication Management Consultation

Opening Discussion

The opening should set the tone for the interview. It is particularly important to develop a helping relationship with the patient in order to make him or her feel comfortable and better prepared for a discussion of personal information.

The opening consists of a greeting and introduction by the pharmacist, and a check on the identity of the patient. If appropriate—for example, in a clinic or a hospital setting—the pharmacist might explain that he or she is working together with the physician. A few minutes should be allowed for casual conversation to set the patient at ease and to further develop a helping relationship. Topics such as the weather or the patient's family might be briefly discussed.

The purpose of the interview and the type of information to be gathered should be explained—in terms of benefits to the patient rather than the convenience of the pharmacist. The pharmacist should explain that information about the patient's conditions and medication use will be gathered to get a complete picture of his or her situation and to help the pharmacist ensure that the patient is getting the most effective therapy possible. The pharmacist might also explain that he or she will be checking for any experiences the patient may have had in the past with drug use (such as drug interactions). At this point, it is important to assure the patient that all information gathered is strictly confidential.

The pharmacist should try to impress on the patient the importance of complete and correct information in the interests of an accurate pharmaceutical assessment. The approximate length of the interview should also be mentioned. The pharmacist should then allow the patient to give consent to continue. This sets the stage for cooperation between the pharmacist and the patient because they have mutually agreed to proceed with the interview.

Gathering Personal Information

A certain amount of personal information needs to be gathered, including name, address, and health-insurance information. The patient's age (birth date) and occupation should also be obtained, because this information might affect the selection of treatments in the future. The names of the patient's physicians and other health care personnel, such as a chiropractor or an ophthalmologist, should also be noted. This will help suggest the direction of further questions about all pertinent conditions, treatments, and medications (traditional and nontraditional). The information will be useful if the need arises to contact these other health professionals to gather more complete information or to discuss identified problems. The patient should be asked for consent to allow the pharmacist to contact other health professionals to discuss specific issues identified. In some jurisdictions this may require written consent.

During this questioning, the patient should be asked a general question about any difficulties accessing necessary care (e.g., difficulty reaching the physician, difficulty paying for care, and difficulty getting help at home for health care). This may indicate a source of medication use behaviors or problems.

Discussion of Medical Conditions and Medication Use

To help the patient recall details about conditions and medications, it is suggested that each condition and the drugs associated with it be dealt with together before proceeding to the next condition. The name of each condition or a description of the symptoms associated with it should be ascertained at the outset. Since the patient's knowledge in this area may not be complete, the pharmacist may need to supplement data gathered from the patient with information obtained from other sources, such as the medical record or the physician, if possible.

The patient should also be questioned about the duration of the condition, since this may elicit the patient's concerns or any misunderstandings about the condition.

The patient should then be asked what medications he or she is using for the particular condition, and the following information should be gathered about each medication separately:

1. *Name of the Medication*: If the patient does not know the name of the drug, the pharmacist can ask the patient to describe it or show it. Alternatively, the pharmacist can arrange to telephone the patient later.

2. *Name of the Prescriber*: Obtaining the name of the prescribing physician will help reduce the possibility of duplicate prescriptions by specialists and family doctors.

3. *How the Medication Is Used*: The patient should be questioned about specific details pertaining to dosage, frequency of use on a day-to-day basis, and the times during the day when the medication is taken. Information should also be gathered about food consumption in relation to medication use. If nonadherence is evident from the patient's responses to these questions, the pharmacist should probe to determine how frequently doses are missed or improperly taken.

4. *Duration of Use*: The patient may find it difficult to remember exactly when a medication was first prescribed. It helps to relate this to a life or family event or in relation to the condition diagnosis.

5. *Efficacy of the Medication*: The patient should be asked whether, in his or her opinion, the medication is helping to alleviate the symptoms. If the patient perceives the prescribed drug to be ineffective, the pharmacist should ask the patient how the drug is ineffective and whether there are any times or circumstances that seem to make the drug more or less effective.

6. *Adherence Investigation*: If information about the use of medication points to nonadherence, it is important to determine its possible causes. As discussed in Chapter 4, the reasons may be varied, and careful but thorough probing may be required to uncover them. The patient may be asked directly (but in a nonconfrontational manner) about his or her failure to take the medication in the dose and frequency recommended. Suggested dialogue is provided in Appendix A.

7. *Side Effects and Adverse Effects*: The patient should be asked about any experiences with medication use. A general question may be followed by probing for specific symptoms (reported in the literature), the details of which—severity, frequency, duration, actions taken, and other related factors—should be gathered.

After all medications used for a particular condition have been ascertained, the patient should be asked about past medications used for this condition. If possible, the pharmacist should try to determine the names of the medications and the reasons why they were discontinued. The patient may not recall this information, and other sources of data may need to be used. This information will help the pharmacist make recommendations to the physician about alternative therapies, if necessary.

The pharmacist should proceed in sequence with each condition and its associated medications. Then ask generally whether any other prescription medications are being used. This provides a check for things forgotten and for any medications the patient may be taking that aren't necessarily related to a particular condition (such as prescribed vitamins).

Discussion of Self-treatment

It is important to gather information about self-treatment by the patient, because nonprescription medications and alternative treatments may interact with prescribed drugs or interfere with diagnostic tests. In addition, the patient may be using them to treat previously undisclosed side effects of prescribed medications such as stomach upset.

The patient should be asked a general question about the use of the medications that he or she purchases, followed by probing to prompt his or her memory. For example, the pharmacist might mention the categories of nonprescription drugs or their uses—medicine to treat coughs and colds, upset stomach, and so forth.

The same details should be gathered about nonprescription medications as prescribed medications, including the name of the drug, the reason for use, the dosage and frequency of use, duration of use, effectiveness, and any possible side effects.

Vitamins, herbal, and homeopathic remedies should also be investigated. Patients may neglect to provide this information to medical personnel because it is often frowned upon. There should be no judgment made by the pharmacist about the effectiveness of these treatments while gathering the information.

Discussion of Alcohol and Tobacco Use

Since alcohol and tobacco use can affect certain medications and conditions, it is important to include information pertaining to them in a medication management consultation. This topic is more personal than that of medication use, and therefore should be introduced with tact, in a nonjudgmental manner. Suggested wording is provided in Appendix A. The pharmacist should explain that this information is important since alcohol or tobacco may affect therapy. If the patient is taking medications that have the potential to interact with alcohol, the pharmacist should also inquire whether medication use is altered when the patient consumes alcoholic beverages.

Discussion of Drug Sensitivity

The pharmacist should inquire whether the patient knows of any medications to which he or she may be allergic. Since the patient may not be aware of specific allergies, he or she should also be asked more generally if he or she has ever experienced an unpleasant reaction to a medication.

If the patient reports an allergy or adverse reactions, the pharmacist should ask for a description of the effects experienced. This will allow him or her to evaluate whether the reaction was a genuine sensitivity to the medication or simply a side effect. For example, although people often report that they are allergic to aspirin (ASA), further questioning reveals that what they experience is stomach discomfort—a side effect of acetylsalicylic acid rather than an allergic reaction to it. In addition, the pharmacist should ask whether the patient has informed his or her prescribing physician of the problem, and if not, recommend he or she do so.

Discussion to Develop a Care Plan and Resolve Problems

Having gathered a considerable amount of information from the patient, the pharmacist must next assess the data in order to develop a care plan and resolve identified problems. As discussed earlier in this chapter in relation to a new prescription, this involves thought by the pharmacist and discussion with the patient.

Each medication should be evaluated to detect any existing or potential problems with current or new medication. In particular, the pharmacist should evaluate medication appropriateness and effectiveness. The data should also be reviewed for evidence of drug-related problems such as nonadherence, drug–drug interactions, drug–disease interactions, side effects, adverse effects, or history of drug sensitivity.

If necessary, the pharmacist should consult reference texts to evaluate these problems and to determine the appropriate course of action. On reflection, it may be apparent that certain additional data are necessary, such as results of laboratory tests, in which case these data should be retrieved.

The results of this assessment should then be documented by the pharmacist noting specific problems, possible causes, recommended action, and treatment plan. It is generally recommended that these notes should follow the SOAP format used in medicine for the problem-oriented medical record system.

The pharmacist should also assess the patient's need for further counseling and education. If nonadherence has been detected, the information gathered concerning reasons associated with it must be considered, along with possible ways to treat the problem, as discussed in Chapter 4. If the patient has raised certain concerns or questions or has demonstrated a lack of understanding about his or her condition or medication, plans to provide information should be made.

The content of the discussion should include that suggested in the earlier section of this chapter, "Developing a Care Plan for a New Prescription." Issues to be discussed are summarized in Table 5-2. This should involve negotiation and discussion with the patient in a way that allows the patient to play a significant role in his or her medication management.

Whether or not it is deemed necessary to discuss issues with the physician during the development of the care plan, there should always be a report to the physician documenting that a medication management review was conducted and any findings and recommendations. It is preferable that this should be accompanied by a verbal discussion with the physician (in person or by telephone) although the report may be mailed or faxed. A suggested Health Care Professional Communication Report is provided in Appendix B.

Discussion with the physician may include the following:

1. Confirmation of the patient's conditions and treatments (prescription and nonprescription, herbal, and so forth).
2. Drug-related problems detected.
3. Recommendations regarding drug-related problems.
4. Outcomes of therapy desired by the patient.
5. Recommendations made to the patient.

TABLE 5-2	**Issues Discussed When Developing a Care Plan in a Medication Monitoring Consultation**

1. Inform the patient that there are some important things to discuss
2. Negotiate the order of importance
3. Establish desired pharmacotherapeutic outcomes for each real or potential problem
4. Recommend ways of using the medication that will improve adherence and, consequently, the effectiveness of the therapy (e.g., suggesting the use of memory aids)
5. Use various techniques to overcome nonadherence (e.g., discussing the importance of the medication to the outcome of the condition)
6. Recommend methods for reducing side effects (e.g., taking the medication with food)
7. Discuss treatment options if changes to medication are recommended including choice of drug, dose, formulation, and regimen
8. Arrange for further consultations as needed to educate the patient about the condition or medication use
9. Discuss a follow-up monitoring plan with the patient

Any actions taken by the pharmacist with the physician and patient should be documented and the outcomes of those actions documented (e.g., discussion with the physician concerning the patient's experience of side effects resulted in a reduction of the dose to a specific level).

Closing Discussion

In closing the medication management consultation, the pharmacist should offer the patient an opportunity to add any information that might not already have been covered. The pharmacist might simply ask, "Is there anything else that you'd like to tell me about?"

The pharmacist should explain to the patient that the information will be included with his or her patient record for future reference and that it may be discussed with the physician as needed with the patient's consent. Confidentiality should be stressed.

If a medication is being dispensed at this time, the pharmacist may assess the data immediately and proceed with the drug counseling. If the need for further consultations was identified during the care plan development, arrangements should be made.

At this time, or at a later date when all the information is accumulated, a report of the consultation should be given to the patient for his or her records. A suggested Patient Consultation Report to give to the patient is provided in Appendix B. The pharmacist should also give the patient his or her business card and offer to answer questions or discuss concerns at any time. Finally, the patient should be thanked for his or her time.

ALTERNATE COUNSELING SITUATION 5.2

Using the preceding suggestions, the pharmacist in Counseling Situation 5.1 discussed at the beginning of this chapter would have been more successful in his task as illustrated in Counseling Situation 5.2.

COUNSELING SITUATION 5.2: Using the Phases of Counseling

Pharmacist: Hello, Mrs. Hampton. Is this your first time here at our pharmacy?

Patient: Yes, I usually go to the pharmacy close to my office.

Pharmacist: Well, we're happy to help you here today. Do you live nearby? *Greeting, Small talk*

Patient: Yes, just down River Street.

Pharmacist: Oh, yes, I know that street. It's a nice area. Well, I hope we'll see more of you. Before I get your prescription ready, I want to explain to you that in this pharmacy we keep records about you and the medications you *Explains* take to help ensure that you get the most benefit from them. To start your *Educates* record, I'd like to ask you for some information about your health conditions *benefits* and any current medication use. Of course, this information is strictly confidential. To save time, perhaps you could fill out this patient history form while we prepare your prescription. Then, I'll discuss it with you when your prescription is ready, in about 10 minutes.

Patient: Yes, all right, but doesn't my doctor have this information?

Pharmacist: Your doctor may have some of this information, but we don't *Explains* have access to that information. We need to check for any concerns with certain medications, for example, allergies or interactions between medications.

Patient: Oh, I see. I'll have to think for a minute to remember all this.

Pharmacist: Take your time. It's important that the information is as accurate as can be.

. . . 10 minutes pass.

Pharmacist: Mrs. Hampton. Your prescription is ready now. Will you come in *Provides privacy* here where we can speak more privately *(indicates counseling booth)*.

Patient: *(comes into booth and hands over the patient history form)* Here's the form.

Pharmacist: Thanks for completing that for me. As I said, this will help us to *Educates* provide the best care for you. I'll just take a few minutes to review it.

Patient: OK.

Pharmacist: Now, let me see. *(reads over the patient history form)* You've filled in just about everything. *(confirms with patient that there are no other chronic or acute conditions or prescription medications)* You didn't list any *Verifies* nonprescription medications. Sometimes people don't think of things like vitamins as nonprescription medications. Do you take any vitamins?

(handwritten margin note: Takes med rx)

Patient: Oh, yes, you're right. I didn't think of that as medication. I take those calcium tablets over there *(indicates a particular brand and strength)* to prevent bone loss when I'm older.

Pharmacist: That's good. And can you tell me how you take them?

Patient: Two tablets every morning like clockwork.

Pharmacist: Good for you. Now, how about anything else, like... *(proceeds to explore each category of nonprescription drug and discovers that the patient uses a popular antacid occasionally. The pharmacist proceeds to ask about the purpose, dosage, and frequency and is satisfied that it is appropriate. Following that, the pharmacist asks a few more questions to fill in gaps in data, then closes the discussion)* Well, I think I have the complete information now. Is there anything else that you'd like to mention?

Patient: No, I don't think so.

Pharmacist: OK then, thank you for helping me. I'll be keeping that information in our records so we can refer to it when you come in for any other medications. In fact, it has been helpful already in showing me how I can help you get the most benefit from your new medication. Let's talk about that now.

Patient: *(sounding interested)* Yes, all right.

Pharmacist: What did the doctor tell you about your prescription?

Patient: She told me it's an antibiotic and to try it for a few weeks. I've taken antibiotics before for a cold.

Pharmacist: That's right, it is an antibiotic. You just need to take it once daily.

Patient: Oh, I'm glad you said that. I was expecting to take it 4 times a day like before.

Pharmacist: Did the doctor explain how it will help you?

Patient: Not really. It's for my skin. I seem to be going through a second puberty, because pimples are breaking out on my face and back.

Pharmacist: This is an antibiotic that helps to cut down on the number and severity of pustules developing. You need to take it regularly to keep the pimples under control.

Patient: Oh, I see.

(handwritten margin note: Educate about interaction)

Pharmacist: *(proceeds to explain how to take it in relation to meals, and so forth)* Now, I noticed from the form you filled out that you take calcium and antacid tablets. These can interfere with how well the minocycline is absorbed into your body from your stomach and decrease how well it works. You should not take them within 1 hour of the minocycline.

Patient: Oh, really?

Pharmacist: *(proceeds to discuss scheduling these medications to avoid problems)* Do you see any difficulty in taking your medication like this?

Patient: No, I guess that would be OK.

Pharmacist: Good. This is a very helpful medication for acne, but occasionally people experience unwanted effects. I want to discuss this with you so you know what to look for and what to do if you notice anything unusual. Did the doctor tell you anything to watch out for while you're on this?

Patient: No, not that I can remember.

Pharmacist: Sometimes people find these medications make them more sensitive to the sunlight. Do you take part in any outdoor activities?

Patient: I go for walks some evenings and on the weekend.

Pharmacist: Just avoid the sun by wearing protective clothing or a sunscreen.

Patient: I always do anyway.

Pharmacist: You're very wise. There are a few other things you should read about here on this information sheet *(points to appropriate section on an information sheet)*. People very rarely experience these side effects and they probably won't happen to you, but if you should notice anything unusual, let your doctor or a pharmacist know right away. *(points out a few of the most common effects, how to recognize them, and what to do if they occur)*

Patient: OK.

Pharmacist: There are a few other things here about how to store the medication, and so forth. You can read this information when you get home.

Patient: OK.

Pharmacist: You mentioned that you have acne. Did the doctor discuss any other things you can do to help with this?

Patient: She said it happens to some people even when they get older. She said I could get something to wash with.

Pharmacist: Yes, you should use a mild facial wash. I can show you some products when you have time. Here is a pamphlet about skin care and acne that will help you with this.

Patient: Great, I'll look at that and talk to you later about the wash.

Pharmacist: The doctor hasn't indicated any further refills. Did she explain what to do when you finish the medication?

Patient: Yes, I have an appointment to see her in about 1 month, when these pills are gone.

Pharmacist: You should be seeing an effect by then. Do you have any questions about all this?

Patient: No, I think it's clear.

Pharmacist: Good. I'll call you in 1 week to see how things are going. *(arranges a convenient time)*

> ● COUNSELING SITUATION **5.2:** (Continued)
>
> **Patient:** That would be good.
>
> **Pharmacist:** Thank you for your time today. Call me if you have any questions or concerns or if you would like to discuss the information in the pamphlets I gave you. Here's my card.
>
> **Patient:** OK. Thank you. *(walks away thinking, "This is great! I'll come to this pharmacy from now on since the pharmacist is so helpful and they have my record on file now." When she gets home she reads over the information sheet and posts the pharmacist's business card on the bulletin board by the phone for future reference)*
>
> **Pharmacist:** *(documents the session and makes note of the time for the monitoring follow-up call)*

In this situation, the pharmacist was able to investigate medication use and counsel the patient as well as establish a relationship with the patient for the future. By introducing the need for the medication management consultation, as well as introducing the medication counseling, the pharmacist gained the cooperation of the patient and was able to complete her task successfully, identifying potential drug-related problems and dealing with them appropriately.

SUMMARY

The protocols for patient counseling suggested in this chapter are a guide to help pharmacists organize their thoughts, and to be as efficient and effective as possible. Often it is difficult or perhaps inappropriate to follow these protocols. The types of situations where adjustments may be needed and the ways that counseling content may be tailored to the individual will be the subject of Chapter 8.

Since these protocols suggest that the patient and the pharmacist should be involved in the counseling discussion, pharmacists require skills in communication to engage the patient as well as to be sure that both the patient and pharmacist understand each other.[34] Communication skills for patient counseling will be reviewed in Chapter 7. Suggested pharmacist dialogues to assist the pharmacist in phrasing introductions and questions during counseling are provided in Appendix A.

The counseling protocols suggested often involve presenting the patient with large amounts of information. Using various educational techniques and counseling aids can assist pharmacists to be efficient and effective in counseling. This will be the topic of the following chapter.

REFLECTIVE QUESTIONS

1. If there is insufficient time available to conduct a complete medication management consultation when filling a new prescription, what could the pharmacist do to ensure that sufficient information is gathered?

2. Lisa G. is an 18-year-old patient with asthma returning to the pharmacy for a refill of her inhaled salbutamol. What information should be gathered from her by the pharmacist at this point?
3. Why is it important to obtain previous treatment information when advising patients about self-care and nonprescription drugs?
4. When a medication has common and severe side effects, what can the pharmacist do to help the patient understand and deal with this information?

REFERENCES

1. Dyck A, Deschamps M, Taylor J. Pharmacists' discussions of medication side effects: A descriptive study. Patient Educ Couns. 2005;56(1):21–27.
2. Schommer JC, Doucette WR, Worley MM. Processing prescription drug information under different conditions of presentation. Patient Educ Couns. 2001;43:49–59.
3. Norris P, Rowsell B. Interactional issues in the provision of counselling to pharmacy customers. Int J Psychoanal Psychother. 2003;11:135–142.
4. Morrow D, Leirer V, Altieri P, et al. Elders' schema for taking medication: Implications for instruction design. J Gerontol Psychol Sci. 1991;46(6):378–385.
5. Cipolle RJ, Strand LM, Morley PC. Pharmaceutical Care Practice, McGraw-Hill, New York, 1998.
6. Feegel K, Dix Smith M. Counseling and cognitive services for Medicaid patients under OBRA-'90. Pharm Times. 1992;9(Suppl):1–9.
7. Anonymous. The pharmacy patient's Bill of Rights. US Pharm. 1992;(5):61–68.
8. Airaksinen M, Vainio K, Koistinen J, et al. Do the public and pharmacists share opinions about drug information. Int J Pharm. 1994;8(4):168–171.
9. Ziegler D, Mosier M, Buenaver BS, et al. How much information about adverse effects of medication do patients want from physicians. Arch Intern Med. 2001;161:706–713.
10. Berry D, Knapp P, Raynor T. Is 15 percent very common? Informing people about the risks of medication side effects. Int J Pharm Pract. 2002:10:145–151.
11. Edwards A, Elwyn G, Mulley A. Explaining risks: Turning numerical data into meaningful pictures. BMJ. 2002;324:827–830.
12. Levin LS. Self-medication: The Social Perspective. Self-Medication: The New Era. A Symposium. The Proprietary Association, Washington, DC, 1980.
13. Srnka QM. Implementing a self-care consulting practice. Am Pharm. 1993;NS33(1):61–69.
14. Anonymous. Fact sheet: The use of over-the-counter medicines. National Council on Patient Information and Education. Available at: www.bemedwise.org/press_room/sep_2003_fact_otc.pdf (accessed January 2005).
15. Anonymous. Executive summary. The attitudes and beliefs about over-the-counter medicines: A national opinion survey conducted for the National Council on Patient Information and Education. Available at: www.bemedwise.org/survey/summary_survey.pdf (accessed January 2005).
16. Boyce R, Herrier R. Obtaining and using patient data. Am Pharm. 1991;NS31(7):65–70.
17. Segal M. Rx OTC: The switch is on. FDA Consumer, 1991.
18. Covington T. Self-care and Nonprescription Pharmacotherapy. In: Handbook of Nonprescription Drugs, 12th Edition. American Pharmaceutical Association, Washington, DC, 2000, p. 3–14.
19. Koren G, Pastuszak A, Ito S. Drugs in pregnancy. N Engl J Med. 1998;338:1128–1137.
20. Holt GA, Hall EL. The Self-care Movement. In: Handbook of Nonprescription Drugs, 9th Edition. American Pharmaceutical Association, Washington, DC, 1990.
21. Rantucci M, Segal HJ. Hazardous non-prescription analgesic use by the elderly. J Soc Admin Pharm. 1991;8(3):108–120.

22. Anonymous. Executive summary. Uses and attitudes about taking over-the-counter medicines: Findings of a 2003 national opinion survey conducted for the National Council on Patient Information and Education. Available at: www.bemedwise.org/press-room/summary_survey-findings.pdf (accessed January 2005).
23. Colt H, Shapiro A. Drug-induced illness as a cause for admission to a community hospital. J Am Ger Soc. 1989;37(4):323–326.
24. Salerno E, Ries D, Sank J, et al. Self-medication behaviors. Fla J Hosp Pharm. 1985;5(7):13–28.
25. Wilkinson I, Darby D, Mant A. Self-care and self-medication: An evaluation of individual's health care decisions. Med Care. 1987;25(10):965–978.
26. Simon HK, Weinkle DA. Over-the-counter medications: Do parents give what they intend to give? Arch Pediatr Adolesc Med. 1997;151:654–656.
27. Singh G. Recent considerations in nonsteroidal anti-inflammatory drug gastropathy. Am J Med. 1998;105:31S–38S.
28. Klein-Schwartz W, Hoopes JM. Patient Assessment and Consultation. In: Handbook of Nonprescription Drugs, 9th Edition. American Pharmaceutical Association, Washington, DC, 1990.
29. Penna R. Introduction. In: Handbook of Nonprescription Drugs, 5th Edition. American Pharmaceutical Association, Washington, DC, 1977.
30. Handbook of Nonprescription Drugs, 13th Edition. American Pharmaceutical Association, Washington, DC, 2002.
31. Anonymous. APhA Drug Treatment Protocols. Self Treatable Conditions. American Pharmaceutical Association, Washington DC, 1999.
32. Isetts B, Brown L. Patient Assessment and Consultation. In: Handbook of Nonprescription Drugs, 13th Edition. American Pharmaceutical Association, Washington, DC, 2002, p. 17–36.
33. Betz Brown J, Adams M. Patients as reliable reporters of medical care process. Med Care. 1992;30(5):400–411.
34. Covington T, Whitney Jr. H. Patient-pharmacist communication techniques. Drug Intell Clin Pharm. 1971;5(11):370–376.
35. Gurwich E. Comparison of medication histories acquired by pharmacists and physicians. Am J Hosp Pharm. 1983;40:1541–1542.

6 Information Provision and Educational Methods and Resources

Objectives

After completing the chapter, the reader should be able to

1. discuss opportunities for pharmacists to use the following methods of patient education: Lectures, dialogue and discussion, print materials, computer-assisted learning, and decision aids.
2. select an educational method or methods appropriate for individual patients or situations.
3. be aware of the various counseling aids available.
4. be prepared to develop a patient education program.
5. evaluate the quality of patient education materials.

As discussed in Chapter 2, one of the prime goals of patient counseling is to provide information and educate the patient. This involves enhancing skills and knowledge about medication and health conditions in order to bring about changes in related attitudes and behaviors.[1] Patients have varied wants and needs regarding information and education about their medications.

When pharmacists think about educating patients and providing information, they generally think of talking to the patient (often in a lecture format rather than a discussion) or providing written information. In some jurisdictions, verbal and/or written information provision is mandated, and so pharmacists use the materials they are provided with to meet requirements. They don't often think about how the individual patient receives this information or the patient's abilities to learn and understand. They may also not consider different methods for imparting knowledge or ways to assist patient behavior change with that knowledge.

There is a vast array of literature about learning and education that pharmacists can apply to patient counseling. It provides information on a variety of different methods and counseling aids that are available to provide counseling and education. Pharmacists need to be able to identify patients' learning needs and abilities, and develop a plan for each patient, using a selection of the available counseling methods and aids. This will assist pharmacists in conducting effective and efficient patient counseling that will improve adherence and outcomes for patients.

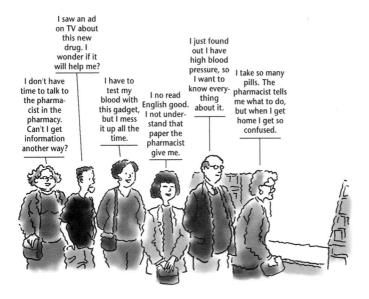

Patients come in all shapes and sizes, just like their learning and counseling needs.

LITERACY AND HEALTH

As the health care community has come to understand patients as individuals and their needs for shared decision making, there has been recognition of adult literacy issues and the concept of health literacy. Literacy is "using printed and written information to function in society, to achieve one's goals, and to develop one's knowledge and potential."[2] According to the World Health Organization, "health literacy represents the cognitive and social skills which determine the motivation and ability of individuals to gain access to, understand and use information in ways which promote and maintain good health."[3] It involves the ability to perform basic reading and mathematical tasks necessary to comprehend and act on health information such as prescription labels, appointment cards, and hospital forms.[4] Skills required include reading, writing, arithmetic, oral communication, conceptual knowledge of health-related topics such as biology, and cultural knowledge (values and approaches to health and health care).[4]

A U.S. Department of Education Survey of health literacy found that 40 million Americans are functionally illiterate and 55 million are marginally literate.[5] But even better-educated people may have poor health literacy. More than 90 million Americans cannot adequately understand basic health information.[5] There is a widespread problem for patients reading appointment slips (26% cannot) and prescription labels (42% do not understand) and understanding terminology (96% could not characterize the term *atherosclerosis*).[6–8] Poorer general health, increased hospitalizations, and increased rates of medication nonadherence are related to functional health literacy.[4] Patients are less likely to be adherent with medication and appointments or to seek an early diagnosis for a condition.[9] Poor anticoagulation and glycemic control and poor metered-dose inhaler (MDI) technique have been attributed to low literacy.[10–12] It has been estimated that this problem costs $73 billion per year in the US in misdirected or misunderstood medical advice.[5,7]

Health literacy has been included as an objective in the US blueprint document used for state and national planning, "Healthy People 2010."[13] Further, the Joint Commission on Accreditation of Health Organizations (JCAHO)—the agency that inspects health care facilities and establishes minimum standards for hospitals and health care institutions in the United States—requires that instructions be given to patients at an understandable level, and that instructions and education be provided that are specific to patients' assessed needs, ability, and readiness.[13] Canada, Australia, and Britain as well as developing countries are also recognizing this issue.[13]

Faced with the issue of health literacy, pharmacists need to approach the task of educating and counseling patients in a comprehensive way, identifying patients' level of understanding, and selecting appropriate educational methods.

EDUCATIONAL METHODS

Many possible methods exist for facilitating learning other than the traditional lecture-style presentation. As patient counseling has gained acceptance as a role for pharmacists, more and better materials and resources have become available. Pharmacists can employ a range of educational methods with their patients, from lectures, dialogue and discussion, and print information, to audiovisual methods, demonstrations (and practice) of techniques, video simulations, and computer-assisted learning. With the advent of the Internet, there are now many sources of health information which add to the resources available to pharmacists and patients.

Lectures

Lectures represent the traditional style of presenting information.[14] Although pharmacists often employ this approach on a one-to-one basis, lectures should really be limited to larger groups, for example, community groups, where individual discussion is not possible.

Although not all pharmacists are comfortable with the idea of lecturing to the public, pharmacists should attempt to promote themselves to their communities as public speakers on health and medication topics. Speaking to community groups is one of the best ways to gain public trust for the profession and to serve clients.[15] Involvement in lecturing will not only promote the profession of pharmacy, and the individual pharmacist in the community, but may also provide the pharmacist with greater confidence in speaking to patients on an individual basis. Pharmacists in institutional settings are often called on to address groups of patients or health professionals, and therefore should become comfortable with this method.

Various books and courses are available to assist pharmacists in developing their public-speaking skills and lecturing techniques.[15–18] Tips for planning, organizing, preparing for, and presenting a speech should be reviewed by pharmacists planning such presentations. This will be discussed in more detail later in this chapter.

Because lecture material is often considered boring and knowledge retention is generally fairly low, lectures should incorporate other educational techniques such as audiovisual aids and group discussion (e.g., a question-and-answer period at the end of the presentation). Descriptions of personal experiences and discussion of particular cases help audiences identify with the material being presented and may increase the impact on behavior and attitude.[16]

Since the learner/patient is passive in the lecture situation, there is little opportunity for the pharmacist to address individual concerns or to have much effect on understanding or attitudes. Because the pharmacist wants to improve the patient's behavior and attitudes as well as his or her knowledge, a lecture is not recommended for counseling individual patients.

Dialogue and Discussion

Although lecturing is a useful skill to develop, one-on-one dialogue with the patient through a patient-counseling protocol as described in the previous chapter is the essence of the pharmacist's regular duties. The discussion may be guided by the pharmacist, but should allow for as much participation as possible by the patient. It has been said that "when pharmacists consult with patients it's like they push a button, turn on the tape recorder, and recite the prescription directions like a machine."[19] Preferably pharmacists should use techniques that allow the patient to be involved in the patient-counseling discussion so that the pharmacist can find out what the patient knows and/or needs to know.[19] Communication techniques to encourage discussion during patient counseling will be discussed in Chapter 7, and suggested dialogues for patient counseling that promote discussion are shown in Appendix A.

Although the dialogue-and-discussion approach may be more time-consuming than simply lecturing to the patient, it is more effective in improving the patient's understanding of medication use and in altering his or her attitudes. In one study of various counseling methods, one group of patients received information via the standard instructions and accessory labels simply read by the pharmacist, whereas another group of patients received the same instructions plus a personal consultation with the pharmacist.[20] Patients receiving the consultation not only had a greater understanding of their medication (identifying appropriate administration times, special instructions, side effects, what to do if they missed a dose), but were also more likely to adhere to medication regimens.[20]

Patients' ability to comprehend and recall information provided verbally can, however, be an issue. Because patients can suffer from information overload, it has been recommended that interaction over multiple points of time may be preferable.[21] Patients apparently forget or ignore much of what is provided verbally by the physician. This is possibly owing to anxiety, or the fact that recall deteriorates as the amount of information increases. It can also be attributed to the use of medical or technical jargon.[22] In studies, 40% to 60% of patients could not remember what the physician's expectations were 10 to 80 minutes after the interaction, and 60% misunderstood directions.[23,24] Although these studies involved physicians, it can also apply to information provision by pharmacists. These statistics warn us against trying to provide too much information in one session. They also illustrate the importance of pharmacists providing counseling in addition to the physician, to reinforce the information provided in the physician's office.

Dialogue and discussion do not necessarily have to occur face to face; but can be conducted over the telephone. In the above study, patients who received no oral consultation at the time of dispensing received telephone consultation as a follow-up on the fourth or fifth day of therapy. This improved adherence to the same degree as the face-to-face consultation had in the other group.[20] Telephone consultation may be particularly useful for certain groups of patients such as palliative care patients who cannot reach the pharmacy, or for embarrassing situations or those requiring privacy if not available in the pharmacy. It is also a good way of providing follow-up monitoring, which has been found to reduce nonadherence and medication-related problems as well as improve satisfaction.[25]

A discussion may include more than one learner—perhaps the patient's family members or several patients with similar problems. Involvement of friends or family members in the patient education discussion may help them to support the patient and as a result, enhance the patient's medication attitudes and behaviors as discussed in Chapters 3 and 4. Discussion among patients with similar concerns can also improve their medication attitudes and behaviors. Group education programs will be discussed later in this chapter.

Print Information

Print information is frequently used by pharmacists. Some jurisdictions require pharmaceutical manufacturers to provide print information along with their products; pharmacists are often required to provide written information, either alone or as an adjunct to verbal instructions.[26] The U.S. Food and Drug Administration instituted an action plan requiring manufacturers to include package inserts so that up to 95% of patients should receive useful written information by 2006.[27] It has been recommended that information leaflets be distributed with all prescription medications; it is likely that leaflets for over-the-counter (OTC) medicines would also be beneficial.[27]

Studies show that pharmacists provide written information quite frequently, but do not always discuss it. In a study of community pharmacies in eight US states in 2002, it was found that 89% of shoppers received written information leaflets, but only 5% of those patients were also provided with some oral review of it, 8% were encouraged to read the information, 21% were told they would receive written information but with no review or encouragement to read it, and 66% were given information with no further mention.[26]

Although patients appreciate receiving information leaflets, they report that they want more information, particularly about side effects and warnings and about how their medicines work.[27] They prefer more breadth and depth to what is often available and report that this tends to decrease their uncertainty about medication use.[21] However, this desire must be balanced with information overload, which can increase patient anxiety.[21] Patients also do not like it when they feel print information is a substitute for personal attention.[28]

It should also be considered that, as noted earlier, 40 million Americans are functionally illiterate and 55 million are marginally literate.[5] In addition, 9% of adult Americans experience vision trouble (trouble seeing, even with glasses or contact lenses) that hinders reading.[29] As a result print material may not be appropriate for all people.

When used alone, print information about specific drugs or conditions is of limited effectiveness in improving patients' knowledge or affecting attitudes and behavior because of variations in the quality of written information and patients' varied needs and abilities.[30,31] Print information alone does not appear to improve adherence.[22] It may in fact create certain misunderstandings through ambiguous language that requires further explanation (e.g., avoid prolonged exposure to sunlight; take plenty of fluid).

However, print information is valuable as an adjunct to dialogue and discussion. Together, print information and dialogue and discussion have been found to be more effective than verbal methods alone.[32] Discussion allows the pharmacist to clarify written language and to receive feedback from the patient regarding his or her level of understanding. The print information can then be taken home and read at the patient's leisure. In the pharmacy, the patient often feels rushed or overwhelmed with information or emotions. Elderly people, in particular, often feel the need for more time to absorb the information provided by the pharmacist.[33] After reading the print information, the patient is generally able to identify areas that need clarification, which can then be achieved through further dialogue with the pharmacist.

Studies find that the majority of patients prefer written and verbal information in combination, although it is an individual decision.[34,35] In one study, although 45% of patients preferred both a leaflet and pharmacist counseling, 30% preferred counseling alone, and 20% preferred the leaflet alone; younger patients (31 to 55 years of age) were more likely to prefer the leaflet.[34]

It is recommended that oral counseling accompany the dissemination of medication information leaflets.[27] Print information may be provided to the patient in a variety of forms, including the required prescription label, auxiliary labels, information sheets, pamphlets, or booklets. As well as preprinted information resources, pharmacy software programs are available that can print medication information at the time of dispensing and personalize it for the patient.[36,37]

Any print information given to the patient should be scrutinized by the pharmacist to ensure that it contains appropriate information that reflects and reinforces the information provided verbally. It should be customized as much as possible to the patient's situation to avoid misunderstanding (e.g., men or older women do not need warnings about use in pregnancy). The quality and quantity of print information should be assessed with consideration of literacy and language level, layout, and print size. It is recommended that written material be at about the fifth or sixth grade reading level. In spite of this, only 3% of materials generated by national health authorities, professional agencies, and pharmaceutical companies are written at this level.[38]

Some guidelines for preparing and evaluating patient education materials will be provided later in this chapter.

Audiovisual Aids

Many people find learning easier when they can see or hear information.[14] Information presented in the form of diagrams or pictures can, therefore, improve the patient's understanding of the method of application or ingestion of medications. Audiotapes or videotapes may also improve understanding and help alter attitudes about medication use and illness. For example, a video simulation of a patient using an inhaler may be helpful in changing other patients' attitudes about the need for correct use, and in improving their confidence about using the medication properly. Seeing patients similar to themselves develop skills or wrestle with concerns and problems with medication similar to their own may be more persuasive than having a health professional present information.

Patients may find audiotapes more interesting or easier to comprehend than reading material, particularly if they are vision impaired. In addition, the professional presenter in an audiotape or videotape may be a more persuasive speaker than the pharmacist.

Audiovisual aids may be used with one patient or with small groups of patients.

A growing selection of audiovisual materials are available, including videotapes, audiotapes, and even comic books covering a wide range of topics on specific drugs, diseases, and devices (e.g., inhalers and injection devices). Added to this is the use of interactive video consultations and video conferencing through video and audio connections whereby video pictures and audio and text from patients can be stored and sent via a dedicated telephone line. This has been used by the US armed forces for events such as "telepain" clinics; in northern Canada it connects rural communities and small regional hospitals with health professionals.[39]

Although these materials may be expensive to produce initially, they are used repeatedly, and may be cost-effective in terms of saving pharmacist or physician time.[40] Reports of the use of audiovisual programs for patient counseling suggest that they are well received by patients and can indeed be effective in improving patient knowledge and skills as well as patient satisfaction.[41–46] Interactive video has also resulted in savings in travel, time, and expense and were felt to provide a higher quality of care.[40]

Some studies show audiovisual materials to be equivalent to verbal counseling in improving patient knowledge; however, like print information, these aids tend to be most effective when combined with discussion with the patient before or after the presentation.[39,41]

A viewing area for audiovisual materials can be set up in the pharmacy, in the waiting area, or preferably in an area with some privacy. Patients may also be allowed to take audiovisual material home and upon return to discuss it with the pharmacist to clarify and discuss any new issues.

As with print information, audiovisual materials should be reviewed and evaluated by the pharmacist to determine if the material is appropriate for the particular patient. Criteria for evaluating patient education videotapes will be presented later in this chapter.

Demonstrations and Practice of Techniques

When a medication requires a particular technique of administration, such as inhalation or injection, demonstration by the pharmacist or by videotape is an effective method of patient education. This approach clarifies procedures, since it is easier to follow than verbal instruction alone. When patients are also given the opportunity to practice the technique, they can develop the requisite skill. By observing the patient practicing, the pharmacist can detect possible errors and subsequently correct them.

Studies show demonstration and practice to be superior to written instruction in this type of situation. In a study of patients given MDIs for the first time, patients were personally instructed by a pharmacist using a placebo inhaler and an instruction sheet, or by videotape, and then allowed a further 5 minutes to become familiar with inhaler use. These patients performed significantly better than those provided only with written instructions when asked to demonstrate inhaler use 10 minutes and 2 weeks later.[41]

The Internet and Computer-assisted Patient Education

As early as 1986, computer software was available for use by patients in the United States.[47] With the increased availability and ease of development of software and the Internet, computers have become another educational method to aid pharmacists in providing patients with general health information as well as information about specific health and medication topics. Hospitals in particular are increasingly relying on computer-mediated information systems for patients and more Internet health sites are appearing everyday.[13] The Internet has become one of the largest suppliers of health information, with over 100 million Americans reporting that they will search online for health-related information and more than 70% reporting that such information has influenced a decision about treatment.[48]

Topics may include good health habits, poison information, specific disease information, drug information on common medications, and deciding when to seek medical care.[47] Computer-assisted programs have been used for education in chronic diseases such as diabetes, with alcoholics, and for occupational rehabilitation patients. They have also been used to do health-risk assessments and to provide support networks for patients.[49]

Computerized educational interventions may be more effective than other educational methods for some patients.[49] Computers are most helpful for patients with chronic diseases because of the high degree of self-management required. They help patients with access to information, increase understanding of their disease, and create positive attitudes by increasing feelings of control and confidence.[49] Studies also show patients are more willing to confide in computers than human interviewers, and so health assessments and history taking can be done with more privacy and confidentiality.[49]

Although the age of participants in studies of computerized education does not appear to affect acceptability, reading and comprehension levels may be an issue. A study of adolescents using online Internet health information resources in the United Kingdom and the United States found that spelling names of medicines and conditions, constructing questions for searches, managing the volume of information, and judging its quality presented difficulties.[50] In another study, patients in hard-to-reach categories such as low literacy, speaking another language, with physical disability, or belonging to a cultural community were found to neither use nor want to use computers.[13]

The most reliable Internet health information sites are those associated with government sources or government-affiliated organizations.[51] Although most health information on the Internet is apparently reliable and beneficial to the health consumer, many people would have difficulty comprehending the technical terminology and statistical information provided.[52] An assessment of the readability of three popular sites found reading level to be on average over the ninth grade.[48] It has been suggested that those developing materials for computers and the Internet provide materials with readability in mind and that they develop frequently asked question to help patients organize their learning.[48,50]

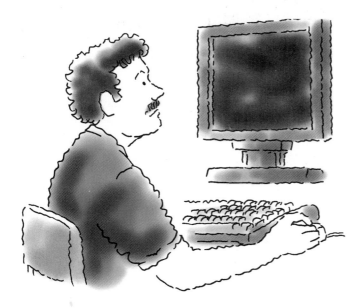

The Internet is a great source of health information, but it can be confusing to find and interpret quality information.

While pharmacists may make use of Internet and computer resources to educate patients, they should be aware that patients will use these resources independently and may get misleading or inaccurate information. Patients should be asked about sources of information they use and appropriate resources should be provided to them by the pharmacist for self-study. They should be advised to check multiple sites and use a "trusted brand" site (such as government health sites).[50]

Decision Aids

Since the model of patient care has moved to shared decision making, it has become important to provide patients with resources to assist them with this. Traditional types of information that generally provide information about the disease and medications are often not sufficient to assist patients in making decisions. Patients need a variety of help not only in learning about their condition and treatments, but also in interpreting that information, assessing risk information, choosing between treatments, weighing pros and cons, and making decisions in light of their own needs, values, and preferences.

Decision aids are defined as "interventions designed to help people make specific and deliberative choices among options (including the status quo) by providing (at the minimum) information on the options and outcomes relevant to a patient's health."[53] Decision aids can help patients by providing information on options, outcomes, diseases and conditions, exercises to clarify values, others' opinions and guidance, or coaching in the steps of decision making and communicating with others.[53]

These can be print-based or computer-based materials, tapes, or videodisks. There are also resources on the Internet such as DIPEx Personal Experiences of

Health & Illness, a database of patient experiences; and Collaborative Care, an online service of the Foundation for Informed Medical Decision Making that has audiovisual presentations and text overviews of evidence-based information on decision making for breast cancer and prostate disease.[54–56] Decision aids often also include discussion with health professionals and sometimes other patients. Compared with usual care with simpler aids, decision aids have been found to produce higher knowledge scores, lower decisional conflict, and more active patient participation in decision making without increasing anxiety, although they did not seem to affect satisfaction.[53]

Miscellaneous Methods

Other educational methods are available to use in patient counseling. Patients can be provided with a diary to monitor their progress and determine if the medication is working by recording their symptoms daily. The pharmacist can help the patients clarify their concerns, as well as improve physician–patient communication by helping patients develop a list of questions to ask their physicians. This tends to improve adherence as discussed earlier.

Pharmacists should keep a list and refer patients where appropriate to various patient support groups that are often available in the community for conditions such as epilepsy, diabetes, psychiatric problems, and alcohol and drug addiction. These types of groups may improve the patient's understanding and attitude toward his or her condition and medication use.

Community groups and community networks have also proved useful in health education. Health care professionals such as pharmacists can become facilitators to educate peer-helpers and community volunteers.[13] This was used in a 1994 study and found to be a more effective way to reach older, low-literate women than traditional and educational approaches.[13]

A contract (written or verbal) between the pharmacist and patient can also help motivate the patient to comply as discussed in Chapter 4.

Telephone consultations via medical help line services provide another avenue for patient education and counseling usually available to the general public 24 hours a day.[40] Although most services initially provided nurses to answer patients' questions and direct patients to appropriate further care, pharmacists have been included in such services in many instances. This has been found to be very beneficial in providing immediate care and in avoiding problems with medications.[40]

With the use of mobile phones, a further means of education has become available, with text messaging being used in one British service to contact patients with health care advice while at work or at home.[40]

Because the family is often an influence on the patient's health attitudes and behavior, family members may also benefit from any of the discussed educational methods as well as involvement in support groups that have been specifically geared to patients' families.

SELECTION OF THE EDUCATIONAL METHOD

Faced with this variety of educational methods for use in counseling, pharmacists must select which to use with their patients. For patient counseling to be most effective, the educational methods used should be appropriate to the context and the objectives of the learning.[14,57] These involve the setting; the patient's stage of behavior change; the patient's personal learning style; the patient's health literacy level; the objectives of the learning based on the needs and goals of the patient; and the patient's physical and mental state.

The Setting

The educational methods used by the pharmacist may vary with the setting in which the counseling interaction takes place. The educational methods used may be somewhat limited by the setting for patient counseling, which is often fairly restrictive. Interactions generally occur at the pharmacy counter or in a more private booth or office setting.

In a more private setting, more discussion is possible. In addition, it is easier to provide demonstrations, have the patient practice administering medication, or present audiovisual materials in a private area. Counseling may be more effective (in terms of patient knowledge and adherence) when it takes place in a private setting (e.g., in an office adjacent to the waiting area) as opposed to a low-privacy area (e.g., across a counter adjacent to a crowded waiting area).[58] This may be a result not only of the patient's greater ease in a private setting, but also of the approach to counseling that privacy makes possible—one in which the pharmacist and the patient tend to ask more questions and engage in more dialogue.[58] Pharmacists have been found to spend more time interacting with patients when they have a private counseling area.[59]

The lack of complete privacy need not, however, limit the pharmacist to the lecture-style presentation or print information. For example, the pharmacist may be able to find a quiet area in the pharmacy to demonstrate the use of an inhaler, or he or she may schedule an appointment with the patient at a quieter time in the pharmacy, or at the patient's home. Alternatively, the patient might be allowed to take written or audiovisual materials home, or be referred to a good Internet resource, and then discuss them later on the telephone with the pharmacist. The telephone is a useful medium for pharmacists to aid in privacy. The setting for patient counseling will be discussed in more detail in Chapter 9.

The Patient's Stage of Learning and Behavior Change

It is important to recognize that education and counseling often need to take place over a period of time with multiple interactions between the pharmacist and patient.[57] Over time, patients pass through different stages of learning. A patient first learning about inhaler use may need to learn what the medication is for through dialogue and print information, and to learn skills to use the inhaler correctly through demonstration and practice. Once he or she has started using the inhaler, the same patient may have to deal with remembering to have the inhaler available at work or during recreational activities. At another point, this patient may also have to deal with personal concerns about having to use an inhaler or about the seriousness of his or her asthmatic condition. These new concerns require a different approach to learning—a more patient-centered approach. The educational method should involve discussion with the patient to help him or her discover where the problems lie and how they may be overcome.

Patients may also pass through stages of behavior change in regard to his or her medication use and/or health behaviors.[60] As discussed in Chapter 4, the Transtheoretical Model of Change, also known as Stages of Change, developed by Prochaska et al., describes how people make decisions to change behavior in stages of emotion, cognitions, and behaviors that facilitate change, including precontemplation, contemplation, preparation, action, maintenance, and relapse prevention.[61,62] Educational and counseling methods that can help move patients toward the action stage include discussion in person or by telephone as well as information resources, training, and practice as shown in Table 6-1.

TABLE 6-1 Educational Methods to Encourage Stages of Behavior Change		
Stages of Change	**Purpose**	**Educational Method**
Precontemplation	To increase patient readiness for counseling To help patient move toward the action stage	Discussion
Precontemplation	To give direct and simple recommendation that the patient take prescribed medication as directed To discuss pros and cons of the treatment To encourage the patient to think about this To let the patient know that help is available when he or she is ready to change	Lecture, dialogue, reading, audiovisual methods
Contemplation	To bolster patient confidence to take the next step To help patient articulate pros and cons	Discussion
Preparation	To reduce adverse effects or to make administration of medication easier To praise and encourage that the patient has the ability	Provide tools and skills to help take action, e.g., memory aids, dosing schedules, and techniques Demonstrations, practice Discussion
Action	To reassess adherence when the patient gets refills of medication	Discussion in person or by telephone
Maintenance	To monitor the patient To prevent relapse or deal with it in a positive way if it does happen	Discussion in person or by telephone Encourage attendance at support groups

Based on information presented in Zimmerman G, Olsen C, Bosworth C. A stages of change approach to helping patients change behavior. Am Fam Physician. 2000;61:1409–1416. Available on line www.aafp.org/afp/20000301/1409.html (accessed 11/2/2004).

The Patient's Personal Style and Orientation

People take in information, make sense of it, and ultimately make use of it to solve problems, make decisions, and create new meanings.[14] The characteristic ways in which people go through these processes are referred to as cognitive and learning styles.[14] Cognitive style refers to the manner in which a person organizes experiences into meanings, values, skills, and strategies.[14] Learning style refers to the manner in which a person's meanings, values, skills, and strategies undergo change.[14] Learning and cognitive styles are relatively stable traits related to personality structure and are distinct from ability or performance in learning.[14]

One of the most commonly used models of learning is that described by David Kolb.[63,64] His theory of experiential learning proposes that there are four elements of learning: Concrete experiences, reflective observation, abstract conceptualization, and active experimentation (Figure 6-1). These elements are based on two dimensions of learning, perception and processing, that are continuums with two extremes. Individuals will have preferences along these two dimensions.

In relation to perception, learners may prefer concrete experience so that they look at things as they are in raw detail, or at the other extreme, prefer abstract conceptualization, looking at things as concepts and ideas. In relation to the processing dimension, people may take the results of their perception and process it through active experimentation, taking what they have concluded and trying to prove that it works; or at the other extreme, process it through reflective observation, taking what they have concluded and watching to see if it works.[63,64]

People will have preferences along both these dimensions, so that there are four types of learners: Accommodators (concrete experiencer/active experimenter); divergers

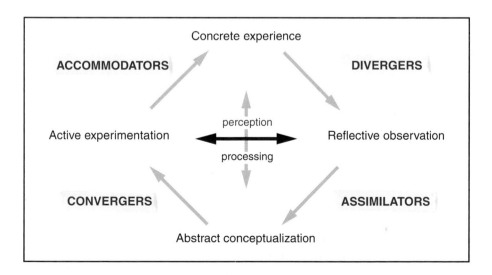

Figure 6-1 Experiential Learning, Learning Styles and Preferences. (Source: Kolb's learning styles. ChangingMinds.org, available online at changingminds.org/explanations/learning/kolb_learning.htm [accessed March 2005].)

TABLE 6-2	Most Effective Educational Methods for Different Learning Styles	
Learning Style	**Learning Preferences**	**Educational Methods**
Diverger: Concrete experiencer/reflective observer	Takes experiences and thinks deeply about them Likes to ask "why?" Influenced by others in a group	Logical instruction or hands-on exploration Discussion Group programs
Converger: Abstract conceptualizer/active experimenter	Thinks about things, then tries out ideas Likes to ask "how?" Likes facts Prefers individual rather than group instruction	Computer-based learning Print materials
Accommodator: Concrete experiencer/ active experimenter	Doing rather than thinking Likes to ask "what if?" and "why not?" Prefers individual rather than group instructions	Hands-on learning Demonstration and practice Individual counseling
Assimilator: Abstract conceptualizer/reflective observer	Prefers thinking to acting Likes to ask "what is there I can know?"	Lectures with demonstrations Discussion Print materials

Based on information presented in Kolb's learning styles. ChangingMinds.org, available online at changingminds.org/explanations/learning/kolb_learning.htm (accessed March 2005)

(concrete experiencer/reflective observer); assimilators (reflective observer/abstract conceptualizer); and convergers (abstract conceptualizer/active experimenter).[63,64] Because of these preferences, individuals respond better to some educational methods than others as shown in Table 6-2.

Although different people prefer to learn via the different steps in the process, all are necessary for successful learning. One person might prefer to learn by abstract conceptualization (understanding how an inhaler propels drugs out of the device and how that combines with inspiration to deposit the drug in the airways), but he or she will have to experiment with how to use an inhaler, experience it, and then reflect on the trials to see if it was done right.[63,64] Because of this and because pharmacists cannot know what patients' individual learning styles are, it is best to use a variety of educational methods, for example, providing demonstration and practice, discussion and print information for a patient receiving a prescription for an inhaler. As noted earlier, patients reportedly prefer a combination of counseling methods to one method alone.

Literacy Level

As discussed earlier, many patients may have low literacy and many more may have low health literacy. Although it is a poorly understood phenomenon, people with low literacy apparently use different communication processes.[12] They report difficulty communicating with their physicians and recall less, especially regarding explanations of their condition and the process of care.[12]

There are tests of health literacy such as Test of Functional Health Literacy in Adults (TOFHLA) and the Rapid Estimate of Adult Literacy in Medicine (REALM).[13] REALM can be administered in 5 minutes and involves the individual pronouncing three lists of 66 medical terms of increasing difficulty ranging from fat and flu to osteoporosis and impetigo, with scores coordinating to achieved school grade level.[13]

Since most pharmacists do not have the training or the time to do such assessments, they must attempt to identify patients with low literacy through other means. Speaking English as a second language, being a senior citizen, not completing high school, and living in conditions of poverty are risk factors for low literacy, and pharmacists should be sensitive and concerned for patients with these characteristics.[65] They should be alert for warning signs that patients are experiencing difficulty with written information such as avoiding filling out forms or questionnaires, relying on others to read material for them, never referring to written information received in the past, asking a lot of questions or none at all, and ignoring or misunderstanding instructions. Nonverbal signs of low literacy may also be apparent such as frustration or anxiety while reading.[66]

When low literacy is identified, print materials should either not be used or selected for easy reading. Educational methods using audiovisual aids and demonstrations may be most helpful. Oral communication may also need to be adapted to use simpler language and slower presentation. Tailoring counseling to patients with literacy or language difficulties will be discussed further in Chapter 8.

Objectives of Learning and Patients' Needs

Counseling may involve a variety of objectives, which will vary with the patient and the situation. Different learning objectives should be based on the patient's needs so that counseling one patient can involve more than one learning objective because of a variety of patient needs.[67]

Patients must acquire knowledge about their medications and the manners in which they are to be administered. They must understand how the medications are used and how they improve their conditions. Patients may also need help in comprehending how their medications can relieve or prevent symptoms and what the implications of their illnesses or medications use might be with respect to their lifestyles.

They must not only receive this information but must have the opportunity to internalize it and understand how to apply the information provided.[67] For example, a patient may have the knowledge that alcohol will interact with his or her medication, but may need help in understanding how alcohol use can be curtailed during social or business events.

Patients must also develop skills in administering the medication such as adhering to a complicated regimen or using an inhaler. The pharmacist can help the patient to develop new skills by demonstration and encouragement to practice the required techniques, both in the pharmacy and at home.[67]

Patients may also need to alter their attitudes in order to get the most benefit from treatment.[67] They may need to develop more positive feelings about their medication use or their conditions, and to become motivated to adhere. For example, consider a patient who refuses to accept his or her diabetic condition and sees no need for regular medication

TABLE 6-3 Educational Methods to Address Patient's Needs	
Patient's Need	**Most Appropriate Methods**
To improve knowledge	Lecture, dialogue, reading, audiovisual methods
To improve understanding	Demonstrations, discussions
To develop skills	Encourage the patient to practice techniques
To change attitudes	Discussion, video simulations

Based on information presented in Knowles, MS. Designing and Managing Learning Activities. In: The Modern Practice of Adult Education: From Pedagogy to Andragogy. Rev. and Updated, 1980. Cambridge Adult Education. Prentice Hall Regents, Englewood Cliffs, NJ:240.

use or lifestyle modifications. The objective of learning for this patient will be the alteration of these attitudes and motivation to change his or her behavior in regard to treatment.

Pharmacists must identify the specific counseling needs and objectives of each patient, and then select the educational and counseling methods best suited to that purpose as shown in Table 6-3.

Patient's Mental and Physical State

Pain, discomfort, and stress can interfere with the patient's concentration and memory, as does the patient's mental state (e.g., possibly confusion, denial, extreme emotions, and hearing or visual disturbances).[68] As a result of these factors, patients forget up to 50% of physicians' statements immediately following their visits.[68]

Patients with disabilities such as sensory or cognitive impairments may find it easier to comprehend information when presented in some formats than others. For example, a vision-impaired patient may prefer verbal information, whereas a hearing-impaired patient may prefer print materials.

It may also be appropriate to delay education and counseling until a patient is in an appropriate state of physical or mental being. Having materials that can be taken home and reviewed at leisure and reviewed repeatedly may be helpful in these cases, with follow-up by telephone or home visit. These issues will be discussed further in Chapter 8.

COUNSELING AIDS

In the discussion of nonadherence in Chapter 4, it was suggested that the pharmacist could make use of a variety of counseling aids to assist the patient. Counseling aids such as calendars and various packaging methods may reduce nonadherence by simplifying multiple drug regimens and by helping overcome difficulties resulting from cognitive or physical impairments.[69]

Currently available counseling aids effectively address nonadherence that arises from difficulties in taking medication, confusion over dosing times, and forgetfulness. However, supplying these counseling aids will not address the many other possible causes of nonadherence discussed in Chapter 4 and therefore should not be seen as a quick fix.

Medication-Reminder Cards and Charts

Patients who have difficulty remembering to take medications or coordinating several medications may find medication-reminder cards and medication charts helpful. These can also be helpful for caregivers and other health professionals to monitor medication use and to be apprised of medication use in the case of an emergency.

A medication-reminder card or chart can be prepared on an individual basis by the pharmacist. It may simply consist of a calendar on which each day is divided into sections according to the number of doses to be taken. Patients can mark off each day's squares as they take doses. If multiple doses are taken each day, daily squares can be subdivided to indicate this. If more than one medication is used, different markings or colors can be adopted as codes (e.g., an asterisk for one drug and an X for another). The pharmacist can indicate the names of the drugs, the dosing schedule, and any coding used on the calendar.[70] Some computer software programs are capable of producing a calendar but these generally apply to individual medications only. A sample medication-reminder card appears in Figure 6-2.

Patient Name:							
Month of:							
	Sat.	Sun.	Mon.	Tues.	Wed.	Thurs.	Fri.
Name of medication and directions for use							
Name of medication and directions for use							
1. Pharmacist completes name of medication and instructions for use.							
2. Patient checks off squares as doses are taken.							

Figure 6-2   Medication-Reminder Card. (Based on information presented in Pritchard R, Senders H. Patient adherence aids. On Continuing Practice. 1989;16(3):25–29.)

Although some patients may find these useful, Ascione and Shimp found that patients using a medication-reminder calendar along with verbal instructions were not more adherent than those receiving only verbal instructions.[71] In addition, patients viewed the calendars negatively, probably because most reported they were already using some sort of reminder system such as keeping drugs in a visible place.[71]

Assisted Labeling

All prescriptions are accompanied by written labels bearing instructions, and print information is often supplied in addition. Some patients, however, may need additional assistance with interpreting or reading labels and print information because of illiteracy, cultural or language problems, poor vision, or confusion over interpreting or coordinating dosing instructions. As discussed earlier, approximately 40 million Americans are functionally illiterate and 55 million are marginally literate.[5] In addition, 9% of adult Americans experience vision trouble (trouble seeing, even with glasses or contact lenses) that hinders reading.[29]

Studies of patients' ability to read prescription labels indicate that in addition to reading or vision problems, a high percentage of patients misinterpret prescription-label instructions. In one such study, 73% of the respondents 64 years of age or under and 93% of those 65 years of age or over misinterpreted label instructions such as "Take one on an empty stomach."[72] Confusion also occurred with instructions that involved coordinating several different medications with different dosage schedules.[72]

For patients with reading difficulties, the use of a chart with a circular diagram of a 24-hour clock has been suggested, as shown in Figure 6-3.[73] The pharmacist can indicate the number of tablets and the dosage times in the section beside each number on the clock. Color or marking codes could be used to distinguish different types of medications. Patients who have impaired vision might benefit from a medication-instruction clock with embossed dots.[73] A picture of the moon and sun can be added beside "A.M." and "P.M." to further assist nonreaders.

Prescription and auxiliary labels can also be adapted for patients with impaired vision. Some computers can be adapted to provide labels with larger print, and some auxiliary labels are available with large print, symbols, and braille.[70]

A recent evaluation of auxiliary labels in community pharmacies found that auxiliary labels were the prime source of information on storage instructions and instructions to shake suspensions; however, labels were sometimes overlooked because of poor color, small font size, or poor placement on the package.[74] Alarmingly, for 24% of prescription bottles the pharmacy had incorrectly placed auxiliary information or did not place all necessary information.[74]

Pictograms may also be useful as an adjunct to prescription and auxiliary labels. Pictograms are available free of charge to professionals and patient information providers from the United States Pharmacopeial Convention Inc. Web site (USP).[75] There is some indication, however, that some pictograms convey meaning poorly, possibly due to their design or because the message is too complex.[76] Understanding of pictograms may also be culture dependent, making them of limited use where language difference is the issue.[76]

| Patient Name: |
| Medication and Code: |

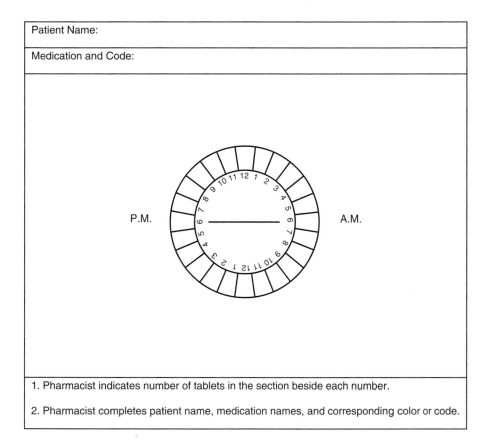

P.M.   A.M.

1. Pharmacist indicates number of tablets in the section beside each number.

2. Pharmacist completes patient name, medication names, and corresponding color or code.

Figure 6-3   **Medication-Instruction Clock. (Adapted with permission from Eustace CA, Johnson GT, Gault MH. Improvements in drug prescription labels for patients with limited education or vision. Can Med Assoc J. 1982;127(8):301.)**

Pill-reminder Containers

Pill-reminder containers assist patients in remembering to take their medications. These containers may be filled by the pharmacist, the patient, a family member, or anyone else involved in the patient's care. They are commercially available, but the pharmacist can also show patients how to devise their own.[70]

Commercially available pill-reminder containers, such as the one shown in Figure 6-4, come in a variety of sizes for daily or weekly scheduling. Some pill-reminder containers actually remind patients to take medication by way of an alarm mechanism, while other pill reminders assist patients by allowing them to keep track of when their medication was taken.[37,77]

Alternatively, patients can make pill-reminder containers out of egg cartons or paper cups that can be filled with medications daily or weekly.

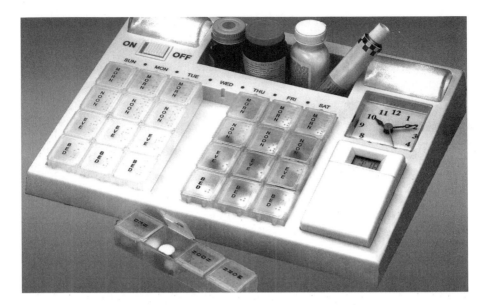

Figure 6-4 Weekly Medication Organization Center. Available from Active & Able. (Picutre courtesy of Active & Able, www.activeandable.com.)

Unfortunately, most only provide one compartment per dosing time, so that several different types of medications must be combined in each container. Another shortcoming of commercially available pill-reminder containers is that some do not include spaces for written instructions to be applied by the pharmacist.[37] They also have no childproofing mechanism so pharmacists should warn patients and advise them to keep their pill-reminder containers out of the reach of children.[70]

The usefulness of these types of counseling aids has been tested. One study found that most patients did not use the pill reminders, and that patients who were organized already had a system for taking medication whereas those who were not found the boxes useless.[78] However, another study found that elderly patients provided with counseling in addition to a medication-reminder package reported improved adherence compared to those receiving only counseling or counseling plus a calendar.[72] Patients also believed that the reminder packages were useful.[72]

Unit-of-use Packaging

Various packaging methods can be used that assist patients by providing one dose of medication at a time, such as blister packaging or individual medication cups.

Medication adherence was found to be significantly better among a group of elderly patients provided with unit-of-use packaging (2-oz plastic cups with snap-on lids containing all drugs to be taken at morning or evening).[78]

In another study, the use of a calendar blister-pack system by a group of ambulatory geriatric clinic outpatients resulted in increased adherence over a 3-month study period.[69]

Unit-of-use packaging provides a continual intervention that demands little involvement by a health professional once it is set up. It provides reinforcement and cuing, supplies easy instructions, and simplifies medication administration for the patient.[69] There are also a number of disadvantages to some unit-of-use packaging, including inability to add or delete drugs once a pack is set up; minimal flexibility for complex regimens; lack of portability; and higher costs of labor and time in preparation. In addition, some are difficult for certain patients to open, whereas most lack child resistance.[69]

Dosing Aids

Patients sometimes have difficulty following exact dosing directions because of problems in making accurate measurements. Directions for fractions of tablets or for liquid measurements may be more accurately followed with the help of dosing aids.

Devices that accurately divide tablets of all sizes and shapes are available on the market, as are various pill crushers.[37] Patients should be advised, however, that these devices cannot be used for sustained-release or long-acting medications or for tablets with enteric or protective coating.

Calibrated spoons or various liquid dispensers such as syringes (without needles) are available for administration of liquid medications. This assists in accurate dosing since household teaspoons can range in volume measure from 4 to 7 mL.[70]

Aerochambers and masks that help direct inhaled medication into the mouth are also available. These assist in using inhaled medication for patients who often fail to get complete doses because they are unable to operate an inhaler (e.g., a baby), or find it difficult to press the inhaler and inhale simultaneously.

Medication Refill-reminder Systems and Telephone Follow-up

As discussed in Chapter 4, increased contact time or supervision by health care professionals can increase medication adherence. This has led to the concept of increasing patient supervision through reminding patients when refills of their medications are due, either by postcards or by telephone calls (either personal or computerized). Follow-up telephone calls to monitor patients also help increase adherence.

Computerized systems that link to patient records and telephone patients automatically are available. Some systems include the ability to calculate drug usage, determine refill dates, initiate a telephone call using the actual voice of the pharmacist, and remind the patient that the drug needs to be refilled, allow for additional comments by the pharmacist and accept the patient's response.[37,77]

Studies evaluating telephone or postcard refill reminders find a significant increase in adherence and patient satisfaction and reduction in medication-related problems.[20,25,79]

The advantages of such programs include not only their effectiveness in improving adherence, but also their ability to recover the lost revenue from prescriptions not refilled each year. However, the disadvantage can be customer dissatisfaction if the patient has not given permission, as well as the risk to patient confidentiality.[77] One pharmacy chain found that 60% of its customers did not want a phone call or reminder postcard, because they thought it was an invasion of privacy or simply an attempt by the pharmacy to make another sale. The pharmacy chain subsequently switched to using a brochure to explain the service, and a form for patients to fill out if they prefer a telephone call or a postcard.[77]

DEVELOPING PATIENT EDUCATION MATERIALS AND PROGRAMS IN THE PHARMACY

In order to develop and implement a pharmaceutical care plan to overcome drug-related problems, pharmacists often need to develop patient education materials and programs or make presentations. To ensure maximum effectiveness of their efforts, pharmacists should consider the various educational principles and patient needs and utilize a variety of resources.

Developing an Individual Patient Education Program

Pharmacists can increase the effectiveness of the various educational methods and counseling aids discussed above by going through a planning process that individualizes the education to the patient's needs, abilities, and personal resources.[80] A decision-making process should be used in a similar manner to the development of a pharmaceutical care plan described in the counseling process discussed in Chapter 5. This should include the following steps, summarized in Table 6-4:[80–82]

1. *Identifying the Educational Needs of the Patient and Family*: Through the information-gathering and problem-identification stages of the patient-counseling protocol, the pharmacist should evaluate the patient's present knowledge level as well as any problems that require educational intervention. As discussed in Chapters 3 and 4, various factors need to be considered to affect the patient's health behavior. These include the patient's perceptions of severity and risk of his or her condition; modifying factors such as age, personality, and knowledge; triggers to action such as advice or support from family; and evaluation of perceived benefits against barriers such as costs and accessibility to care.

   The pharmacist should also ask the patient to evaluate his or her own educational needs. Although the family is often not included in this discussion, family members can have a significant influence on the patient's attitude and behavior and therefore should be considered for inclusion in any educational interventions.

   As noted earlier, educational needs identified for the individual patient may involve knowledge, understanding, skills, attitudes, or beliefs.

TABLE 6-4   Developing an Individual Patient Education Program

1. Identify the educational needs of the patient and family
2. Establish educational goals
3. Select appropriate educational methods
4. Implement the educational plan
5. Evaluate

Based on information presented in Witte K, Bober K. Developing a patient education program in the community pharmacy. Am Pharm. 1982;NS22(10):28–32.

2. *Establishing Educational Goals and Objectives*: The goal of the program is stated as a broad description of the desired outcome. For example, one educational goal may be: To provide the patient with information about high blood pressure so he or she will understand how to self-treat effectively and safely.[81]

Objectives further explain specific behavior that the education should change with respect to knowledge, skills, and attitudes.[81] They should be stated in a way to highlight this, for example:

- *Objective to Change the Patient's Knowledge*: "By the end of the program the patient will be able to list reasons why medication is needed and state proper dose and times of medication use."

- *Objective to Change the Patient's Attitudes*: "The patient will believe the consequences of high blood pressure are serious, and that he or she can take action to control blood pressure by complying with medication."

- *Objective to Change the Patient's Skills*: "The patient will take medication regularly."

These goals and objectives should be discussed with the patient to be sure that they are understood and accepted. In addition, various constraints must be considered so that objectives are realistic. For example, it cannot involve drastic changes in the patient's lifestyle to be accomplished overnight.

3. *Selecting Appropriate Educational Methods*: Together with the patient, the pharmacist should consider possible educational options. As discussed above, the selection of the most effective educational methods should take into consideration the objectives as well as the context of learning. In addition to the effectiveness, another more practical consideration will be the efficiency in terms of costs and time for patient and pharmacist.

4. *Implementing the Program*: The selected educational methods and materials should be synthesized into a program, and a plan should be made as to when the program should start, how long it will be used, and when it will be assessed.[80,81] The outcomes specified in the objectives should be reviewed and a time agreed on for achieving the objectives and evaluating them. Follow-up should be arranged and carried out.

5. *Evaluating the Program*: Plans and methods to evaluate the program should be made early and discussed with the patient. The evaluation should be specific to the goals—for example, if one goal of the program is to change attitude, then some way must be found to ascertain that attitude change has indeed occurred. Clearly stated goals and objectives make evaluation easier.

Evaluation should be ongoing, and may involve observing the patient (e.g., using his or her inhaler); interviewing the patient (during refill counseling or follow-up counseling); or asking the patient to complete a questionnaire.

In a study of pharmacists using this systematic process in developing patient education for individual patients, pharmacists spent an average of 81 minutes per patient in the total process.[83] This time included providing a consultation letter to the physician, performing a number of separate patient interactions (patient history, patient assessment, patient education session, feedback telephone call), and planning and documenting.

Developing a Patient Education Program for Specific Patient Groups

Although patients are all individuals, some similarities in the medication-related problems that they face allow programs to be developed to target specific groups of patients. As discussed above, individual program planning can be time-consuming, and therefore, costly. Some benefits can be accrued by selecting specific patient groups for whom a general educational plan could be developed (e.g., diabetes patients). This plan could then be adapted for use with small groups or with individual patients.

Examples of patient groups who will likely benefit most from planned education programs include patients on drug therapy with a high iatrogenic potential, such as patients on warfarin or digoxin; patients for whom adherence is particularly critical, such as those with diabetes or hypertension; patients with conditions or taking medications requiring significant lifestyle modification, such as smoking cessation or weight loss.[81-83] Alternatively, pharmacists can select groups of patients who are common among their pharmacy clientele, such as caregivers of young children or the elderly.

Developing the plan should involve the same elements as for the individual patient, except that the initial step will involve selecting the target group and identifying common problems they may face. Common problems can be identified from reading journal reports, local hospital-admission reports, discussion with other health professionals, observation during practice as well as from questionnaires conducted within the pharmacy clientele, and discussion with patients from the target group. The patients' perceptions of the need for education should be included with clinical evidence of need, since this will help the pharmacist determine the best way to approach patients for involvement in the program (i.e., there may be a need to overcome initial resistance or raise awareness of problems and the need for education).

When selecting material appropriate to the target population, the pharmacist should select a variety of educational methods and materials so that the program can address a variety of patients' needs. As discussed previously, multiple methods are most effective, and no single strategy is effective for all patients under all circumstances.

Even though the program has been planned for a group, each patient's specific needs should be considered to ensure that his or her needs would be met by the program. If necessary, changes should be made to the program to accommodate the individual.

Individual programs should be conducted by the pharmacist, but some group programs can be provided by facilitators trained to provide all or part of the program, including pharmacy technicians, other health workers, or lay members of the community with referral to the pharmacist for individual questions.

An example of such a program is the Arthritis Self-Management Program presented in California.[84] It included six weekly 2-hour sessions by pairs of trained lay-leaders to groups of 10 to 15 participants. Benefits were still apparent up to 4 years after participation, including decreased pain, physician visits, and reduced costs. The main benefit, however, was felt to be increased perceived self-efficacy to cope with chronic arthritis.[84]

Educational Presentations

Presenting various topics about medication use to various groups can be a worthwhile educational intervention for pharmacists. It not only provides a good source of information to the public, but also raises the public's awareness of the availability of the pharmacist for individual counseling.

TABLE 6-5	**Planning an Educational Presentation**

1. Offer services to local groups
2. Select topics to meet the audience's wants and needs
3. Gear the information and style of presentation to the audience's level
4. Be knowledgeable on the topics presented
5. Use a variety of resources
6. Organize the speech carefully
7. Include humor judiciously
8. Use handout materials, props, audiovisual aids
9. Involve the audience as much as possible
10. Ask for feedback

Based on information presented in Pritchard R. The pharmacist as a public speaker. On Continuing Practice. 1988;15(1)15–18.

When preparing a presentation, pharmacists need to carefully plan and organize. A series of steps for planning an education presentation are summarized in Table 6-5. The first step involves the pharmacist offering his or her services to local groups.

Starting small and informally with local community groups or groups of patients gathered in the pharmacy will help the pharmacist gain confidence. Often the pharmacist is invited by a group, but pharmacists should also contact groups to offer this service. Some potential audiences include senior citizens, women's groups, religious groups, schools, service clubs, special interest groups (e.g., diet groups), drug treatment centers, schools, community centers, and health clubs.[18]

Sometimes the pharmacist is asked to present a particular topic, but it may be left up to the speaker. It is important for the pharmacist to be comfortable with the topic and very knowledgeable, although the level of material will vary with the audience. The depth of information, language level, and style of presentation should be adjusted for the expected audience.

Sources of information for talks include journal articles, pharmacy organizations, government organizations such as the National Institutes of Health, and disease-specific organizations such as the American Heart Association.[85,86]

When writing the presentation, the old adage "tell them what you're going to tell them, tell them, then tell them what you told them" should be kept in mind. The use of appropriate and tasteful humor as well as props such as examples of medications or pamphlets can add interest, as can audiovisual aids such as computerized presentations and videotapes. It is preferable not to read a speech as such, but to speak extemporaneously as much as possible, with a few note cards and props as memory aids.

It is also advisable to involve the audience as much as possible, asking questions and inviting their input. It may be necessary to change the order of topics or to repeat some information to suit the audience's questions.[15] There should be an opportunity for individual audience members to speak with the pharmacist after the presentation, since some people feel uncomfortable asking questions in public. The pharmacist should ask for feedback or distribute a short evaluation questionnaire at the end of the presentation to help in future presentation planning.[15]

Developing Written Educational Materials

There has been considerable study about the development of appropriate and effective written health information. The type and level of language, readability, the print size and layout of the material, the content, and the way that concepts are delivered should all be considered when a pharmacist is developing or using existing print materials for patients. A summary of the following suggestions for preparing more understandable written information is shown in Table 6-6.

1. *Use of Language*: The language should be clear, and free of vague instructions such as "plenty of water." The language should be free of jargon or technical terminology, and the layout and print size should be easy to read.

   Certain medical words may not be well understood. Words such as "void" and "topical" have been found to be comprehended by less than 50% of people, and required 12th and 13th grade education level, respectively.[87] In another study, 25% of patients interpreted "every 6 hours" as meaning "three times a day"; and "as needed for water retention" as meaning "pill would cause water retention."[88] Words such as "follow-up" and "workup" reportedly need further explanation.[89]

   Four kinds of words cause misunderstanding in health care: Medical words (e.g., lesion), concept words used to describe an idea (e.g., option), category words used to describe a group (e.g., generic), and value judgment words (e.g., moderately).[90] These need to be expressed differently for clearer meaning. Some suggestions of these misunderstood words are shown in Table 6-7.[90]

   The word "drug" has been found to have four meanings by the public (medicine, put to sleep, habit forming, and knock out or poison). It has therefore been recommended that "medication" be used rather than "drug" since it is generally taken to mean "healing drug."[87]

2. *Readability*: As noted above, literacy and health literacy should also be considered. People generally read at one or two grade levels below their last completed grade at school so that the average American reads at about the grade eight or nine level.[90] As a result, it is recommended that written material be at about the fifth or sixth grade reading level.[38] This can be accomplished by keeping the wording and sentence structure simple and minimizing the number of multiple syllable words. However, it has been noted that efforts to simplify the readability should not sacrifice the amount or order of information, or the inclusion of important risk information.[27] As noted above, patients want full information, and need it in order to make health care decisions. When preparing materials, pharmacists should assess readability using various available formulas as discussed later in this chapter. Computer spelling and grammar checking programs often include the capability to assess readability of material composed on the computer.

   It should be noted that when reader interest is high, readability indices may overestimate the difficulty.[68] On the other hand, pain, discomfort, and stress interfere with the patient's concentration and memory, as does the patient's mental state (e.g., possibly confusion, denial, extreme emotions, and hearing or visual disturbances).[68]

3. *Organization and Layout*: The text organization can also affect readability.[68] It is important to provide an introduction that explains the purpose of the material and a summary of information at the end. Font should be at least 14 point, with larger print where necessary.[91] It is helpful to use headings and varied formats such as

TABLE 6-6	Suggestions for Preparing Written Patient Education Materials
Wording	Use common words, preferably one or two syllables, and define medical or technical words
	Use a readability index and adjust to result in grade 5–6 reading level
	Use both brand and generic names and provide a pronunciation guide
	Use active sentences most of the time (e.g., *swallow each capsule with water*)
	Use affirmative sentences most of the time unless referring to avoiding an action (e.g., *Take with food* rather than *Do not take on an empty stomach*)
	Be specific (e.g., *Drink at least 8 oz of water* rather than *Drink plenty of fluid*)
Layout	Use headlines and subheadings rather than numbering
	Group or "chunk" similar bodies of information using brief, clear titles
	Use margins and plenty of empty spaces
	Emphasize points with different type face, bold face, underlining, boxing, columns
	Use color
	Use Arabic numbers rather than Roman numerals for letters and lists
	Use upper and lower case rather than blocks of capitals which are more difficult to read
	Keep pictograms simple, close to corresponding text
	Use at least 14-point font size and use larger print where appropriate
Content and delivery of concepts	Address specific audience needs
	Use accurate, objective, and unbiased material
	Present risk with comparative frame of reference
	Individualize risk where possible
Structure and organization	Use short, simple sentences
	Keep sentences and paragraphs short (10 words or less per sentence)
	Introduce one idea per sentence, and limit the number of ideas per page
	Provide reasons for instructions
	Precede information with an advance organizer (e.g., *Things that may reduce back pain are . . .*)
	Use objectives (e.g., *The following information will help you use your inhaler*)
	Use questions followed by information (e.g., *What should I do if I feel dizzy?*)
	Use simple checklists, diagrams, and charts

Based on information presented in Dolinsky D, Gross S, Deutsch T, et al. Application of psychological principles to the design of written patient information. Am J Hosp Pharm. 1983;40(2):266–71; Hilts L, Krilyk BJ. W.R.I.T.E. Write readable information to educate. Chedoke-McMaster Hospital, Hamilton Civic Hospitals, Hamilton General Division, 1989; USP, Optimizing patient comprehension through medicine information leaflets. A final report submitted by University of North Carolina at Chapel Hill and Duke University. 1999. Available online at www.uspdqi.org/pubs/other/PatientLeafletStudy.pdf

TABLE 6-7 Alternatives to Misunderstood Words in Health Care	
Term	**Alternative**
Benign	Will not cause harm: Is not cancer
Lesion	Wound; sore; infected patch of skin
Inhibitor	Drug that stops something that is bad for you
Gauge	Measure; get better idea of; test
Factor	Other thing
Generic	Product sold without a brand name
Adverse	Bad
Adequate	Enough
Adjust	Fine-tune; change
Progressive	Gets worse (or better)
Significantly	Enough to make a difference

Adapted with permission from Partnership for Clear Health Communication. Words to Watch-Fact Sheet, AskMe3, available online at www.AskMe3.org (accessed March 2005)

numbered points, diagrams, and charts. Pictograms can be helpful but should be simple and placed near to appropriate text, with additional explanatory notes.[27]

4. *Content*: The material should address the needs of the specific audience it is aimed at, such as teenagers or newly diagnosed diabetics. Material should be objective and unbiased, and of course accurate. As much as possible, material should be practical and useable by the public. The focus should be on providing useful information to not only improve knowledge, but also develop skills and change behavior.

   Including resources for further information such as Web sites will widen the audience of the material to more advanced learners.

5. *Delivery of Concepts*: Considerable effort has been made to find appropriate ways to present detailed information about concepts such as risk for use in decision aids. Graphical displays of information have been found to increase the effectiveness of information about risks, with simple bar charts preferred over representations such as stick figures.[56] Comparisons of treatment choices should be done in ways to inform, not to manipulate or convince. For example, providing positive comparisons of choices such as information about chance of survival rather than negative comparisons such as chance of death is more likely to persuade people to choose risky options.[56]

   Risk is best presented with a comparative frame of reference to everyday familiar risks such as having a car accident. Where possible, risks should be individualized—for example, calculating an individual's risk of coronary heart disease by using information on risk factors (age, hypertension, cholesterols, and smoking) from available data and charts.[56]

There are many excellent resources to use when developing print materials. The Harvard School of Public Health has a list of resources for creating print materials on its Web site including specific resources for use with patients with low literacy and with seniors.[92] A Health and Literacy Compendia with a bibliography of print and web-based health materials for use with limited-literacy adults is also available online.[93]

TABLE 6-8 Readability Tests

Fog index:

Count about 100 words. Stop at the nearest sentence end

Count the number of sentences in the 100 words sample, S

Count the number of hard words (three syllables or more), A

Calculate the grade reading level using the formula: GL = (100/S + A) × 0.4

If the piece is long, repeat this for several 100-word sections and average the results

SMOG formula:

Select 30 sentences

Count words containing three or more syllables

Find nearest perfect square root

Add 3 = grade level

Based on information presented in Spadaro D, Robinson L, Smith LT. Assessing readability of patient information materials. Am J Hosp Pharm. 1980;37(2):215–21; Bernier MJ. The SMOG formula. In: Developing and evaluating printed education materials: A prescriptive model for quality. Orthopedic nursing, 1993;12(6). Available online at www.depts.washington.edu/pfes/pdf/Worksheet-smog.pdf (accessed March 2005)

Disease-specific organizations such as the American Diabetes Association are also an excellent source of disease-related information for use with patients.[94]

Evaluation of Patient Education Materials

Although pharmacists can develop their own materials, an ever-increasing variety of prepared materials are available. Before embarking on development of materials or programs, pharmacists should check to see what is already available to avoid wasted effort, time, and money. However, not all materials are equal, and it is important for pharmacists to evaluate prepared educational materials before using them.

The same principles that were discussed above regarding the development of written materials can also be applied to evaluating existing written materials (Table 6-6). In order to ensure materials are at an appropriate reading level, a readability formula can be applied. This is a mathematical equation that describes the relation between the reader's skill and the author's style of writing to result in a score depicting the level of reading skills needed by the intended reader.

A number of readability tests are available (Table 6-8).[95] One such test, Gunning's Fog index, is one of the easiest methods for calculating achieved school grade-level readability.[95] Another similar measure, Simple Measure of Gobbledygook (SMOG), is also frequently used.[96]

Audiovisual materials should also be assessed prior to using them with patients. Criteria for selecting patient education videos have been suggested as follows:[97]

1. Uses a vocabulary that is not above the reading level of your patient.
2. Has graphics to help simplify complex medical terminology.
3. Presents the information concisely and in an appropriate sequence so progressive patient learning can be accomplished.
4. Contains practical information appropriate for the individual patient.

5. Displays high-quality audio and visual clarity.
6. Is no more than 10 minutes long in order to maintain the patient's attention.
7. Additional considerations in selecting materials are cost and availability.

Internet information sources and computerized patient education programs should also be reviewed for accuracy of information and readability.

Materials that do not adhere to the above standards do not necessarily need to be rejected. Since it is advisable to use written or audiovisual materials in conjunction with verbal counseling, any shortfalls can be overcome through discussion with the patient to identify misunderstandings, and verbal reinforcement can be provided. If materials are to be viewed or read by the patient at home, the pharmacist should be sure to follow up (in person or by telephone) to answer any questions or concerns raised by the material.

SUMMARY

Pharmacists have many resources available to educate individuals and groups of patients. Studies show that no single strategy is effective for all patients under all circumstances.[98] In addition, patients' attitudes toward pharmacists have been found to be more positive when any information was provided, regardless of the method used.[99] Many of the educational methods and counseling aids discussed in this chapter were found to be more effective when verbal counseling was a component of patient education. It is therefore essential that pharmacists gain expertise in verbal counseling. Good communication skills are critical to effective verbal counseling. This will be discussed in the following chapter.

REFLECTIVE QUESTIONS

1. Describe the elements a pharmacist should consider when selecting an appropriate method of learning for a 16-year-old male patient recently diagnosed with diabetes.
2. Create a medication-instruction clock for an elderly patient with a prescription for furosemide 20 mg tablets and instructions to take 40 mg in the morning and 20 mg in the afternoon.
3. What can a pharmacist do to address the fact that different patients have different learning styles?
4. Prepare a chart showing the pros and cons of the different educational methods presented in this chapter.

REFERENCES

1. Knowles MS. What is Andragogy? In: The Modern Practice of Adult Education. Prentice Hall Regents, Englewood Cliffs, NJ, 1970, p. 40–62.
2. Government of Canada. Good Medicine for Seniors: Guidelines for Plain Language and Good Design in Prescription Medication. Canadian Public Health Association/National Literacy and Health Program, Ottawa, Canada, 2002, p. 1–79.
3. World Health Organization. Health Promotion Glossary. Health Promot Int. 1998;13(4):349–364.
4. Andrus MR, Roth MT. Health literacy: A review. Pharmacotherapy. 2002;22:282–302.

5. Kirsch I, Jungeblit A, Jenkins L, et al. Adult literacy in America. A first look at the results of the National Adult Literacy Survey. US Department of Education. National Center for Educational Statistics. Educational Testing Service, Princeton, NJ, 1993.

6. Williams MV, Parker RM, Baker DW, et al. Inadequate functional health literacy among patients at two public hospitals. JAMA. 1995;274(21):1677–1682.

7. Anonymous. Fact sheet: The use of over-the-counter medicines. National Council on Patient Information and Education. Available at: www.bemedwise.org/press_room/sep_2003_fact_otc.pdf (accessed January 2005).

8. Tabor PA, Lopez DA. Comply with us: Improving medication adherence. J Pharmacy Pract. 2004;17:167–181.

9. Malveaux JO, Murphy PW, Arnold C, et al. Improving patient education for patients with low literacy skills. Am Fam Physician. 1996;53(1):205–211.

10. Estrada CA, Hryniewicz MM, Higgs VB, et al. Literacy and numeracy skills and anticoagulation control. Am J Med Sci. 2004;328:88–93.

11. Williams MV, Parker RM, Baker DW, et al. Inadequate literacy is a barrier to asthma knowledge and self-care. Chest. 1998;114:1008–1015.

12. Schillinger D, Piette J, Grumback K, et al. Closing the loop. Physician communication with diabetic patients who have low health literacy. Arch Intern Med. 2003;163:83–90.

13. Shohet L. Health and Literacy: Perspectives in 2002. Centre for Literacy of Quebec, Montreal, Quebec, Canada. Available at: www.staff.vu.edu.au/alnarc/onlineforum/AL_pap_shohet.htm (accessed March 2005).

14. Brundage DH, MacKeracher D. Characteristics of the Adult Learner. Adult Learning Principles and Their Application to Program Planning. Ontario Ministry of Education, Ontario Institute for Studies in Education, Toronto, Canada, 1980.

15. Nelson M. Our guest for tonight is . . . Pharmacists and public speaking. Am Pharm. 1993;NS33(3):59–62.

16. McKay M, Davis M, Fanning P. Public Speaking. In: Messages: The Communication Book, New Harbinger Publications, Oakland, CA, 1983.

17. Gondin W, Mamman E. The Art of Speaking Made Simple. Rev. Ed. Doubleday & Co., Garden City, NY, 1981.

18. Pritchard R. The pharmacist as a public speaker. On Continuing Practice. 1988;15(1):15–18.

19. Anonymous. U.S. Indian services to rethink Rx counseling. Drug store news for the pharmacist. 1991;1(5):21.

20. Garnett W, Davis L, McKenney J, et al. Effect of telephone follow-up on medication adherence. Am J Hosp Pharm. 1981;38(5):676–679.

21. Schommer J, Doucette W, Worley M. Processing prescription drug information under different conditions of presentation. Patient Educ Couns. 2001;43:49–59.

22. Mottram DR. Comparative evaluation of patient information leaflets by pharmacists, doctors and the general public. J Clin Pharm Ther. 1997;22:127–134.

23. Svarstad B. Physician-patient communication and patient conformity with medical advice. In: Mechanic D, ed., The Growth of Bureaucratic Medicine, John Wiley & Sons, New York, 1976.

24. Ley PN, Spellman MS. Communication with the Patient. Staples Press, London, 1967.

25. Clifford S, Barber N, Horne R, et al. Evaluation of a pharmacist-delivered intervention to improve patients' adherence and reduce their problems with medicines. Health Services Research & Pharmacy Practice Abstracts, 2003. Available at: www.hsrpp.org.uk/abstracts/2003_47.shtml (accessed March 2005).

26. Svarstad B, Bultman D, Mount J. Patient counseling provided in community pharmacies: Effects of state regulation, pharmacist age, and busyness. J Am Pharm Assoc. 2004;44(1):22–99.

27. Anonymous. United States Pharmacopeia. Optimizing patient comprehension through medicine information leaflets. A final report submitted by University of North Carolina at Chapel Hill and Duke University, 1999. Available at: www.uspdqi.org/pubs/other/PatientLeafletStudy.pdf (accessed March 2005).

28. Norris P, Rowsell B. Interactional issues in the provision of counselling to pharmacy customers. Int J Psychoanal Psychother. 2003;11:135–142.
29. Anonymous. Summary Health Statistics for U.S. Adults: National Health Interview Survey, 2002, Vital and Health Statistics, Series 10, Number 222, DHHS Publication No. (PHS) 2004–1550, U.S. Department of Health and Human Services Centers for Disease Control and Prevention National Center for Health Statistics, Hyattsville, MD, 2004. Available at: www.cdc.gov/nchs/data/series/sr_10/sr10_222acc.pdf (accessed March 2005).
30. McBean BJ, Blackburn JL. An evaluation of four methods of pharmacist-conducted patient education. Can Pharm J. 1982;115:167–172.
31. Morris LA, Halperin JA. Effects of written drug information on patient knowledge and compliance. A literature review. Am J Public Health. 1979;69:47–52.
32. Mullen PD, Gren LW. Measuring Patient Drug Information Transfer: An Assessment of the Literature. Pharmaceutical Manufacturers Association, Washington, DC, 1984.
33. Chermak G, Jinks M. Counseling the hearing-impaired older adult. Drug Intell Clin Pharm. 1981;15(5):377–382.
34. Harvey J, Plumridge RJ. Comparative attitudes to verbal and written medication information among hospital outpatients. DICP. 1991;25(9):925–928.
35. Culbertson V, Arthur T, Rhodes P, et al. Consumer preferences for verbal and written medication information. Drug Intell Clin Pharm. 1988;22(5):390–396.
36. Cataldo R. OBRA-'90 and your pharmacy computer system. Am Pharm. 1992;NS32(11):39–41.
37. Anonymous. Resources Showcase. Talk About Prescriptions Month. Planning Guide. National Council on Patient Information and Education, Washington, DC, 1992.
38. Jacobson TA. The forgotten cardiac risk factor: Noncompliance with lipid-lowering therapy. Medscape Cardiol. 2004;8(2):1–10. Available at: www.medscape.com/viewarticle/496144 (accessed March 2005).
39. Marshall WR, Rothenberger MA, Bunnell SL. The efficacy of personalized audiovisual patient-education materials. J Fam Pract. 1984;19(5):659–663.
40. Phul S, Besseell T, Cantrill J. Alternative delivery methods for pharmacy services. Int J Psychoanal Psychother. 2004;12:53–63.
41. McElnay JC, Scott MG, Armstrong AP, et al. Use of video for patient counseling. Pharm J. 1988;241(Suppl 6508):R28.
42. Olsenk MS, Du Bé JE. Evaluation of two methods of patient education. Am J Hosp Pharm. 1985;42(3):622–624.
43. Soflin D, Young WW, Clayton BD. Development and evaluation of an individualized patient education program about digoxin. Am J Hosp Pharm. 1977;34(4):367–371.
44. Darr MS, Self TH, Ryan MR, et al. Content and retention evaluation of an audiovisual patient education program on bronchodilators. Am J Hosp Pharm. 1981;38(5):672–675.
45. Putnam GL, Yanagisako K. Skin cancer comic book: Evaluation of a public educational vehicle. J Audiovisual Media Med. 1985;8(1):22–25.
46. Mahoney C, Jeffrey L, Powlina A. Recorded medication messages for ambulatory patients. Am J Hosp Pharm. 1983;40(3):448–449.
47. Ascione F, Fish C. Computer health/medication information software-compilation for pharmacists. Am Pharm. 1986;NS26(2):45–50.
48. Gottlieb R, Rogers J. Readability of health sites on the Internet. Int Electron J Health Educ. 2004;7:38–42. Available at: www.aahperd.org/iejhe/template.cfm?template=2004/rogers.html (accessed March 2005).
49. Krishna S, Balas A, Spencer D, et al. Clinical trials of interactive computerized patient education: Implications for family practice. J Fam Pract. 1997;45(1):25–33.
50. Gray NJ, Klein JD, Sesselberg TS, et al. Health literacy and the Internet: Implications for pharmacy practice. Health Serv Res Pharm Pract Abstr. 2003. Available at: www.hsrpp.org.uk/abstracts/2003_46.shtml (accessed March 2005).

51. Rippen HE. What every viewer and developer should know about site standards. Med Mark Media. 2000;35(5):53–57.

52. MacColl GS, White KD. Communicating Educational Research Data to General, Nonresearcher Audiences. Office of Educational Improvement, Washington, DC, 1998.

53. O'Connor A, Rostom A, Fiset V, et al. Decision aids for patients facing health treatment or screening decisions: Systematic review. Br Med J. 1993;319:731–734.

54. Personal Experiences of Health & Illness. DIPEx. Available at: www.dipex.org (accessed March 2005).

55. Collaborative care, foundation for informed medical decision making. Available at: www.collaborativecare.net (accessed March 2005).

56. Edwards A, Elwyn G, Mulley A. Explaining risks: Turning numerical data into meaningful pictures. Br Med J. 2002;324:827–830.

57. Simpson EL. Adult Learning Theory: A State of the Art. In: Moore J, Lasker H, Simpson E, eds., Adult Development and Approaches to Learning. US Government Document, Washington, DC, 1980.

58. Beardsley R, Johnson C, Wise G. Privacy as a factor in patient counseling. J Am Pharm Assoc. 1977;17(6):366–368.

59. Laurier C, Poston J. Perceived levels of counseling among Canadian pharmacists. J Soc Admin Pharm. 1992;9:104–113.

60. Mullen PO, Green LW, Pessinger GS. Clinical trials of patient education for chronic conditions: A comparative meta-analysis of intervention types. Prev Med. 1985;14:753–757.

61. Prochaska JO, Velicer WF. The transtheoretical model of health behavior change. Am J Health Promot. 1997;12:38–48.

62. Zimmerman G, Olsen C, Bosworth C. A stages of change approach to helping patients change behavior. Am Fam Physician. 2000;61:1409–1416. Available at: www.aafp.org/afp/20000301/1409.html (accessed November 2, 2004).

63. Anonymous. Kolb's learning styles, Changing minds.org. Available at: changingminds.org/explanations/learning/kolb_learning.htm (accessed February 2005).

64. Kolb DA. Experiential Learning. Prentice-Hall, Englewood Cliffs, NJ, 1984.

65. Gillis DE. Beyond words. The health literacy connection. Canadian Health Network, Public Health Agency of Canada, 2005. Available at: www.canadian-health-network.ca/servlet/ContentServer?cid=105968393879&pagename=CH-RCS%2FCHNResource%2FCHNResourcePageTemplate&c=CHNResource (accessed March 2005).

66. Baker DW, Williams MV, Parker RM, et al. Development of a brief test to measure functional health literacy. Patient Educ Couns. 1999;38:33–42.

67. Knowles MS. Designing and managing learning activities. In: The Modern Practice of Adult Education: From Pedagogy to Andragogy. Prentice Hall Regents, Englewood Cliffs, NJ, 1980.

68. Hilts L, Krilyk BJ. W.R.I.T.E. Write Readable Information to Educate. Chedoke-McMaster Hospital, Hamilton Civic Hospitals, Hamilton Geriatric Division, Hamilton, Ontario, Canada, 1989.

69. Wong B, Norman D. Evaluation of a novel medication aid, the calendar blister-pak and its effect on drug adherence in a geriatric outpatient clinic. J Am Geriatr Soc. 1987;35(1):21–26.

70. Pritchard R, Senders H. Patient adherence aids. On Continuing Practice. 1989;16(3): 25–29.

71. Ascione F, Shimp L. The effect of four educational strategies in the elderly. Drug Intell Clin Pharm. 1984;18(11):926–931.

72. Hurd P, Butkovich L. Adherence problems and the older patient: Assessing functional limitations. Drug Intell Clin Pharm. 1986;20(3):228–230.

73. Eustace CA, Johnson GT, Gault MH. Improvements in drug prescription labels for patients with limited education or vision. Can Med Assoc J. 1982;127(8):301.

74. Ellington A, Barnett C, Nykamp D. Effectiveness of auxiliary labeling in community pharmacies. US Pharm. 2003;28(4):56–62.

75. USP Pictograms, United States Pharmacoepia. Available at: www.usp.org/drugInformation/pictograms/form.html (accessed February 2005).
76. Price S, Raynor DK, Knapp P. Developing effective medicine pictograms for the UK. Health Serv Res Pharm Pract Abstr. 2003. Available at: www.hsrpp.org.uk/abstracts/2003_41.shtml (accessed February 2005).
77. Clepper I. Nonadherence the invisible epidemic. Drug Topics. 1992;136(16):44–50, 56–65.
78. Cramer J. Adherence: Uncovering the hidden problems in practice. Drug Topics. 1992;Suppl 136(13):6–10.
79. Murray M, Birt J, Manatunga A, et al. Medication adherence in elderly outpatients using twice-daily dosing and unit-of-use packaging. Ann Pharmacother. 1993;27(5):616–621.
80. Strodtman LA. Decision-making process for planning patient education. Patient Educ Couns. 1984;5(4):189–200.
81. Witte K, Bober K. Developing a patient education program in the community pharmacy. Am Pharm. 1982;NS22(10):28–32.
82. Bond W, Hussar D. Detection methods and strategies for improving medication adherence. Am J Health Promot. 1991;48(9):1978–1988.
83. Opdycke RA, Ascione F, Shimp L, et al. A systematic approach to educating elderly patients about their medications. Patient Educ Couns. 1992;19:43–60.
84. Lorig K, Mazonson, Holman H. Evidence suggesting that health education for self-management in patients with chronic arthritis has sustained health benefits while reducing health care costs. Arthritis Rheum. 1993;36(4):439–446.
85. National Institutes of Health website, National Institutes of Health. Available at: www.health.nih.gov
86. American Heart Association website. Available at:www.Americanheart.com
87. Wilson J, Hogan L. Readability testing of auxiliary labels. Drug Intell Clin Pharm. 1983;17(1):54–55.
88. Mazullo JM III, Lasagna L, Griner PF. Variation in interpretation of prescription instructions: The need for improved prescribing habits. JAMA. 1974;227:929–931.
89. McKinney JB. Who is really ignorant—physician or patient? J Health Soc Behav. 1975;16:3–11.
90. Anonymous. Words to watch—fact sheet. AskMe3, partnership for clear health communication. Available at: www.askme3.org (accessed March 2005).
91. Morrow D, Leirer V, Sheikh J. Adherence and medication instructions. Review and recommendations. J Am Geriatr Soc. 1988;36:1147–1160.
92. Anonymous. Recommended resources for creating print materials. Health Literacy Studies, Harvard School of Public Health. Available at: www.hsph.harvard.edu/healthliteracty/how_to/resource_create.html (accessed March 2005).
93. Irvine C. Health and Literacy Compendia. An annotated bibliography of print and web-based health materials for use with limited-literacy adults. Health and Literacy Initiative, World Education, Boston, MA, 1991. Available at: www.worlded.org/us/health/docs/comp/index.html (accessed March 2005).
94. American Diabetes Association website. Available at: www.diabetes.org (accessed March 2005).
95. Spadaro D, Robinson L, Smith LT. Assessing readability of patient information materials. Am J Hosp Pharm. 1980;37(2):215–221.
96. Bernier MJ. The SMOG formula. Developing and evaluating printed education materials: A prescriptive model for quality. Orthop Nurs. 1993;12(6):39–46. Available at: www.depts.washington.edu/pfes/pdf/Worksheet-smog.pdf (accessed March 2005).
97. Blouch D. Tuning into patient videos. Pharm Pract. 1993;9(4):38.
98. Anonymous. Researcher calls Rx package inserts ineffective. Drug Store News. 1984;6(22):62.
99. Kimberlin C, Berardo D. A comparison of patient education methods used in community pharmacies. J Pharm Market Manag. 1987;1(4):75–94.

7 Human Interactions and Counseling Skills in Pharmacy

Objectives

After completing the chapter, the reader should be able to

1. describe the many variables that affect human interactions in pharmacy.
2. list strategies pharmacists can use to enhance relationships with patients.
3. describe the counseling skills necessary for effective patient counseling.
4. suggest solutions to common causes of poor relationships with other health professionals.
5. be prepared to practice interacting verbally, in writing, by telephone, and by e-mail using techniques discussed.

Human interactions and counseling skills have become important issues for health professionals. Interest in health professionals' interactions grew out of concern over patient nonadherence to therapeutic regimens.[1] As discussed in Chapter 4, providing information alone does not necessarily improve adherence, particularly over the long term. Information is only useful to patients if they notice, understand, and remember it.[2] Investigations involving patient–health professional interactions suggest that communication is needed to accomplish this and therefore improve patient care.[3-5]

The trend to shared decision making has further emphasized the need for interaction between patients and their health care providers so that patients can understand their conditions and treatment options and come to well-thought-out decisions about their health care. The nature of pharmaceutical care makes the development of a therapeutic relationship a necessity for pharmacists.[5]

Research has shown that when a trusting relationship is established between patients and their health professionals, patients recover more quickly, experience less pain and a greater variety of physiological, psychological, and behavioral gains as compared to patients who do not have this relationship.[6]

Building such a relationship requires both quantity and quality in the interaction, participation of both patient and pharmacist, and the use of counseling skills by the pharmacist.[5] It involves becoming familiar with the patient, establishing a feeling of trust, and making the patient feel sufficiently comfortable to discuss personal matters and to express himself or herself.[7] This in turn leads to a cooperative and harmonious interaction.[7]

In the course of providing pharmaceutical care, pharmacists also need to be able to interact effectively with other members of the health care team in order to gather more detailed information about the patient and to discuss the patient's medication-related problems. They must be able to interact effectively with other pharmacists and pharmacy personnel, working cooperatively both within the pharmacy and with other pharmacists in the community or hospital for the benefit of the patient.

UNDERSTANDING HUMAN INTERACTION

As a basis for understanding interactions in pharmacy and the skills used in patient counseling, we need to consider the many variables and theories that are involved. This will provide insight into communication as an exchange of messages, psychological aspects, the interactionist approach, and consideration of human needs, values, and culture.

Communication as an Exchange of Messages

One way to view human interaction is as a communication process in which information is exchanged between two individuals (the pharmacist and the patient in the case of patient counseling).[8,9] An idea (message) is formed in the mind of the sender and is translated into a form that can be transmitted by spoken or written words or by body language (e.g., an extended hand to greet a person). The intended message is transmitted by the sender (pharmacist), perceived by the receiver (patient) through hearing or seeing, and then translated to determine the meaning of the message (e.g., the extended hand was a greeting).

Unfortunately, the perceived meaning by the receiver is often not identical to the intended meaning transmitted by the sender, and the result is a misunderstanding between the pharmacist and patient. This is apparent through a feedback message provided by the patient as to how the message was perceived. The pharmacist must be alert to this feedback and be prepared to modify and clarify the message as necessary.[10] The pharmacy environment can affect the message and a variety of barriers to communication can distort the message or inhibit feedback.[8] The pharmacy environment and barriers will be discussed further in Chapter 9.

Since the purpose of the communication in patient counseling is to form a relationship as well as to educate, it is important that the pharmacist recognizes the importance of the message received back from the patient. It should become the basis for the next question or action of the pharmacist so that it is not just a lecture but the start of a relationship.[9]

Psychologic Theories

Human interaction is further complicated by the complexities of individual personalities. Various psychologic types have been described to help explain how people interact.[11] Although this may appear to stereotype people, it does acknowledge that even though no two people are totally alike, there are identifiable similarities in each of us. Jung described these commonalities as pairs of opposing aspects of personality that describe a person's preferences with respect to interest in the outer world, perception, decision making, and approach to life.[11]

The two extremes of attitude toward life are extroversion and introversion. Extroverted behavior involves turning outward to act, looking forward to socializing, being energized by people and events. Introverted behavior involves turning inward, being energized more by inward reflection rather than by socializing.[11]

People also have different perception styles that affect how they take in information through sensing or intuition. Sensing involves being systematic and detail conscious, able to see the big picture. The other extreme is intuition, which involves using insights and hunches rather than concrete details.[11]

People also vary in the way that they make decisions about information ranging from thinking to feeling. Those who use thinking to make decisions tend to be objective, considering causes and outcomes in an impersonal manner. Conversely, people who use feeling to make decisions are more likely to be subjective and personal, weighing the values of choices and how others may be affected.[11]

People tend to approach life in different ways, tending to rely mainly on judgment or perception. Those who rely on judgment aim to control events and live in a decisive and planned way. Those who rely more on perception tend to be more spontaneous and flexible, aiming to understand and adapt to life rather than to control it.[11]

People can generally identify themselves within a continuum between these sets of opposite psychologic types. One end is no better than the other; it simply helps us see a different perspective in the way people communicate.

In order to provide a more complete picture of personality, these eight different ways of dealing with information have been combined by Myers-Briggs to describe 16 personality types as shown in Table 7-1.

The personality traits of both pharmacist and patient will be involved when they interact. Although the pharmacist cannot know the personality of each patient, the pharmacist can recognize that it will affect interactions. If aware of his or her own personality type, the pharmacist can modify behavior to become more effective in patient counseling, for example, to be slightly less extroverted, or to use a little more intuition during patient counseling.

One study considered pharmacists' personality types as it related to nonprescription counseling.[12] Patients counseled by pharmacists who were more extroverted were less likely to change their purchase decision. The authors suggested that the patients may have perceived these pharmacists as more unreliable and untrustworthy.

Transactional Analysis Theory

The transactional analysis (TA) theory further helps us understand the way people interact during counseling. Eric Berne observed that everyone's personality consists of three distinct ego states that describe consistent patterns of feeling, experiencing, and behaving: The parent, adult, and child.[8,13] People of all ages can react in these ego states, and Berne suggests that during communication, a transaction occurs between people's ego states.

The parent state incorporates attitudes and behavior taught by an individual's parents and often causes people to respond automatically in the manner their parents or other authority figures would have (nurturing or critical).[8] The child ego state contains the feelings an individual had as a child, and tends to emerge with an emotional response, often in response to another person's parent state (either free and irresponsible, or adapted and obedient).[8] The adult ego state causes people to respond more analytically, gathering

TABLE 7-1 Myers-Briggs Personality Types

	Sensing (S)		Intuition (N)	
	Thinking (T)	Feeling (F)	Feeling (F)	Thinking (T)
Introversion (I)	ISTJ	ISFJ	INFJ	INTJ
Judgment (J)	Quiet, practical, realistic, careful	Cautious, friendly, thoughtful, gentle	Warm, reserved, polite, thoughtful	Curious, aloof, autonomous, innovative
Introversion (I)	ISTP	ISFP	INFP	INTP
Perception (P)	Logical, quiet, aloof, autonomous	Empathetic, thoughtful, humble, friendly	Reserved, quiet, sensitive, kind	Private, quiet, skeptical, curious, independent
Extroversion (E)	ESTP	ESFP	ENFP	ENTP
Perception (P)	Talkative, curious, impulsive	Warm, gregarious, talkative, impulsive	Talkative, outgoing, curious	Friendly, outgoing, humorous, flexible,
Extroversion (E)	ESTJ	ESFJ	ENFJ	ENTJ
Judgment (J)	Energetic, outspoken, friendly	Active, friendly, outgoing, talkative	Friendly, outgoing, enthusiastic	Friendly, outspoken, strong willed, logical

Based on information presented in Myers-Briggs Type Tables, Myers & Briggs Foundation. Available online at www.myersbriggs.org (accessed 4/19/2005); Hilliard D, Learning styles and personality types, Western Nevada Community College, 2001. Available online at www.wncc.edu/studentservices/counseling/styles_types/2_16_personality_types.html (accessed 4/20/2005).

information, reasoning out a decision, or predicting consequences of actions.[8] It is less automatic than the parent or child states.

Generally, it is ideal for both parties in an interaction to be communicating in the adult state. Sometimes, people have a preferred ego state or find that they react in particular ego states in certain kinds of situations. Also, communication between two people often involves unconscious and destructive ways of relating (games). Health care professionals often use the parent ego state, and as a result, patients often respond in the child state (free or adapted), or critical parent, resulting in problems in communication.

Example:

Pharmacist (parent ego): You must take these pills, or you'll have a heart attack.

Patient (adapted child ego): Yes, all right.

Or (free child ego): I don't want to take those horrible pills, and you can't make me.

Or (critical parent ego): You can't tell me what to do. Of course I'm not going to have a heart attack.

None of these are desired responses, since they either create friction or encourage dependence by the patient rather than self-responsibility. The desired transaction is "adult" to "adult."

Example:

Pharmacist (adult ego): It would be in your best interest if you followed the instructions carefully for this heart medication for the reasons I've explained.

Patient (adult ego): Yes, I understand that. I'll do my best to take them as you suggested.

This approach to understanding human interaction has been used in the health care field, particularly with respect to solving problems and in encouraging self-responsibility by the patient.[14]

Human Needs

All humans have the same basic needs, and these needs motivate a person's behavior.[8] These five basic needs as described by the psychologist Abraham Maslow include: (a) physiologic needs (to eat, sleep, breathe, avoid pain, and so forth); (b) safety needs (to be free from physical harm); (c) belonging needs (to be loved and to belong); (d) esteem needs (to feel good about oneself, independence, achievement); (e) self-actualization (to creatively fulfill your potential).[7] This is a hierarchy, so that physiologic needs must be met before an individual will be concerned with safety, and so forth. People strive to satisfy these needs, so that when a need is perceived (e.g., hunger), an individual's goal will be to satisfy that need.

During an interaction, each individual will be attempting to satisfy his or her needs. For example, a patient's attempt to satisfy physiologic needs might cause him or her to ask for analgesic prescription in a hurry to relieve the pain, while the pharmacist's need for esteem and self-actualization (fulfilling his or her potential as a health professional) will cause him or her to try to discuss the medication with the patient regardless of this pain. The result may be frustration for both parties, unless the pharmacist recognizes the patient's needs and attempts to find a way to satisfy both of their needs.

Individual Values

Individuals have preferences for certain activities, characteristics, or ways of being and for a particular way of life—these are their values.[8] For example, a pharmacist may have chosen to be a pharmacy owner because he or she likes to be independent, likes status in the community, wants to help others who are ill, and has a duty toward his or her parent to take over the business.

As with an individual's needs, the patient and pharmacist may have different values that affect interactions. For example, the pharmacist may value authority and want to dictate to the patient regarding adherence, but the patient may value independence and want to take the medication in his or her own way. The opposing values will lead to conflict in an interaction between the patient and pharmacist.

Although people's values do not change readily, pharmacists can at least become aware of their own values and how they may affect their interactions. Pharmacists should also be aware that others may have different values from theirs, and respect those values.[8] This awareness of values will serve to improve relationships in pharmacy.

Culture

Ethnicity and culture can also affect human interactions in relation to communication and counseling. Culture is defined as a "shared learned behavior, transmitted from one generation to another, to promote individual and social survival, adaptation, growth, and development."[15] Culture has both external (e.g., artifacts and roles) and internal (e.g., values, attitudes, beliefs, cognitive/affective/sensory styles, consciousness patterns, and epistemologies) representations.[15] Culture is elaborate and multidimensional, encompassing language, nonverbal behavior, and how you relate to others. It helps us determine our beliefs, values, and worldview.

Culture is learned through conscious or unconscious conditioning from various sources.[16] Each of us belongs to a culture identifying strongly with a particular group or combining practices from several groups, although individuals vary in the degree to which they adhere to a set of cultural patterns. Humans tend to be ethnocentric; we see other cultures from the perspective of our own culture. This can impede intercultural communication and sensitivity.

Cultural differences occur internationally (some countries have immigrants from many countries) and domestically (in the United States there are African-Americans, Native Americans, and so forth), and can have influence to varying degrees through successive generations. Depending on where a pharmacist practices, the patient population may comprise immigrants from many different cultures, second-generation immigrants, and possibly aboriginal people (e.g., in the United States, Canada, Australia, and New Zealand). Individual pharmacists themselves also belong to varied cultural groups. Added together, these result in a complex situation.

The effect of culture and racial differences on counseling and adherence is complex. Culturally based issues may affect treatment choice (from the patient's and health professional's clinical and personal perspectives), reaction to illness and treatment, and communication—all of which can affect adherence. As a result, providing pharmaceutical care may be affected at many points by culture and race. This will be discussed further in Chapter 8. Pharmacists need to become "culturally competent," acknowledging and respecting cultural diversity, in order to develop relationships with patients in which health and medication use can be discussed.[17]

Effect of Culture on Perceptions and Values

Our individual culture tends to affect how we perceive and make sense of the physical and social world. It affects how credibility is perceived. For example, Americans view expressing opinion openly and forcefully as admirable. They see people who are direct and confidant as credible, and place only moderate importance on social status. The Japanese admire quiet people who listen more than speak and view indirect, sympathetic, and humble people as more credible. They also place major emphasis on social status.[18]

Beliefs, attitudes, and values are also affected by cultural perception. Culture conditions us to hold certain beliefs to be true and worthy, and discourages us from questioning those beliefs.[18] Cultural values determine what is worth dying for and what is frightening. A number of theorists including Hofstede, Kluckhohn and Strodtheck, and Hall and others have suggested different sets of cultural values (Table 7-2).

The effect of differences in cultural values is seen in the ways that we perceive others, our attitudes toward them, and how we communicate.

TABLE 7-2	Dimensions of Cultural Values
Dimension	**Description of Cultural Values**
Individualism—collectivism	Independence and uniqueness of person in culture vs. greater emphasis and dependence on the group
Uncertainty–avoidance	Extent to which persons in a culture are made nervous by unstructured, unclear, or unpredictable situations
	High-avoidance cultures maintain strict codes of behavior and beliefs to avoid uncertainty
Power–distance	Distances among members of society with and without power
	Cultures with large power–distance believe people are not equal, everyone has rightful place, rigid value system
	Cultures with small power–distance minimize inequality and de-emphasize rank and status
Masculinity–femininity	Degree to which masculine and feminine traits are valued and revealed
	Masculine culture values ambition, acquisition of money; men taught to be domineering, ambitious, assertive
	Feminine culture values caring, nurturing; promotes sexual equality; people and environment are important; gender roles are more fluid
Confucian dynamism	Degree of adherence to Confucian values: Long-term orientation, perseverance, status, sense of shame, face-saving
Relationship with nature	May see people as subject to nature, in harmony with nature, or master of nature
Sense of time	Past, present, or future oriented
Value placed on activity	Value being (spontaneity) vs. becoming (spiritual life more than material) vs. doing (accomplishment judged by things you do)
High context–low context orientation	High context: More meaning in gestures, silence; awareness of surroundings, status, and friends
	Low context: Verbal message more important
Level of formality	Emphasis on formality vs. informality in way people address others, dress, conduct themselves
Level of assertiveness	Value assertive and aggressive style vs. harmony and accord

Based on information presented in Samovar L, Porter R. Cultural Diversity in Perception. In: Communication Between Cultures, 4th Edition. Wadsworth, Belmont CA, 2001. p. 52–80.

Cultural Differences in Communication

When dealing with patients from different cultures, pharmacists must contend with English as a second language and the cultural context of language, words, and nonverbal language.

Language, thought processes, and perceptions are intertwined with culture, affecting how people express themselves, how frequently they speak, the meaning of their words and expressions, and how they interpret others' words and behavior. Cultural variations in use of talk, silence, and body language can speak volumes.

Words can elicit many meanings.[19] Linguists estimate that 500 of the most-used words in the English language can produce over 14,000 meanings.[19] In conjunction with different cultural values, language can become even more confusing. For example, the words "pain," "freedom," "sexuality," "wealth," "leadership," and "security" have different meanings in different cultures.[19] In some cultures, there are many meanings for one word. For example, the Sami language in Sweden has 500 words to explain "snow." Some cultures use different words for the same thing. British say "lift" and Canadians say "elevator."

Further complexity is added when you consider how language reflects cultural values (Table 7-3). This can make translation into English difficult, resulting in inaccurate or misleading interpretation because all characteristics of the language cannot be translated.

Cultural differences are also seen in nonverbal communication demonstrated in body behavior, proxemics (space and distance), and use of silence.[20] This will be discussed further later in this chapter.

TABLE 7-3   Culturally Diverse Language Usage

Cultural Characteristic	Language Usage
Directness	Some cultures use more direct language, e.g., North Americans favor explicit, blunt language. Other cultures are less direct to preserve feelings, dignity, and save "face"; many Asian cultures reverse "yes" and "no"
Maintain or enhance social relationships	Expression of formality: Latin languages have formal and informal versions of verbs depending on person being addressed
	Communicate social status: Many languages have different vocabularies when speaking to superiors
Emotive expression	Ability to verbally express feelings: Some cultures avoid strong expression of feelings, restrain emotions vs. frequent expression of gratitude
Enjoyment of language	Some cultures have oral traditions, enjoy verbal play
	Patterns of language may be rich with intonation, repetition, exaggeration

Based on information presented in Samovar L, Porter R. Language and Culture. In: Communication Between Cultures, 4th Edition. Wadsworth, Belmont CA, 2001. p. 136–160.

Culture and Health Care

A patient's health beliefs may be the most important aspect of culture for pharmacists to recognize when it comes to patient counseling. Different cultures understand the cause, treatment, and prevention of illness differently, and this affects how they perceive their health problems and treatments. Culture teaches us what causes people to become sick or injured, what words to use to describe body parts and symptoms, how to behave when we are ill or injured, and what we need (or are allowed) to say or do to feel better.[15] Failure to recognize these health beliefs and match treatments accordingly can result in misdiagnosis, unnecessary procedures and treatments, and failure to treat.[21] The specifics of the effect of culture and health care will be discussed further in Chapter 8.

Complex Model of Pharmacist Interaction

The result of considering these various aspects of human interaction and communication is a complicated picture of pharmacist–patient interaction. In formulating and transmitting a message to the patient, the pharmacist must consider the values, needs, psychologic type, ego state, and culture of self and the patient, and must consider these factors when interpreting the feedback from the patient. In addition, the pharmacist should recognize that various environmental factors can affect the interaction, and can act as barriers to the transmission and feedback of the message. Barriers to patient counseling will be discussed in Chapter 9. Figure 7-1 illustrates this complex model of pharmacist interaction that results.

Pharmacists certainly aren't going to psychoanalyze everyone they deal with; however, they can use their understanding of the complexity of human interaction to realize that the patients they deal with may be very different from one another, and different from the pharmacists themselves. Pharmacists should therefore be prepared to modify and adjust their ways of interacting to suit each patient.

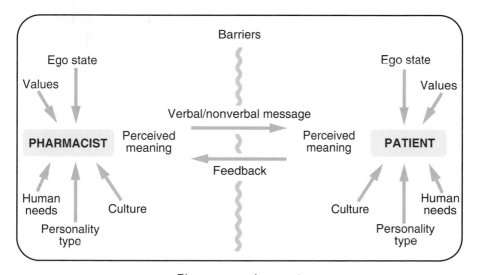

Figure 7-1 Complex Pharmacist Interaction Model

ESTABLISHING A HELPING AND TRUSTING THERAPEUTIC RELATIONSHIP

Since the advent of pharmaceutical care, a great deal of emphasis has been put on the relationship between patients and pharmacists, changing from provider of products to that of concerned partner in a quality, committed relationship with the patient.[5] This has been referred to as a "therapeutic alliance," a psychological term describing a collaborative state in which there is mutual respect, liking, trust, and commitment.[22] Components of a therapeutic alliance between a pharmacist and patient are the pharmacist's reliability as an information resource, trust in the pharmacist, and perception by the patient that the pharmacist cares about his or her medical concerns.[22]

Although patients are not always expecting pharmacists to do more than dispense, they apparently do want aspects of the therapeutic alliance described above. When patients were asked about their interactions with pharmacists in a 2003 study, they reported wanting to feel at ease in the pharmacy; to feel confident in the quality of counseling; to feel included and to understand the counseling; to have privacy respected; and to feel genuine concern from the pharmacy staff.[23] These describe a helping and trusting therapeutic relationship.

Developing a therapeutic relationship involves both skills and aspects of the context in which the encounter takes place.[4] These include building rapport with the patient, demonstrating empathy toward patients, attending to nonverbal communication, being assertive, providing privacy and confidentiality, and displaying clinical objectivity.[70]

To understand the value of establishing a helping and trusting therapeutic relationship, consider the patient–pharmacist interaction in Counseling Situation 7.1.

COUNSELING SITUATION 7.1: The Need to Establish a Helping and Trusting Relationship

Patty Lester is a 24-year-old woman. Her patient profile indicates that she has received several prescriptions over the past few months from the pharmacy where the pharmacist, Joe, is working today. Another pharmacist also practicing at the pharmacy apparently conducted a medication management consultation, and was on duty when Patty's previous prescriptions were filled. Although Joe had seen Patty in the pharmacy looking around in the nonprescription medication aisle just a few days ago, he did not take the opportunity to speak with her. Patty's medication record indicates that she had received cotrimoxazole tablets for a urinary tract infection a few months ago. Today she brings in a prescription for ciprofloxacin modified release tablets.

Pharmacist: OK Ms. Lester, your prescription is ready for you.

Patient: *(stooped shoulders, hanging head, flat voice)* Thanks.

Pharmacist: This is an antimicrobial tablet to treat your infection. Take one tablet every day for 7 days.

Patient: *(looking doubtful)* OK.

Pharmacist: *(noticing her doubt)* It's just the usual dose. Be sure to take it with plenty of water and finish them right up.

COUNSELING SITUATION **7.1:** (Continued)

Patient: *(nods her head)*

Pharmacist: *(handing her a patient information leaflet)* Here's some more information about them. *(points to various sections on the leaflet and reviews the information about adverse effects)* They might also make you more sensitive to the sun, so stay out of the sun or wear a sunscreen.

Patient: *(in a sad voice)* I don't think I'll be doing any sunning.

Pharmacist: Fine. OK, well here's your medication then. Do you have any questions?

Patient: No, I guess not.

Pharmacist: OK. Goodbye then.

The nonresponsiveness of this patient made it difficult for the pharmacist to deal with the situation properly. Although Joe gave Patty all the correct information, he did not gather sufficient information to identify real or potential medication-related problems. In addition, he did not attempt to explore her apparently sad mood or her doubtfulness. In fact, Patty wasn't feeling at all well and was feeling down because she thought the medication would interfere with her plans for a weekend away. She was intending to take the medication, as she had taken a previous cotrimoxazole prescription, one tablet twice daily because she wanted to get better fast. She also worried about having another urinary tract infection.

If the pharmacist had attempted to build rapport with the patient, he would have been better equipped to enter into discussion with the patient and recognize these issues.

Building Rapport

A helping and trusting relationship with a patient is an ongoing process that develops over time, but it must start somewhere. Pharmacists must begin to establish some degree of a relationship during the initial interaction, particularly during the opening phase, in order to proceed through an effective patient-counseling encounter. This involves the skill of building rapport.[24]

Building rapport involves a number of elements (Table 7-4). The friendly atmosphere of the patient–pharmacist interaction helps develop a helping, trusting relationship. The pharmacist should begin each patient-counseling encounter by a friendly, unhurried greeting, calling the patient by name, introducing himself or herself to the patient, and spending a few minutes in general conversation (e.g., discussing the weather, news, and family).[7] This initial "small talk," however, should be kept relatively brief since the patient will probably be anxious to discuss the matter at hand, as well as for reasons of practicality.[7]

It is also important for the pharmacist to be polite, in some cases asking permission to ask questions or apologizing for intervening (e.g., when a patient is self-selecting a nonprescription drug), since to some degree pharmacists do not have a clear mandate to gather personal information.[23] Patients have reported that a friendly and relaxed atmosphere that was not too clinical was preferred; however, they did not like it if it was too casual and off-hand. They preferred the pharmacist and staff to relate to them as equals, not aloof or snobby.[23]

TABLE 7-4	Techniques to Build Rapport
Greeting	Friendly and unhurried
Conversation	Brief general conversation to start
Personal attention	Introduce self and use patient's name
Explain purpose of counseling and questions	Reduces feeling of suspicion
Two-way interaction	Invite questions and respond to questions
Demonstrate genuine interest and concern	Spend time, explain, listen, display empathy, nonverbal language
Demonstrate trustworthiness	Credentials, communication skills, ability, pharmacy and pharmacist attributes

A friendly interaction may occur whenever the pharmacist comes in contact with a patient, even if the patient is just asking the location of a particular product in the pharmacy. The pharmacist who goes out of the way to talk with and become familiar with a patient (regardless of the topic) has started to develop a helping relationship. Future encounters with the patient for medication counseling will likely be more effective as a result of such seemingly unimportant interactions.

Building rapport also involves the actual content of the interaction. With a new patient, the time that the pharmacist devotes to the patient during the medication management consultation and the explanation that patient records are maintained for the patient's benefit will instill confidence in the service quality, and convey interest and concern. During prescription or nonprescription counseling, explaining the purpose of medications and providing information then inviting questions in a two-way interaction further develops a helping relationship by making the patient feel included and involved.[23] By explaining the purpose of the counseling and questioning, the patient will be less likely to feel under suspicion and more likely to interpret it as a show of concern by the pharmacist.[23]

The pharmacist's genuine interest in and concern for the patient will also be apparent if the pharmacist listens and responds empathetically to the patient's concerns ensuring that the patient's real needs are being met.[6]

The pharmacist's nonverbal language can further portray interest, concern, and empathy for the patient. Recognition of the patient's nonverbal messages can assist the pharmacist in identifying and addressing patients' concerns. Listening skills and nonverbal language will be discussed in the following sections.

Trust is an important element of building the therapeutic relationship.[25] Respondents in a 2002 study assessed pharmacist trustworthiness through evidence (credentials, white lab coat, professional dress, diploma on the wall); communication skills (gives attention, greets, involves in one-on-one); ability (documents and provides information, questions about medical history, answers questions, takes time); pharmacy appearance (organized, clean, reference library, plentiful supply, modern technology); attributes of the pharmacist (professional, informative, patient friendly, honest, caring confident, knowledgeable); and pharmacy attributes (well established, professional appearance, good reputation).[25] Patients used different qualities of the pharmacy and pharmacist to perceive trustworthiness in dispensing ability compared to providing pharmaceutical care.[25] When receiving pharmaceutical care, patients focused more on communication skills and information provided to assess trustworthiness rather than on the physical appearance of the pharmacy or pharmacist. They wanted the full attention of the pharmacist and two-way dialogue with full drug information.[25] Overall they wanted the pharmacist to be knowledgeable, honest, and caring.

Using these techniques, Counseling Situation 7.1 could be improved, as shown in Counseling Situation 7.2.

COUNSELING SITUATION 7.2: The Effect of Establishing a Helping and Trusting Relationship

Although the pharmacist had not counseled Patty for a prescription before, he had seen her in the pharmacy just a few days earlier. He took the opportunity to speak with her then by asking if she needed any help. This resulted in a consultation for a sunscreen product that Patty was purchasing. Today when she brings in a prescription for ciprofloxacin modified release 500 mg tablets, Joe can use her name and refer to the earlier encounter.

Pharmacist: OK Patty, your prescription is ready for you. Would you like to come into the booth over here where we can speak more privately about it?

Patient: *(stooped shoulders, hanging head, flat voice)* I guess so.

Pharmacist: I remember speaking with you a few days ago about a sunscreen for your holiday weekend coming up. That lake you were telling me about sounded like a great place. But you look a little down today.

Patient: *(sounding unhappy)* This bladder infection is making me feel so lousy.

Pharmacist: Yes, bladder infections can be pretty uncomfortable. It's a good thing you've got that holiday weekend coming up so you can have a good rest.

Patient: *(brightening a little)* I don't know if I'll be able to go the way I'm feeling. I hope these pills work fast.

Pharmacist: I can see you aren't feeling too good right now but this medication should start making you feel better within 2 to 3 days. I would like to spend a few minutes going over some information to make sure you get the most benefit from them. *(pause)*

Patient: Yes, alright.

Pharmacist: How did the doctor tell you to take them?

Patient: She didn't say much. I guess it's the same as last time, one tablet twice a day for a week.

Pharmacist: Well, actually, these are a little different from last time. You only need to take one tablet daily.

Patient: *(looking doubtful and thinks she might take them twice a day anyway so they'll work faster)* OK.

Pharmacist: *(noticing her doubt)* You look a little doubtful. These will work just as well, probably better than the other ones, but they are a slow release formulation so they last longer.

Patient: Oh really? I guess that will be easier to remember anyway. (*decides to take only once daily as directed*)

Pharmacist: (*hands her a patient-information leaflet*) Here's some more information about them. (*points to various sections on the leaflet and reviews the information about drinking fluids and avoiding antacids*) Do you think you'll be able to take these while you're away?

Patient: I think so. Since it's only once a day it will be easier.

Pharmacist: That's right, it will be. It's important to take them regularly and to finish them right up, to make sure the infection is completely gone.

Patient: I'll be sure to take them all. I don't want this to go on any longer than it has to.

Pharmacist: Good. Now I need to tell you more information. Occasionally, unwanted effects occur with this medication, although they're unlikely to happen to you, it's best if you are aware of what to notice. (*reviews those noted on the information sheet*) If you notice any of these symptoms, let me know right away.

Patient: OK.

Pharmacist: It also mentions here that this may make you more sensitive to the sun. Be sure to wear that sunscreen you bought the other day.

Patient: Yes, I always wear sunscreen.

tion for you. Did she arrange to see you again?

Patient: No, she just said to come back if the symptoms come back again.

Pharmacist: There are some things you can do to try to reduce the chance of getting this kind of infection.

Patient: Oh, really? I've been worrying about this a lot lately and about whether it could affect becoming pregnant later when I'm ready.

Pharmacist: (*proceeds to discuss the patient's concerns, providing information about bladder infections and ways to prevent infections, use of medications in pregnancy and encouraging her to discuss the details of her condition and her concerns further with her physician, then closes the discussion*) We've discussed quite a lot today. Have I made myself clear enough?

Patient: Yes, it's been great. And I have this pamphlet to read at home.

Pharmacist: Here's your prescription then. I hope you're feeling better soon. Give me a call before you go away to let me know how it's going. And feel free to call if you have any questions.

Patient: (*smiling*) OK, I'll do that. It sounds like I'll be feeling well enough to go after all. Thanks for everything. Goodbye.

In this scenario the pharmacist had laid the groundwork for medication counseling by interacting with the patient on a previous occasion. He tried to make her feel relaxed and comfortable in the counseling session by introducing himself and discussing her vacation. He explained the reason for the counseling and questions, making her feel included. The pharmacist observed the patient's nonverbal language, noticing that she was not her usual self. By demonstration of genuine interest and concern, Joe made Patty feel comfortable disclosing her concern about not being well enough to go away for the weekend and her intention to be nonadherent. By inviting questions from the patient, the pharmacist further made the patient feel included, opening up the discussion to more important concerns the patient had about her condition in relation to pregnancy. To further establish the relationship, the pharmacist arranged to follow-up with the patient later in the week.

Demonstrating Empathy Toward the Patient

Since the theories discussed above suggest that much of human interaction involves an individual's feelings and beliefs, pharmacists need to find ways to recognize these aspects of the patient and respond to them. This is the essence of demonstrating empathy.

Empathy is critical to the foundation of the patient–pharmacist relationship and for patient counseling. When the pharmacist demonstrates empathy toward the patient, the patient sees the pharmacist's interest and concern. This improves the patient's sense of worth and dignity, which may have been temporarily diminished as a result of illness. The patient feels encouraged to voice concerns and problems (or anticipated problems) regarding the illness or medication use. The pharmacist is then better able to assess accurately the patient's needs, concerns, motivations, and level of knowledge in order to provide the appropriate information and reassurance.[26] The result will be an effective patient consultation.

To appreciate empathy in a pharmacy situation, consider Counseling Situation 7.3.

COUNSELING SITUATION **7.3:** What is Empathy?

A pharmacist is working in a community pharmacy on a very busy afternoon. He is, as usual, trying to do several things at once, and the pharmacy technician is away for the afternoon. The pharmacist is preparing prescriptions for several waiting patients, but is continually interrupted by telephone calls. He has just taken a prescription over the phone from a dentist, Dr. Jordan. As he puts down the phone, a patient starts banging on the counter and yelling, in a loud and angry voice, "Can't someone help me here? I'm in a hurry and I have to pick up the prescription that Dr. Jordan phoned in for me."

The pharmacist turns quickly toward the patient with a surprised expression, and accidentally knocks over a bottle of antibiotic liquid. He cries out, "Oh no!" and leans on the counter with his hands over his face, shaking his head.

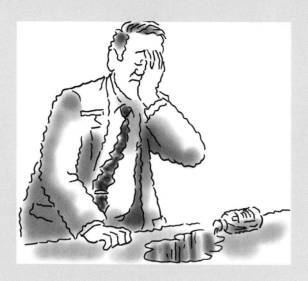

What does the pharmacist's nonverbal language convey?

If you can imagine what the pharmacist is feeling at that moment—his emotions, his concerns, his frustrations—then you are feeling empathy. Empathy involves understanding the world as another person sees it, attempting to "get into his shoes."[11] It is the ability to understand not only the other person's words, but also what those words mean in terms of his feelings.[26] Demonstrating empathy involves communicating this understanding. In order to do this, you must first be able to identify the person's feelings and meanings, then communicate this understanding by responding empathetically.

Identifying Feelings and Meanings

In Counseling Situation 7.3, it may have been easy for the reader to empathize with the pharmacist, because most people have experienced spilling something before. Empathizing with the patient may be more difficult for the reader and for the pharmacist in the scenario. Close observation of the patient, the expression on his face, and other manifestations of nonverbal language may help tell the pharmacist more about the patient's emotion.

Another clue to identifying feelings is to imagine the range of emotions the patient might be experiencing and to try to isolate the one that predominates. The patient who says he is "in a hurry" may be feeling worried, frustrated, or in pain.

The pharmacist must also interpret the patient's words to identify their true meaning.[27] Is the patient saying that he is in a hurry because he is in pain, because he feels he is wasting his time treating an unimportant condition, or simply because he has an appointment to go to? One way to help identify the patient's feelings is for the pharmacist to ask himself, "What one word describes the patient's feeling when he made that statement?"[28] In the scenario, the word may be "anger" or "frustration." That one word or a variation of it can be used in an empathetic response to the patient.

Responding Empathetically

The pharmacist must communicate to the patient, in a nonjudgmental way, that he understands and accepts the patient's feelings and concerns, even if those feelings make the pharmacist feel uncomfortable.[26] The pharmacist must verbally encourage the patient to express concerns and feelings, while conveying an attitude of concern and acceptance.[26,27] This recognition and acceptance helps the patient become less anxious and more open to discussion of his or her problems.[27]

Pharmacists often have difficulty formulating an empathetic response. Sometimes we say, "Yes, I understand how you must feel," and then receive the angry and frustrated retort, "No, you don't! How could you possibly understand?"

In a more complete response, active listening, the pharmacist would reflect the patient's feeling, and then paraphrase the patient's comments to include a possible reason for the feelings. For example, "You sound pretty angry about having to wait here so long."

The pharmacist may not be sure about the accuracy of his interpretations, and should ask the patient for clarification: "Is it because you're in so much pain?"

If the pharmacist happens to misinterpret the patient's feelings or meaning, the patient can correct him, but he will nonetheless have received the message that the pharmacist is interested and concerned.[28] The patient may reply, "I'm in pain, and the dentist didn't even help. He says he can't do anything today until I get rid of the infection."

Empathetic responding may be used alone or in combination in a discussion with a patient, until the patient's emotional state has been resolved.[29]

A formula for an active listening response includes a "feeling reflection" and a "content reflection" as follows:

"You feel_____because_____."[6]

It also helps to vary the introductory phrase such as:[28]

"You think . . ."

"It seems to you . . ."

"As I understand it, you seem to be saying . . ."

"You believe . . ."

"In other words . . ."

"I gather that . . ."

As an illustration of the value of demonstrating empathy in counseling, consider Counseling Situation 7.4.

COUNSELING SITUATION 7.4: The Need for Empathy

Mrs. Miller has adult-onset diabetes, which had been controlled through diet alone until recently. She has undergone testing and has just come from her physician with a new prescription for glyburide 5 mg, one tablet daily. She is a regular customer at this pharmacy and the pharmacist, Alison, knows her fairly well. When the prescription is prepared she calls Mrs. Miller into the counseling booth.

Pharmacist: Hello, Mrs. Miller. How are you today?

Patient: *(in a subdued voice)* Oh, I'm OK, I guess.

Pharmacist: I'll just spend a few minutes discussing your prescription with you to make sure you get the most benefit from it.

Patient: *(looking distracted)* OK.

Pharmacist: This medication is glyburide. What did the doctor tell you about it?

Patient: *(sounding worried)* She told me that the diet I was on for my sugar isn't working, and so I have to take pills now. She says I'm a diabetic, and I know that's really bad. My friend has a son who had all kinds of problems with it.

Pharmacist: Don't worry, Mrs. Miller. Lots of people have diabetes at your age. It's nothing to worry about. As long as you take your pills regularly, you'll be just fine. You must take one tablet every day. You should be testing your blood sugar regularly to check that the pills are working. Here's an information sheet listing the signs of low blood sugar *(refers to a written list)* and here's a list of side effects. *(again refers to written information)*

Patient: *(cutting in, visibly distressed)* All this and side effects too?

Pharmacist: Yes, but don't worry. They don't happen very often. By the way, you shouldn't drink alcohol because it may make you sick. Do you see any difficulties with following these instructions?

Patient: *(stunned into silence, simply shakes her head)*

Pharmacist: Good. Do you have any questions?

Patient: *(in a shaky voice)* No, I guess not.

Pharmacist: Fine, then give us a call when you need a refill. The doctor has authorized six refills for your prescription.

Patient: *(walks away thinking to herself)* I have to go through this six more times? I would rather take nothing and take my chances with the diabetes!

This pharmacist certainly covered all the necessary information, but the effort was probably counterproductive. Rather than helping the patient get the most benefit from her medication, the pharmacist may have increased the patient's concerns about her condition and medication use, and may actually have discouraged her from taking the medication. If she had considered how the patient was likely to be feeling about a serious and chronic condition like diabetes and about potential problems with medication use, and if she had taken notice of her nonverbal behavior, she may have been more effective in counseling. This is demonstrated in Counseling Situation 7.5.

COUNSELING SITUATION 7.5: Demonstrating Empathy

Pharmacist: Hello, Mrs. Miller. How are you today?

Patient: *(in a subdued voice)* Oh, I'm OK, I guess.

Pharmacist: *(noticing the patient is subdued and distracted)* You sound a little down today.

Patient: *(sounding worried)* Well yes, I guess I am. The doctor told me the diet I was on for my sugar wasn't working, and so I have to take pills now.

Pharmacist: *(empathetic tone)* It sounds like you're worried because you're unsure about the need for switching to the pills.

Patient: Yes, I guess it means I'm really a diabetic now, and I know that's really bad. I had a friend whose son had all kinds of problems with it.

Pharmacist: I can see why that would be a worry for you, thinking you might end up with complications like your friend's son. Perhaps it would help if I explained a little about diabetes. *(proceeds to explain about adult-onset diabetes, the potential complications, and the need to keep tight control of blood sugar levels)*

Patient: I see. The doctor did say something about adult diabetes, but I didn't understand. I guess my diabetes must be getting worse if I need this pill now.

Pharmacist: I realize it must seem that way, with the doctor adding the prescription to your diet. Actually, this is a better way of getting control of your blood sugar than diet alone. I'd like to spend a few minutes now to discuss your prescription to make sure you get the most benefit from it.

Patient: *(sounding interested)* OK. That might help.

Pharmacist: This medication is called glyburide. What did the doctor tell you about it?

Patient: That I should take one every day, and be careful to notice if my blood sugar gets too low. First, I have to worry about it being too high, and now I have to worry about it being too low. How am I supposed to know?

Pharmacist: I realize it sounds like a lot to keep track of. Here's an information sheet that has it all written down. You can read it over at home, then keep it for reference if you forget.

Patient: OK, I'll do that.

Pharmacist: There's some other important things you should know about. Along with the effects on your sugar, glyburide may cause some unwanted effects. These are quite rare, but I want you to be able to recognize them so you can call me right away if you notice anything like this. This information sheet lists the things to look out for. *(points to section of information sheet)*

Patient: OK. As long as I know what to look for, I won't worry so much.

Pharmacist: That's good. Now, did the doctor mention anything about testing your blood regularly for sugar?

Patient: Yes, and she told me to buy a machine to test it.

COUNSELING SITUATION **7.5:** (Continued)

Pharmacist: Good, because it's an important part of keeping your condition under control. Let's arrange a time when we can sit down and go over the glucose meter *(proceeds to set up an appointment)* I've covered a lot of information fairly quickly. Do you have any questions?

Patient: No, not right now. I'll read this information when I get home.

Pharmacist: Good. I'll be seeing you in a few days to discuss the glucose meter, and we can discuss this information some more then. You have a refill on this prescription to continue on, so I'll be seeing you again in 30 days. We can discuss this further then.

Patient: Thanks so much. *(thinks to herself)* I guess things aren't quite as bad as I thought, after all. I just have to take these pills regularly and test my blood.

This time, the pharmacist identified the patient's feelings, understanding that diabetes can be very worrisome to patients. Although there was a lot of information to provide about the medication, the pharmacist acknowledged the patient's feelings and concerns before proceeding. The pharmacist realized that the patient would not be very receptive to too much information in her worried state of mind, and arranged for a separate appointment and follow-up counseling.

This identification and response to the patient's feelings was the demonstration of empathy by the pharmacist. By observing the patient's nonverbal language, by listening to the patient, and by identifying her feelings and the meanings of her words, the pharmacist was able to encourage her to discuss her concerns. This in turn gave the pharmacist the opportunity to identify problems and to overcome them. Arranging for follow-up counseling further showed the patient that the pharmacist was genuinely concerned for her welfare. This would encourage further discussion by the patient in future counseling sessions.

Attending to Nonverbal Communication

Nonverbal communication involves all aspects of communication other than spoken or written words, including facial expressions, eye contact, body position, touching, and voice characteristics.[6,10,30,31] Nonverbal communication is actually believed over verbal communication and is hard to control because it is subconscious and automatic, making it difficult for a new English speaker to adjust.[20,31] It has been suggested that the impact of any message comprises 7% verbal, 38% vocal, and 55% facial communication.[32]

Body behavior provides a nonverbal message, including general appearance, attire, body movement, facial expression, eye contact, touch, and paralanguage.[20] Body movements (kinesics), such as posture and how one seats oneself, may illustrate respect and manners while facial expressions convey emotions such as happiness, sadness, fear, anger, disgust, and surprise.[20] Eye contact is used to engage people and show interest, and the gesture of touch sends messages about what you are thinking and feeling.[20] Paralanguage, which includes volume of voice and noises, communicates emotion but can also be used to show assertiveness and can help create a feeling of privacy, although a furtive tone can create embarrassment.[23]

Proxemics refers to the positioning of individuals' bodies while communicating. Different distances covey different levels of intimacy. In North America, 1.5 ft distance is considered intimate; 1.5 to 4 ft is personal (conversation with friends and acquaintances); 4 to 12 ft is social distance for more formal and impersonal interaction; and 12 ft and more is for public communication such as lectures.[33]

The use of silence also has communication implications. Silence may have meaning and some people may feel more or less comfortable in silence. Although pharmacists may try to engage a patient in discussion during the consultation, they may not be comfortable with this, preferring to remain silent.

Pharmacist Nonverbal Language

In Counseling Situation 7.3, the pharmacist had a surprised look on his face when he heard the patient banging on the counter. Then the pharmacist knocked over the antibiotic and leaned on the counter shaking his head. This nonverbal language conveys meaning about the pharmacist and will affect the patient's perception.

Pharmacists' nonverbal language can indicate to patients whether or not they are willing to provide information and help. To truly demonstrate concern and willingness to help, the pharmacist must display a variety of nonverbal cues, including facial expressions, eye contact, body movements and position, voice characteristics, and appearance.[6,10,23,31,32] Since nonverbal messages are generally trusted more than verbal, a pharmacist may verbally express willingness to help the patient while the patient may perceive a nonverbal message of lack of interest. If the pharmacist is rushed, abrupt, condescending, rude, or bored looking, patients do not feel genuine concern.

Of note, patients have said that when pharmacists are focused on the computer, involved in the sales transaction before counseling, give only written information, or sell more than advised, then they doubt the sincerity and caring of the pharmacist.[23]

Appropriate pharmacist nonverbal behavior for effective patient counseling is illustrated in Table 7-5. However, nonverbal behaviors will not be convincing if they are part of an act. Only a genuine feeling of interest and concern for the patient will translate into an effective nonverbal message.

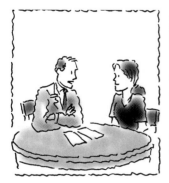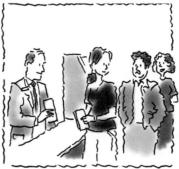

Both patient and pharmacist communicate through nonverbal language.

TABLE 7-5	Pharmacist Nonverbal Behavior for Effective Patient Counseling
Smiling and friendly facial expression	Pharmacist should try to think "pleasant" thoughts before greeting patients because facial expressions reveal feelings
Varied eye contact	Direct contact 50% to 75% of the time to create trust without the discomfort of continual eye contact
Open and warm body gestures	Raised shoulders and erect head to imply pride and self-esteem, leaning forward to suggest warmth and trust, touching where appropriate to express deep feelings
Appropriate distance	1.5 to 4 ft for personal discussion, 4 to 12 ft for impersonal business, avoiding violation of patient's personal space
Level position free of barriers	Sit or stand beside patient with head at same level, avoiding barriers such as desk or counter
Moderate and varied voice	Rate, pitch, volume appropriate to words and varied to keep interest; indicating "permission" for patient to speak through higher or lower pitch at end of a comment or by silence
Professional appearance	Pharmacist and pharmacy should be neat and clean, pharmacy layout should allow access to pharmacist and privacy

Based on information presented in Gerrard BA, Boniface W, Love B. Developing Facilitation Skills. In: Interpersonal Skills for Health Professionals. Reston Publishing, Reston, VA, 1980. Samuelson K. Nonverbal messages can speak louder than words. Health Care. 1986;Apr:12–13; Knapp M. Nonverbal Communication: Basic Perspectives, The Effects of Territory and Personal Space. Chapters 1 and 4. In: Essentials of Nonverbal Communication. 2nd ed. Holt, Rinehart & Winston, New York, 1980.

Patient Nonverbal Language

In the situation described in Counseling Situation 7.3, a patient starts banging on the counter and yelling, in a loud and angry voice. In addition to attending to his own nonverbal behavior, the pharmacist in this scenario also needed to observe the patient's.[7] This would assist the pharmacist in identifying the patient's feelings as well as improve patient satisfaction. Studies have found that patients tend to be more satisfied with health care providers who are skilled at translating nonverbal language to emotional states.[34]

In addition, observation of the patient's nonverbal communication may indicate special needs. For example, a patient with a hearing difficulty may turn his or her head to bring the ear closer, stand closer than normal, or put his or her hand to the ear. Eyeglasses and hearing aids are also nonverbal indicators that a patient may have special communication needs.

When dealing with patients from different cultures, pharmacists may find nonverbal language of patients helpful since much of what is lost in translation is still communicated nonverbally. However, this can be misinterpreted since there are cultural differences in nonverbal communication seen in body behavior and movement, paralanguage, touch, eye contact, proxemics (space and distance), and use of silence.[20] A summary of these aspects of nonverbal communication and the effect of culture is found in Table 7-6.

TABLE 7-6 Patient Nonverbal Behavior	
Body behavior	General appearance may send a message about the value of modesty (use of head and body covering for men or women); religious values (use of turban, yarmulke); and traditional values (wearing traditional costume)
	Different cultures regard different body types as attractive so that being thin or heavy may have different meaning or importance
Body movements (kinesics)	May illustrate respect and manners
	Pointing and beckoning have different meanings, some rude or vulgar
	Different cultures beckon using fingers, hand gestures, or head movements
Facial expressions	Happiness, sadness, fear, anger, disgust, and surprise are universal, but culture will dictate when, how, and to whom they are displayed
	Generally, Mediterranean cultures show exaggerated signs of grief or sadness
	North American white men tend to suppress showing emotions as the Chinese do, in order to save face
	Japanese hide expressions of anger, sorrow, and disgust by laughing or smiling
Eye contact	Highly valued in Western society but is considered an insult in Asian cultures
	Latin American, Caribbean, and African cultures tend to avoid eye contact as a sign of respect[12]
Touch	Kissing, hugging, and shaking hands are used more or less in different cultures and may be misconstrued to have a sexual meaning
	Cultures with more emotional restraint are less likely to touch (English, German) while others encourage signs of emotion and touch (Latin American, Middle Eastern, southern European)
Paralanguage	A loud voice communicates strength and sincerity for Arabs, strong belief for Israelis, authority for Germans, impoliteness for Thais, and lack of self-control for the Japanese
Proxemics	Cultures that stress individualism demand more personal space than collective cultures which may view the violation of personal space as aggressive
	Africans, Arabs, and Mexicans tend to stand much closer when speaking than Western and European cultures
	Asians use extended space to denote deference and esteem
Use of silence	Some cultures, such as Eastern, Indian, and Native American, believe silence has meaning and feel less uncomfortable in silence
	North Americans, Arabs, and Europeans consider talking an important activity and often avoid silence

Based on information presented in Samovar L, Porter R. Nonverbal Communication. In: Communication Between Cultures, 4th Edition. Wadsworth, Belmont CA, 2001. p. 164–195.

Being Assertive

Another important skill involved in establishing a helping and trusting therapeutic relationship in pharmacy practice is the pharmacist's assertiveness. Some pharmacists find it difficult to participate in patient counseling, feeling awkward initiating involvement with their patients. Although they will answer patients' questions, they are reluctant to take the first step in communicating. Such pharmacists tend to take comfort in the physical barrier of the pharmacy counter and often allow auxiliary staff to deal with patients. This essentially describes the passive pharmacist.

Conversely, pharmacists who are anxious to get involved in patient counseling sometimes become too aggressive. They insist on counseling each patient regardless of the situation, and tend to force their beliefs and values about medication use and illness on the patient. This kind of behavior inhibits the pharmacist's effectiveness in counseling. As illustration of this, a study of pharmacists during nonprescription counseling observed that pharmacists who were extroverted and aggressive were less likely to persuade the patient to use the product they recommended.[12]

Patient Counseling Situation 7.6 demonstrates the need for assertiveness.

COUNSELING SITUATION 7.6: Lack of Assertiveness

Bill Gregson is a middle-aged man who is a regular patient at this pharmacy. He has been getting a regular prescription for hydrochlorothiazide 50 mg daily. Today he is receiving a new prescription for atenolol 50 mg daily.

Pharmacist: Hi, Bill! Your prescription is ready. How are you today?

Patient: *(clipped tone)* Fine. How much is it?

Pharmacist: *(ignoring his hurried tone)* I'll just spend a few minutes to go over it with you.

Patient: *(looking irritated)* I'm in a real hurry.

Pharmacist: It'll just take a few minutes. This is a medication for high blood pressure, atenolol . . .

Patient: *(cuts in, sounding more annoyed now)* Look, the doctor told me all this, and I really have to go. How much is it?

Pharmacist: *(persisting in an authoritative tone)* Did he tell you about precautions?

Patient: *(sounding frustrated and angry)* No, but I really must go. I've got a job interview across town in 15 minutes. I have to leave right now. Just take my money or give me my prescription back and I'll go elsewhere!

Pharmacist: *(feeling frustrated)* OK. The cashier will take care of you now. Goodbye.

The pharmacist in this situation began by being aggressive with patient counseling, and thereby aggravated the patient; then the pharmacist became passive, giving up on any attempt to provide important information. The pharmacist was right to attempt to counsel the patient, since it is his responsibility to provide pharmaceutical care. However, an aggressive approach to patient counseling is unlikely to be successful, because counseling requires the patient's cooperation and consent to enter into a two-way discussion. Even if he had managed to give all the necessary information, the patient would not have benefited, since proper discussion to identify and resolve medication-related problems would have been inhibited by the patient's preoccupation, as well as his increasing feelings of frustration and anger.

The passive approach to patient counseling, which the pharmacist finally opted for, was equally ineffective. The patient left without important information and the pharmacist was unable to attempt to discuss real or potential problems with the patient.

The most effective way for the pharmacist to become involved with patients falls somewhere between these two extremes of passivity and aggression: Assertiveness.

Assertiveness "involves standing up for legitimate rights without violating the rights of others or having bad feelings in the process."[35] This allows the pharmacist to express his or her ideas and advice about medication use to patients and other health professionals without infringing on their rights to believe and do what they wish. The result of such an approach is a win-win situation, in which the pharmacist and the other person feel respected and a trusting and mutually respectful relationship can develop.

Although the win-win situation resulting from assertiveness is desirable for all, many pharmacists find it difficult to behave assertively.[35] One reason a pharmacist may avoid patient counseling is fear of the patient's rejection of his or her assistance or the patient's anger at being given advice. The assertive pharmacist realizes that although some patients may be unprepared for, or in some way angered by, receiving assistance, he or she can overcome the problem by approaching these patients with empathy and concern, and by explaining the purpose of counseling.

Another concern of the passive pharmacist is that it is a sign of respect to avoid interfering in the patient's affairs. The aggressive pharmacist, on the other hand, believes he or she is doing patients a favor by "telling" them what to do and feels that everything about a patient is his or her business. The assertive pharmacist, however, recognizes that although it is a must to consider the patient's point of view and be sensitive to the patient's need for privacy, he or she has a responsibility to "help" the patient get the most benefit from the medication.

Pharmacists may also lack assertiveness as a result of fear of imperfection in themselves.[35] Perfectionist standards can cause them to avoid patient counseling—because it can't always be carried out perfectly. But assertive pharmacists realize that they have a responsibility to help patients, even though they may not always be able to do it exactly as they would wish.

Nonassertive individuals often continue to be passive or aggressive in the belief that their behavior is rooted in an inherent trait. However, individuals can learn to be less passive or less aggressive in their dealings with others through assertiveness training. Assertive behavior will not only improve pharmacists' interactions with patients, but also with employees or employers, co-workers, and other health professionals.

Assertiveness Techniques

The essence of assertive communication is to solve problems in a way that allows both parties to "win." Its aim is not to manipulate people or situations, but to encourage the honest and direct expression of what each party feels and wants. This involves a number of techniques.[35]

1. *Confrontation:* This skill involves letting another person know that he or she is being aggressive, that it is hurting you, and that you will not tolerate it. This can

involve simply stating how you feel about another's behavior and the results of that behavior. For example: "When you arrive late for your shift, I feel angry because then I'm late picking up my son."

This can be expanded by a specific request of what you want to happen to resolve the situation: "I'd appreciate it if in future you could call if you can't make it on time. This would allow me to make other arrangements."

This can be softened by the use of an empathetic statement to start, for example, "I realize that you find it difficult to get here on time."

2. *Saying No*: When another person's request is unreasonable or not possible, the assertive response is to politely refuse. This can be softened by offering an alternative solution. For example, a patient demanding a prescription might be told, "Your doctor is not available to authorize the repeat right now. If your pain is severe, perhaps you could get some treatment in the hospital emergency department."

3. *Making Requests*: When things aren't to your liking, rather than suffering silently, or blowing up and making demands, you are more likely to create a win-win situation if you simply ask someone for what you want.

4. *Expressing Opinions*: Sharing your beliefs and ideas with others can prevent missing out on being involved in a decision or activity. It does not mean that your opinion is forced on others. Opinions should not be forced on others and should preferably include the mention of alternative views.

5. *Initiating Conversations*: Conversation can be initiated with a warm and tactful introduction rather than an abrupt beginning, for example, "Hi, I'm the pharmacist, Susan. I see you're looking at the cough medicines. Can I help you select one?"

6. *Self-disclosing*: Although pharmacists expect their patients to give them personal information, they often neglect to act similarly. Building a relationship with a patient can be enhanced by disclosing personal feelings where appropriate (e.g., "I'm sorry your prescription isn't ready; I'm a little slower today because I'm feeling a little under the weather"). This is not to say that excuses should be made regularly, but pharmacists can let patients know that they are people too.

If the pharmacist in Counseling Situation 7.6 discussed earlier had used these assertiveness techniques, he might have been more effective in counseling, as shown in Counseling Situation 7.7.

COUNSELING SITUATION 7.7: Using Assertiveness

Pharmacist: Hi, Bill! Your prescription is ready. How are you today?

Patient: *(clipped tone)* Fine. How much is it?

Pharmacist: *(recognizing hurried tone)* It's $39.98. The cashier will look after that for you. It sounds like you're in a real hurry.

Patient: *(looking agitated)* Yes, I am.

Pharmacist: *(empathetic tone)* I realize you probably have something important to rush off to, but perhaps you could spare just a few minutes. I need to discuss your prescription with you, to make sure you get the most benefit from it.

COUNSELING SITUATION 7.7: Using Assertiveness

Patient: *(sounding calmer, but still hurried)* There's no need. The doctor discussed all that. I've got to get going because I have a job interview across town in 15 minutes.

Pharmacist: *(persisting in an assertive tone)* I understand why you wouldn't want to be late for that. What I have to discuss with you is important too, but some of it can wait until later, perhaps this evening. I'll just give you some printed information for you to read before you take the medication. *(hands over a printed information sheet, pointing to a particular section)* You'll notice that it explains that this medication may cause some dizziness at the beginning due to lowering of your blood pressure. You should probably take it easy for the first few days until your body gets used to it.

Patient: *(sounding interested)* Oh, I didn't realize that. Perhaps I should cancel my tennis game for tomorrow.

Pharmacist: That might not be necessary as long as you are aware. I don't want to hold you up any further, but there's more we need to discuss about your blood pressure and your hydrochlorothiazide together with the new drug atenolol. How about if I call you this evening to go over the information with you?

Patient: Oh, am I supposed to keep taking the hydrochlorothiazide too? I guess we should talk. I would like to understand more about blood pressure and why it seems to be getting worse. Could you call around seven?

Pharmacist: Fine, I'll do that and good luck with the job interview.

Patient: *(rushing off)* Thanks. I'll talk to you tonight.

This pharmacist acknowledged the patient's questions about the price right away, allowing the patient to focus his attention on the medication for a minute rather than on paying for the medication. When he responded empathetically to the patient's hurried tone, the patient was encouraged to explain why he was in such a hurry, allowing the pharmacist to recognize immediately that his need to get to the job interview would have to take precedence over counseling. He used the technique of confrontation to explain what he wanted to happen, and he stressed the importance of counseling as a benefit to the patient, not as something that he needed to do for himself. The pharmacist compromised by providing written information and made a specific request of the patient to arrange to continue counseling by telephone later. Although this took about the same amount of time as the previous situation, it resulted in a win-win situation, and both the patient's and the pharmacist's needs were met.

Providing Privacy and Confidentiality

Privacy is an important aspect of human relations in pharmacy. In many jurisdictions, regulations have been put into place to protect the privacy and confidentiality of patients and their personal information in health care, particularly since the advent of electronic communication methods and records.[36] Patients do not feel comfortable discussing personal topics such as their illnesses in places that they feel others can observe or overhear.[7]

Lack of privacy discourages patients from introducing or elaborating on problems and may distract them from listening to advice.[23] Although complete privacy is not always physically possible, psychological privacy is necessary in which patients can feel that they have the full attention of the pharmacist, and that other patients or pharmacy staff will not be listening.[7] Ways to achieve this will be discussed in Chapter 9.

Patients must also be assured of confidentiality in order to feel comfortable giving the pharmacist information. Assurance of confidentiality should be part of the introduction to information gathering by the pharmacist, and should be stated on any forms used. Pharmacy staff should also be made aware of this issue, and policies and procedures initiated to ensure compliance.

Clinical Objectivity

When attempting to identify the patient's feelings and the meaning of the patient's words, the pharmacist's own biases and distortions may hinder accurate perception.[26] Personal concerns may cause a pharmacist to be less than fully aware of the patient's feelings. The pharmacist may have certain predetermined ideas about the way a patient should feel in a certain situation.

The situation may arouse the pharmacist's own emotions or cause prejudices toward certain characteristics in the patient to surface, interfering with the ability to identify the patient's feelings accurately, e.g., emergency contraception may conflict with a pharmacist's religious or ethical beliefs.

If the pharmacist is aware that such biases may be present, he or she can attempt to compensate for them by making a conscious effort to remain nonjudgmental and impartial.[26]

This is not to say that the pharmacist should be cold and unfeeling.[7] As mentioned above, it is sometimes appropriate and desirable for the pharmacist to disclose his or her feelings to the patient. However, the pharmacist's feelings should not encroach on the patient's ability to express feelings and needs, or on the pharmacist's ability to focus on the patient or provide patient care.[7] If there is a strong conflict such as may occur in relation to the provision of emergency contraception, it may be appropriate to refer the patient to another pharmacist in order to ensure that the patient receives necessary care.

COUNSELING SKILLS

A number of skills have been identified as important in conducting a patient-counseling session. They are sometimes referred to as interviewing skills.

As discussed in Chapter 5, the counseling encounter starts with an opening phase, during which it is important for the pharmacist to set a climate for communication with the patient. This is accomplished through the skills involved in developing a therapeutic relationship discussed above, particularly establishing rapport with the patient and demonstrating empathy.

The second phase of the counseling encounter involves gathering information and identifying problems. Here, the pharmacist needs counseling skills such as listening and probing to fully understand the patient's problems and needs. Other interviewing skills such as paraphrasing, summarizing, transition, and repeating help to keep the discussion flowing smoothly, and encourage the patient to become involved.

In the next phase of the counseling encounter, the pharmacist must resolve problems and provide information or educate the patient. Motivational interviewing, used in situations where behavior change is required, is an approach to interviewing that combines skills in a directed way to motivate patients to change.[37] Skills in risk communication can help the pharmacist provide information in a way that deals with uncertainty while providing reassurance so that the patient is not frightened but is aware of risks.[38]

In the final phase of counseling, it is helpful to use the teach-back technique, in order to ensure that the patient fully understood information and instructions.[39]

Listening Skills

The need to listen to a patient would seem to be an obvious element of developing a therapeutic relationship and communicating. But pharmacists, in their attempt to cover all the necessary information about medication use, often forget to focus their attention fully on the patient and listen to what he or she has to say, and the meaning behind the words. Listening skills fall into four categories: Passive listening, acknowledgment responses, encouragement, and active listening.[6]

Passive Listening

Passive listening simply involves allowing the patient to express himself or herself without interference.[6] Pharmacists are often too quick to jump into conversation, denying the patient the opportunity to speak or to finish speaking.

Before telling a patient the purpose of his or her medication, for example, the pharmacist should allow the patient a chance to tell what he or she already knows. This will make counseling more efficient, since the pharmacist may not need to provide any further information; it gives the patient the feeling of being in charge of the situation (an important element in adherence); it allows the pharmacist to detect any misunderstandings; and it may indicate to the pharmacist the kind of language the patient feels comfortable using to describe his or her medication and condition.

As discussed earlier, an important part of empathic responding involves identifying the patient's feelings. While listening passively, the pharmacist can observe the patient's nonverbal language and "read between the lines" to detect the feelings and meanings behind the patient's words.

Acknowledgment Responses

When listening passively, the pharmacist should respond at intervals to let the patient know that he or she is indeed listening. This may involve simply nodding or uttering expressions such as "Uh-huh."[6]

Encouragement

The pharmacist can also use some words or phrases to encourage the patient to say more about a particular topic.[6] Encouraging phrases may be: "Oh yes." "I see." "Go on." "Tell me more."

Active Listening

Active listening, as the term implies, involves more active participation by the pharmacist. The pharmacist not only makes comments that let the patient know that he or she is listening and understanding, but also takes the opportunity to clarify the patient's feelings and concerns, for self and for the patient. This is an essential component of empathetic responding.

Active listening responses often begin with phrases such as: "You seem to feel . . . ;" "It sounds like you . . . ;" "I get the sense that you . . . ;" "In other words . . . ;" "As I understand it, you seem to be saying . . . ."[28] Such responses must be made in the appropriate tone of concern or interest; if the pharmacist does not genuinely care about the patient's feelings, this will not sound genuine, and the patient will feel patronized.[6,26]

Active listening should generally be preceded and followed by passive listening, allowing the patient to confirm the feelings that have been identified, and discuss concerns at greater length.

Nonlistening Responses

Pharmacists' abilities to listen to their patients are often limited because of behaviors that are counterproductive to listening.[6,7,28] Pharmacists often respond to patients' comments with excessive verbalization, tending to lecture patients rather than engaging them in a discussion, cutting off the patients' expressions of feelings. Pharmacists interrupt patients and monopolize the conversation either because they are in a hurry or because some statement by the patient has caused them to react and interject their own comments. Sometimes, pharmacists simply believe that this behavior constitutes patient counseling and do not realize that the patient may have something to contribute.

Although part of the counseling process involves asking questions, it is inappropriate to ask questions prematurely, before the patient has had an opportunity to express his or her feelings. This tends to remove the focus from the patient and may cause him or her to become defensive. Appropriate questioning should be interspersed with discussion from the patient. This will be discussed in the following section.

Pharmacists sometimes inappropriately evaluate the patient, passing judgment on the situation and the individual involved. This does not help patients; it serves only to discount their feelings and may even make them feel guilty or foolish for having had such feelings or concerns.

A pharmacist's first instinct is often to give advice, since this is an opportunity to show his or her expertise. However, advice is most effective if it is offered after the patient has had an opportunity to finish speaking and explaining the problem. And although giving advice is intended to help, it may not be the recommended course of action. In many cases, it is preferable for the pharmacist to encourage patients to explore various avenues themselves, and then to assist them in making decisions.

In an effort to make the patient feel better, and perhaps to feel comfortable, the pharmacist often ignores the feelings expressed by the patient. The pharmacist may do this by changing the subject or by shifting the focus of the discussion from the patient to someone else—often the pharmacist himself or herself, or other patients in general. Pharmacists may believe that it will encourage the patient to know that others share their problems. In reality, however, shifting the focus from the patient tends to discount the patient's feelings, and may make him or her feel guilty or foolish for having had such concerns.

TABLE 7-7	**Nonlistening Responses**

The pharmacist may make one of the following responses to the patient's statement, "The dentist told me I'd have to come back again next week. I just wonder if he knows what he's doing."

Excessive verbalization	"Well, the prescription the dentist gave you looks fine. It's for an analgesic to help the pain. Take it every 4 hours . . . etc."
Premature questioning	"What were your symptoms when you saw the dentist? Did he take any X-rays?"
Being evaluative	"You're just feeling bad because of the pain. If you had regular check-ups you wouldn't be in such a bad state now."
Advising	"You should see another dentist if you feel that way."
Ignoring the patient's feelings	"Lots of people have problems with their teeth and have to return to their dentists for treatment. I had an abscessed tooth, and it took weeks to clear up."
Reassuring	"I'm sure the dentist knows what he's doing, and everything will be just fine."
Hostile	"Well, that's just plain unfair to the dentist. Anyway, you'd better do what he says or you'll end up losing that tooth."
Active listening	"I guess you're pretty frustrated at having to go back to the dentist again."

Based on information presented in Gerrard BA, Boniface W, Love B. Developing Facilitation Skills. In: Interpersonal Skills for Health Professionals. Reston Publishing, Reston, VA,1980:133–136.

Although an important part of patient counseling may involve reassuring the patient that the treatment is appropriate and safe, this is inappropriate if it is overly optimistic. The pharmacist has no way of being sure if indeed everything will be alright.

Sometimes pharmacists become angry or aggravated with patients' behaviors and respond with hostile comments, sometimes making threatening statements about patients' conditions. Although this understandably happens occasionally, the pharmacist must try to control such feelings. Ways to deal with conflict will be discussed in Chapter 8.

A summary and examples of these nonlistening responses and the appropriate active listening response are shown in Table 7-7. Pharmacists often find it difficult to formulate an active listening response, rather than these nonlistening responses. This takes practice and thought, but can offer the reward of more effective patient counseling and better relationships.

Probing Skills

After having listened to the patient, the pharmacist may need to probe in order to clarify the problem and determine how he or she can help. Also, during the information-gathering phase of the medication management consultation, the pharmacist needs to probe and ask specific questions about the patient's condition and medication use.

The way in which these questions are asked is important because it can build, maintain, or destroy rapport between the pharmacist and the patient.[29,40] To be effective, questions asked by the pharmacist must obtain accurate information, obtain the information efficiently, and involve the patient as much as possible.[29,40]

The skills used in asking effective questions during counseling involve the organization and phrasing of questions. This is the essence of probing skills.[29,40]

Organization of Questions

As noted in Chapter 5, having an organized plan or protocol is more effective for helping patients to remember and understand information.[41] Patients also report that an organized protocol rather than haphazard or vague counseling increases their satisfaction with the interaction, and confidence in the quality of advice.[23]

Questioning should be introduced with a statement regarding the purpose in order to prevent the patient from becoming defensive. For example, to introduce questioning during nonprescription counseling the pharmacist may say, "I need to ask you some questions about your symptoms to determine which medication would be most effective for you." Patients report that they interpret questioning introduced in this way as concern rather than suspicion.[23]

Because patients may feel more comfortable later in the interview once more trust has been developed, the pharmacist should begin with less personal questions and proceed to more personal questions such as details of the patient's alcohol use.

To explore where the questioning should focus, the pharmacist should start with more general questions and become more specific as the direction becomes clear, for example, "What sort of cold symptoms do you have?" "Is there also a cough?" "Is the cough dry?"

Finally, questions should be grouped together by topic to allow both the pharmacist and the patient to focus attention on a particular area, likely resulting in better patient recall. For example, during a medication management consultation, the pharmacist should ask all relevant questions about a particular drug before proceeding to questions about the next drug.

Phrasing of Questions

The way that questions are phrased may also contribute to their effectiveness.[29,40] Open questions, which demand more than a "yes" or "no" answer, encourage the patient to explain his or her point of view, and to express problems in his or her own terms. They are formulated using words such as how, when, where, what, or who.

Open questions are particularly useful at the beginning of the interview to elicit as much information from the patient as possible. They can also assist information gathering by encouraging more discussion by the patient, such as "Tell me more about that."

Closed questions are those that require only a "yes" or "no" response and tend to elicit mostly factual information. They are useful for gathering specific information about a particular problem and fill in the gaps left by the open-ended questions. For example, if the patient has reported that the medication seems to cause an upset stomach, the pharmacist might ask, "Do you take this medication with food?" The judicious use of a variety of open and closed questions will result in the most effective gathering of information.

Questions that begin with "why" should be avoided because they may elicit defensiveness, and are less likely to gather accurate information. "Why" questions tend to elicit what the patient believes to be a socially acceptable answer rather than the truth either because they don't want to reveal the truth or they aren't sure of the answer. For example, when questioning a patient about nonadherence, rather than asking, "Why aren't you taking this medication?" the pharmacist should first ask, "How are you taking this medication?" and then, "What problems are you having taking this medication?"

Certain phrasing of questions may lead to bias in the patient's answers. Leading questions that suggest the expected answer or restrictive questions that dissuade the patient from providing a truthful response should be avoided. Rather than asking, "You do take this medication the way your doctor told you to, don't you?" the pharmacist should ask, "How are you taking this medication?"

Double-barreled questions that solicit more than one item of information should be avoided, since this will lead to confusion. The patient will not know which part to answer first, and the pharmacist may not know which question is being answered. In addition, the other questions will probably have to be repeated or will be forgotten.

Finally, questions should be tactful and never unnecessarily personal or prying. The pharmacist should ask only necessary questions and consider the patient's personal situation (e.g., marital or employment status) so as to avoid embarrassing the patient or putting him or her on the defensive.

A summary of these probing skills is presented in Table 7-8.

Other Interviewing Skills

A number of other interviewing skills can help the pharmacist be efficient and effective in counseling. Paraphrasing is a helpful technique for the pharmacist to verify his or her understanding of the patient.[20] Intermittently, as necessary, the pharmacist might simply restate what he or she believes the patient has said. As well as verifying the facts, restating answers or paraphrasing lets the patient know that the pharmacist has been paying attention. For example, in response to the patient's statement, "This pain in my kidneys is so bad I can hardly stand up," the pharmacist might respond, "Are you saying the pain in your lower back makes it difficult for you to straighten?" Paraphrasing is

---

TABLE 7-8   **Probing Skills**

Organization of Questions

Introduce questions and explain purpose
Proceed from less to more personal
Proceed from general to specific
Group questions together by topic

Phrasing of Questions

Appropriate use of open and closed questions
Minimizing "Why" questions
Avoid questions that lead to bias
Avoid double-barreled questions
Questions should be tactful and should avoid unnecessary prying

---

Based on information presented in Gardner M, Boyce R, Herrier R. Pharmacist-Patient Consultation Program. 1991. U.S.A., U.S. Public Health Service, Indian Health Service; Bernstein L, Bernstein RS. The Probing Response. In: Interviewing: A Guide for Health Professionals. 4th ed. Appleton-Century Crofts, New York, 1985.

also part of empathetic responding, which was discussed earlier, and can help calm and focus the patient's thoughts.

Summarizing is a useful technique to end a series of probing questions.[29] This helps the pharmacist to clarify what problems have been identified before going on to discuss those problems. For example, "It seems from what you've told me that you find the medication is helping with your arthritis pain, but that it upsets your stomach a little." If this summary is incorrect, the patient can then inform the pharmacist and provide additional information as necessary.

Repeating the patient's words in the form of questions is another technique that encourages the patient to talk more about a particular topic.[24] For example, in response to the patient's comments about pain in the kidney, the pharmacist might say, "A pain in your kidneys?" This should not be done too frequently or it could become annoying.

Sometimes the pharmacist needs to use a transition statement to switch the discussion to a different topic, for example, from discussion of the patient's conditions to the medications used.[24] This is also useful when the patient intervenes with comments on another topic. After discussing that briefly, the pharmacist needs to return to the topic at hand. For example, the pharmacist might say, "Your holiday sounds like it was terrific, but now I'd like to talk about how you managed to take your heart pills while you were away."

Motivational Interviewing Techniques

As discussed in Chapter 4, motivational interviewing is a client-centered counseling technique used to motivate behavior change such as in the case of weight loss, or smoking cessation, or adherence to medication. The four counseling techniques used are empathy, developing discrepancy, rolling with resistance, and supporting self-efficacy.[37] It begins with relationship building techniques discussed above of establishing rapport and developing a trusting relationship to facilitate the process.

Communication with the patient is directed to drawing out arguments for change by exploring the patient's feelings and concerns, values, perspectives, and goals. This is done primarily by using empathy and active listening along with open questions that direct the patient to the desired end.[42]

To move the process along, the pharmacist must help the patient develop discrepancy between the current behavior and the desired goals and values. This is done by helping the patient list the pros and cons of change.

During this process, the pharmacist will meet with resistance as the patient tries to resolve the discomfort of ambivalence—knowing they should change but not wanting to, or feeling unable. The pharmacist will need to use the technique known as rolling with resistance. Rather than arguing with the patient, resistance must be approached by acknowledging the reluctance to change, asking the patient directly—but in a nonconfrontational manner—about reasons for reluctance, and countering the patient's reasons with questions about how the patient feels, and what they think they can do to change.

The pharmacist must then raise the patient's level of confidence in his or her ability to change by supporting the patient's belief in his or her self-efficacy. The pharmacist supports this by offering help, giving alternatives, and providing role models who have made similar changes so that the patient will feel empowered and be able to take responsibility for change.[37]

Risk Communication

As discussed in Chapter 5, there is controversy about how best to discuss the risk of treatments. The wording is important as discussed earlier, so that actual numbers if available are preferable to vague terms such as "sometimes," "possibly," or "might occur." In many cases, however, we don't really know with any accuracy what the chances are of adverse effects or of one therapy being better than another. The issue becomes how to express this uncertainty while being reassuring.

Some suggestions have been made by Sandman as to how to do this.[38] The key for the pharmacist is not only to acknowledge uncertainty up front, but also to communicate as precisely as possible what he or she thinks is accurate so far. This may include what is for sure, what is probable, what is a toss-up, and what is possible but unlikely.[38] The pharmacist can show distress at having to be tentative, but express hope of desired outcomes. The pharmacist should of course suggest precautions because of uncertainty, but should not go too far with uncertainty, appearing timid or bumbling. Although expressing uncertainty in this way tends to decrease competence of the speaker in the patient's view, it will increase trust.[38] This is preferable to the outrage that patients might express when they feel they have been misled.

Teach-Back

A simple and efficient technique for reducing errors and improving communication is the teach-back method, also knows as show-me or closing the loop. In order to ensure that the patient fully understood information and instructions the pharmacist should ask the patient to either tell or demonstrate what the pharmacist had previously explained or demonstrated.[39] This not only elucidates lack of knowledge or understanding, but also often reveals the nature of the misunderstanding, allowing a further communication by the pharmacist tailored to this.

The teach-back should be introduced in such a way as to place blame for any lack of understanding on the pharmacist rather than the patient, for example, "Just so I can be sure that I have made myself clear, could you show me how you are going to measure your blood sugar using the glucose meter." This will avoid embarrassment or reluctance on the part of the patient. If necessary this process can be repeated several times until clear understanding is apparent, completely "closing the loop."[39]

This technique has been found to be particularly important for patients with limited health literacy who are unlikely to ask questions or admit that they do not fully understand instructions.[39]

INTERACTING WITH HEALTH PROFESSIONALS AND OTHERS IN PHARMACY

During the course of their daily activities, pharmacists interact not only with patients, but also with other pharmacy personnel such as pharmacists, pharmacy technicians, clerks, delivery people, sales representatives and order-desk clerks. Pharmacists also interact regularly with other health professionals such as physicians, dentists, nurses, and various community health workers (home-visiting nurses, public health nurses, social workers, and home care workers). In order to provide optimal pharmaceutical

TABLE 7-9   Development of a Physician–Pharmacist Collaborative Working Relationship

Stage	Characteristic	Strategies to Develop CWR
Stage 0: Professional awareness	Minimal exchange of short, discrete interactions, e.g., refill requests and alerting about ADR Little thought to developing relationship	—
Stage 1: Professional recognition	Pharmacist asks physician for referrals to new pharmacy service Necessary for pharmacist but not for physician Physician may not see value in service or relationship Efforts to develop relations instigated by pharmacist	Inform physicians of interest in CWR Identify services to complement physician's practice and patient group Discuss and refine ideas Schedule regular face-to-face meetings
Stage 2: Exploration and trial	Pharmacist initiates Physician considers risks and benefits and evaluate pharmacist's skills and competence Physician identifies patients needing services and both share information in a formal communication	Make high-quality recommendations Get physician feedback Document outcomes Discuss preferred method of communication
Stage 3: Professional relationship expansion	More bilateral communication Fine-tune relationship through performance assessments Physician comes to expect service as the norm and values it Pharmacist given more responsibility, e.g., dosage adjustments	Communicate outcomes to physician Be consistent in provision of service Continue making high-quality interventions Meet regularly with physicians Discuss conflicts and strategies to overcome
Stage 4: Commitment to the CWR	More physicians collaborating Physician views less risk and higher value Physician and pharmacist on more equal footing with high input by both More consistent, longer term Face-to-face meetings, feedback, discussions of issues Formalized CPA	Continue providing high-quality services and regular communication with physicians

Based on information presented in McDonough R, Doucette W. Dynamics of pharmaceutical care: Developing collaborative working relationships between pharmacists and physicians. J Am Pharm Assoc. 2001;41(5):682–692.

care as well as to find the time to counsel patients, pharmacists need to communicate well with all of these people.

The ability of various health care providers to work together is critical to patient care, increasing drug therapy monitoring, more timely exchange of patient information, and more effective and efficient resolution of drug therapy problems.[43] In recent years, pharmacists have begun entering into more formal relationships with physicians known as collaborative practice agreements (CPAs) in order to integrate their services with physicians.[43] Many jurisdictions have regulations addressing collaborative drug therapy management, but in order to engage in this level of relationship, pharmacists must form successful collaborative working relationships (CWR).[43]

A model describing the development of CWR between physicians and pharmacists has been suggested by McDonough and Doucette.[43] It describes five stages as shown in Table 7-9, from stage 0, professional awareness, which reflects traditional practice, through to stage 4, commitment to the collaborative working relationship, with a formalized CPA.[43]

In order to develop through these stages, pharmacists must come to understand the nature of peer and physician relationships, and develop better ways of working together.

Factors Affecting the Development of Collaborative Working Relationships

Although physicians are generally cooperative when pharmacists contact them to recommend another product or strength, ask for clarification, or correct an error (96% of the time in one survey), they are less accepting of pharmacists' recommendations regarding drug-related problems identified in pharmaceutical care (76% of the time in a recent survey).[44,45] Pharmacists find physician–pharmacist relations increasingly strained as they become more involved in the patient's therapy and treatment outcomes.[46]

The development of a collaborative working relationship between pharmacists and other health professionals has been proposed by McDonough and Doucette to be affected by the health professionals' personal and professional characteristics, the context of their practices, and the nature and extent of exchanges (including monetary, communication, information) that occur between the health professionals.[43] These are described in Table 7-10.

The main sources of pharmacists' difficulties dealing with other health professionals have been found to include struggles for power, poor communication, lack of trust, and an unsatisfactory communication environment.[1] Some of these difficulties can equally apply to problems between pharmacists and other pharmacy personnel.

Struggles for Power

Struggles for power and autonomy have been identified as the main barriers to communication between pharmacists and other health professionals.[1] Cooperation may be hindered by the possibility that pharmaceutical care represents an expansion into the traditional roles of physicians and nurses. Physicians are gradually becoming more accepting of pharmacists providing pharmaceutical care, but do not believe pharmacists have the required knowledge and skills to offer many of the proposed nontraditional pharmacy services.[47] Although a majority of physicians apparently support pharmacists catching prescription errors (88% in one survey)[48] and community-based health

TABLE 7-10   Factors Affecting the Development of Collaborative Working Relationships

Health Professionals' Personal and Professional Characteristics

Individual characteristics	Younger ones may be more receptive
	Education included interdisciplinary experiences
Knowledge, attitudes, beliefs	Familiarity with other professional's abilities
	Confidence in the benefits of the collaboration
Professional experience	Specialists may need knowledge of pharmacists in areas outside their fields of expertise

Context of Their Practices

Proximity	Being closer geographically, same organization, or associating socially will increase number and ability of interactions
Volume of exchanges	More opportunities to meet face-to-face increases comfort level with competence
Practice features	Having the same pool of patients, e.g., in a rural setting
	Resources available (personnel, finances, facilities, contracts)
	Patient mix with higher need for pharmacy services
Health care system	Organizational structure may facilitate or hinder, e.g., rules, opportunities to interact, and payment models

Nature and Extent of Exchanges

Communication	Ability for face-to-face, two-way communication
	Content of communication is clear and concise, focused on the patient
Power and justice	Fairness of cost and benefits of relationship
	Balance between physicians' legal ability to prescribe and pharmacists' expertise needed
	Ability to influence each other
Development of norms and expectations	As services are provided more frequently over time physicians become more comfortable with competence and develop trust
	Opportunity to assess each other's performance and build trust and see the value

Based on information presented in McDonough R, Doucette W. Dynamics of pharmaceutical care: Developing collaborative working relationships between pharmacists and physicians. J Am Pharm Assoc. 2001;41(5):682–692.

promotion (74%),[47] providing patient education (65%)[48] and offering health screening such as blood pressure or cholesterol testing (69%)[49] are less popular, and conducting call-backs to monitor adherence, side effects, and efficacy are supported by still fewer physicians (53%).[47–49] Specifically, physicians have complained that pharmacists sometimes provide inappropriate information, or that pharmacist counseling conflicts with advice, scares patients, or sometimes infringes on the physician's role.[48,50]

Pharmacists need patients' medical information in order to provide pharmaceutical care services, but physicians are often not in agreement with pharmacists receiving this.[47]

Relationships with hospital pharmacists appear to be better as physicians consider hospital pharmacists to be their primary source of drug information, but do not generally identify community pharmacists in this role.[51]

Poor Communication Between Professionals

Pharmacists often engage in discussions with other health professionals, particularly physicians, under difficult circumstances (e.g., when a patient outcome has been negative or when the pharmacist has detected a problem involving the physician's prescribing). Studies suggest that pharmacists are aware of this problem.[52,53] Part of the problem simply may be that too little communication occurs. In a recent study, 25% of physicians had personal contact with a pharmacist regarding patients' medication four or more times daily, but 20% reported rarely having this type of contact.[48]

The nature of the communication that does occur constitutes another aspect of the problem. Other health professionals have different issues, priorities, and concerns that may differ from those of pharmacists, or so they believe.[52] Physicians sometimes perceive that pharmacists are only concerned with reducing costs rather than optimal patient care.[52] Greater exposure to services by pharmacists tends, however, to improve physicians' attitudes toward pharmacists.[53]

Communication between pharmacists and their peers often occurs over the telephone, and this medium tends to accentuate the distance between the parties involved. Physicians dislike waiting on the telephone or getting busy signals, and pharmacists are irritated by having to deal with receptionists and having to make unnecessary phone calls to physicians.[51]

Written communication between physicians and pharmacists occurs mostly through prescriptions. Surprisingly, physicians seem to be more sensitive about problems involving this than pharmacists: 50% (compared with only 10% of pharmacists) report that their illegible handwriting is one source of the problems they experience with pharmacists.[51] Written forms and notes are also used between pharmacy personnel, and between pharmacists and other health professionals. These forms can sometimes be perceived negatively, because they are impersonal, and often poorly worded so that recommendations are perceived as demands, or reports of problems are perceived as blame.

The communication between physicians and pharmacists is generally initiated by the pharmacist and often one way (written or telephone messages left with nurse or receptionist). The development of two-way communication has been found to be a distinguishing characteristic of late-stage collaborative relationships between physicians and pharmacists.[54]

The Environment

The hospital and community pharmacy environment often lacks privacy, so that any altercations or reprimands can be overheard by others, adding to the degree of discomfort for the individual involved. There is often interference and background noise, even during telephone conversations, as well as many distractions and the pressure of time.

The health care system in which health professionals work is often fragmented so that information is not shared, and there is little opportunity for health professionals to communicate or work together as teams. Physicians tend to see patients as their prime responsibility, and are reluctant to share this with others in the system.

The proximity of pharmacists to other health professionals improves the collaborative nature of the relationship. When practices are geographically close, opportunities to communicate face to face, interact socially, and care for mutual patients are increased.[43]

Improving Pharmacist-Health Professional Relationships—Developing a CWR

Many of the techniques discussed above for counseling patients apply to interacting with other health professionals. Using empathy, listening, questioning skills, assertiveness, and so forth when interacting with anyone, including family and friends, will improve communication, reduce stress, and improve efficiency.

Strategies suggested by McDonough and Doucette for pharmacists to develop CWR from stage 0 to 4 are shown in Table 7-9. In addition to providing high-quality services to patients with documented outcomes, the most important strategies involve improving frequency and content of communication, dealing with conflict, demonstrating empathy for peers, and being assertive with peers.

Improving Communication

The problem of differing issues, concerns, and priorities for different health professionals and pharmacy personnel can be overcome by bringing the focus to the patient.[43,52,55] Since this should be the concern for all involved, making any suggestion by framing it in terms of how it will benefit patient care will remove the focus from an individual health professional's behavior and reduce confrontation and arguments.

Providing a high level of service to patients and other health professionals will improve health professional relationships by showing the value of pharmacy services, instilling confidence in the pharmacist's competence, and developing new norms of practice.[43]

Pharmacists must also increase the frequency of communication with other health professionals. This can be done by pharmacists actively campaigning to promote pharmacy services, both individually and through pharmacist and health care organizations. Pharmacists should consider meeting regularly with the health professionals with whom they deal. For example, when starting in a new practice, pharmacists should take the initiative to introduce themselves in person (or by telephone as a second choice) to health professionals with whom they will be dealing. New health professionals who move into the area should be contacted. This introduction should include personal information about the pharmacist as well as his or her practice approach, services that will be provided, and an assurance that his or her concerns, like the health professionals, are based on securing the best possible health care for the patient.

Pharmacists can create forums for communication with other health professionals by organizing seminars on drug information or mutually interesting issues. Pharmacy services orientation programs can be organized to improve communication between pharmacy personnel and others such as nurses.[56]

Pharmacists can also communicate with peers through written, facsimile, or telephone consultations. Providing a newsletter and written reports of pharmaceutical interventions can let health professionals know that pharmacists are knowledgeable and are performing a valuable service. Careful attention should be taken, however, when preparing written communication so that the message is not misinterpreted, as this can be a source of problems as discussed earlier. This will be discussed in the next section on written communication.

Since the environment of the communication can contribute to problems, attention should be given to this. Attempts should be made to have conversations in private, or at least away from the mainstream of activities. Regular meetings should be arranged (e.g., staff meetings and pharmacy–nursing meetings) so that concerns can be aired and positive feedback can be given to the group for cooperative work. The move toward health care systems based on primary care, health maintenance organizations (HMOs), and multidisciplinary clinics increases the opportunity for pharmacists to work in closer proximity with other health professionals. Models of practice are developing whereby the pharmacist consults from within the physician practice, or physicians share common space with a pharmacy, increasing opportunities for communication and collaboration.[57]

Pharmacists can improve their frequency and content of communication with health professionals by the following practices:[51,55,58]

1. Using physician's level of language (rather than patient's).
2. Keeping the discussion focused on the patient.
3. Being available to answer questions in a timely and dependable manner.
4. Taking the time to explain problems with data and references to support the advice rather than informing the health professional that an error has been made.
5. Suggesting alternatives rather than one recommendation, allowing the health professional to make an informed decision rather than feeling as if he or she has been dictated to.
6. Providing services such as information about current drug issues, warnings of potential drug abuse/misuse and drug interactions, sharing of patient profiles, medication reviews for patients identified by the physician by referral.
7. Monitoring patient treatment and providing feedback regarding the patient's progress to other health professionals involved.
8. Providing proper documentation of actions taken with patients, preferably using subjective, objective, assessment, plan (SOAP) format used by physicians for charting.
9. Proactively meeting with health professionals to introduce self and offer services.
10. Meeting regularly with physicians to get feedback on services and to discuss issues around communication and collaboration.
11. Creating opportunities for social interaction or joint learning.

Dealing with Conflict

Improving communication will reduce the frequency of conflict, but inevitably conflict will occur from time to time when pharmacists are working with other health professionals. Conflict resolution and negotiation techniques should be used by pharmacists to resolve issues that arise.[59] Conflicts often arise when pharmacists make recommendations, or provide services outside of other health professionals' expectations.[59] Some suggestions for avoiding conflict when making recommendations to colleagues include:[59]

- Reporting factual information in a clear, concise, and organized manner
- Clearly explaining the way in which the recommendation decreases risk or improves care for the patient
- Displaying flexibility and willingness to admit a lack of understanding
- Avoiding criticism of colleagues
- Providing feedback to make sure that others understand and to encourage questions and comments

In addition, keeping the lines of communication open by encouraging regular meetings and making opportunities for social interaction will reduce the chance of conflict occurring. Communicating face to face about issues rather than by telephone or in writing is also helpful, although using the telephone and written reports can be done in ways to reduce chance of conflict, as discussed in the next section.

Empathizing with Health Professionals

Pharmacists can improve relations with peers by demonstrating empathy with health professionals and colleagues in the same way that they do with patients. By letting the other person know that his or her point of view has been understood, the pharmacist can reduce tensions and lead the way to better problem solving together in a more equal partnership.

Consider a nurse telephoning the hospital pharmacist to check on a missing medication. The nurse's first priority is to get the dose to the patient on time. She is probably very rushed, is concerned about the patient, and is worried about being held responsible for any problems resulting from a missed dose. If the pharmacist responds to her query by defensively accusing her of not sending down the order or by complaining that he or she too is busy, conflict is sure to arise. Alternatively, the pharmacist can empathize with the nurse's situation and let her know that her needs will be addressed as soon as possible. The pharmacist can then proceed to ask any questions that might be necessary to solve the problem, and suggest possible solutions.

Being Assertive with Health Professionals

Assertiveness on the pharmacist's part can also help develop better health professional relationships. Pharmacists who are tentative and unsure of themselves in their communications are not likely to receive respect. Recall that assertiveness involves giving and receiving respect and creating a win-win situation.

By being assertive, the pharmacist can ensure that his or her point of view gains recognition while at the same time letting colleagues know that their views are receiving

TABLE 7-11	Good Employee–Employer Relations

- Clear rules set and consistently enforced
- Mistakes admitted
- Employees involved in planning and encouraged to be creative
- Power of decision making and conflict resolution shared where possible
- Individuals not required to do more than they are able
- Employees shown that they are trusted
- Problems identified are a result of an employee's actions, not the individual person
- The good in what the person is doing discussed along with the bad
- Comparisons between employees and favoritism avoided
- Honest expression of feelings encouraged for management and employees
- Kindness and consideration observed
- Regular opportunities for discussion of issues, e.g., staff meetings

Based on information presented in Sepinwell S. Managing to communicate. The Leading Edge. 1992;2(3):8–9.

equal consideration. This too will lead the way to focusing on the patient's problem and solving it together in a rational way, for the patient's benefit. Pharmacists may sometimes need to remind other health professionals that it is the patient who is at issue and on whom the discussion should focus—rather than on any of the colleagues.

Pharmacist-Employee Relations

Because pharmacists are often in a supervisory capacity in the pharmacy, they also need to be aware of communication aspects particular to the employee–employer relationship. Good relationships in this quarter will allow the pharmacist to concentrate on patients' concerns, by freeing up time and mental capacity, as well as reducing stress in the pharmacy environment.

Building and maintaining an effective employee–employer relationship takes time and patience.[60] The communication skills discussed with respect to dealing with patients and with health professionals apply equally here including empathetic responding, active listening, conflict resolution, and assertiveness. Some guidelines to foster good employee–employer relationships have been suggested, as shown in Table 7-11.[60]

OTHER FORMS OF INTERACTION

A significant portion of pharmacists' communication with patients and health professionals is conducted over the telephone, and in writing through notes, e-mail, faxes, and reports. Since these forms of communication do not involve face-to-face contact, there is no nonverbal component to assist in transmitting the message, allowing a greater opportunity for misinterpretation. Pharmacists should be aware of the potential for problems and attempt to overcome them through various techniques.

Telephone Communication

Pharmacists spend a good part of the day on the telephone talking to physicians and patients. Although there are some commonalities, there are specific points to consider when dealing with patients as compared with health professionals.

Telephone Communication with Patients

Although most patient counseling is conducted in person, patient counseling over the telephone can be useful to improve access and speed of care.[61] It is particularly useful for situations where the patient cannot be present in the pharmacy, where the patient or pharmacist is limited by time, or where the situation demands a level of privacy that is not available in the pharmacy. Patients often initiate communication with the pharmacist by calling the pharmacy to ask questions and place orders. Telephone services have been initiated in some regions to provide patients with access to nurses and pharmacists for primary care consultations, resulting in avoidance of problems with medications.[61–63]

Telephone communication has been found to be more efficient for conducting regular medication reviews than face-to-face meetings (on average 10 minutes shorter).[64] When used for monitoring patients in palliative care, telephone communication was found to increase satisfaction with the pharmacist as patients found it to be less stigmatizing and to improve opportunity to ask questions.[65] A study using the telephone for follow-up monitoring found adherence and satisfaction with information were improved, and fewer medication problems occurred.[66]

Mobile phones and text messaging also offer opportunities for new services that can make contacting patients easier, and have been used for patients to report on effectiveness of treatments as well as to consult with their clinicians, resulting in reduced waiting time for the results of investigations and health care advice.[67] Sometimes a telephone call is the patient's first interaction with the pharmacy and a particular pharmacist, and therefore may be important in developing rapport for future interactions. However, there is concern that lack of visual cues when consulting by telephone could result in missing a serious condition. In addition, the lack of nonverbal communication should be considered when communicating over the phone.[61]

The following suggestions and considerations can improve the pharmacist's efficiency and effectiveness in conducting patient counseling by telephone:[68,69]

1. *Be Prepared*: If the pharmacist is initiating a telephone interview, the pharmacist should be prepared with the patient's drug profile and any additional information the pharmacist wishes to provide. If the patient initiates the phone call, then the patient's name should be ascertained and used during the call and the patient's drug profile should be retrieved so that complete information is available during the discussion.

2. *Deal with Patients Promptly*: There should be a prearranged plan of who should answer the telephone with an allowance for backup after two to three rings if that person is not available. If the patient must wait for the pharmacist, the clerk answering the telephone should indicate that the pharmacist is with a patient and will come to the phone as soon as possible. If it appears that it will be a lengthy wait, the clerk should indicate this and if possible arrange for the pharmacist to call the patient back. If the patient must be put "on hold," the patient should be told why and asked to hold, then should be thanked for waiting when the conversation is resumed.

3. *Start with a Friendly Greeting*: The pharmacist should try to smile when speaking on the telephone to transmit a friendly attitude through his or her voice. Whether the pharmacist or patient initiates the phone call, the pharmacist should greet the patient and identify his or her pharmacy, name, and title.

4. *Avoid Interruptions*: The pharmacist should try to ensure that he or she is not interrupted while on the telephone with a patient, and try to remove distractions so that the patient can be given full attention.

5. *Maintain Confidentiality*: The patient's confidentiality should be maintained by ensuring that the telephone conversation cannot be overheard by other pharmacy customers. The pharmacist should also be careful when telephoning the patient that the patient's situation is not discussed with anyone in the household other than the patient.

6. *Follow the Appropriate Counseling Protocol*: As with any patient-counseling session, the interview should follow the appropriate protocol as discussed in Chapter 5.

7. *Compensate for the Decrease in Nonverbal Communication*: Since nonverbal communication is reduced, the pharmacist should be alert for the patient's tone of voice and speech rhythms to detect concerns or lack of understanding. The pharmacist can compensate by using good verbal descriptions and a variety of terms. Also, if a pause is made to write or think, some sound or indication should be made to let the caller know this.

8. *Conclude by Asking If the Patient Has Anything Further to Discuss*: Since the pharmacist cannot see any hesitation on the caller's part, it is particularly important that the interview be concluded by asking if the patient has any questions or anything further to discuss.

9. *Offer to Make a Follow-up Call*: As with the face-to-face counseling protocol, the pharmacist should offer to telephone the caller later for follow-up if necessary to make sure everything was understood.

10. *End on a Positive Note*: To close the telephone call, the pharmacist should try to end on a positive note, particularly if a problem is still unsolved, for example, "I've tried my best to help. Please call again." The pharmacist should not hang up until he or she is sure that the patient is indeed finished speaking.

11. *Document*: Telephone counseling should be documented on the patient's profile in the same way as any patient-counseling interview would be, to note any problems identified and interventions recommended.

Telephone Communication with Other Health Professionals

As discussed above, telephone conversations can be a source of problems between pharmacists and other health professionals. However, if appropriate communication skills are used, telephone communication can be an effective way to increase communication with health professionals.

Some suggestions to make telephone conversations with physicians more efficient follow:[69]

1. *Arrange for a Private Line*: A separate telephone line should be used only for health professionals, and answered by a pharmacist to ensure quick and direct response to telephone calls from health professionals.

2. *Observe Telephone Manners*: Telephone manners as recommended above should be observed when answering the telephone, putting on hold, and hanging up.

3. *Be Prepared*: The pharmacist should be prepared when telephoning a physician by having appropriate patient information and well-thought-out recommendations, alternatives, and supporting data.

4. *Be Brief But Friendly*: Conversations should be brief and to the point, but should not be curt. After clearly identifying himself (e.g., name and pharmacy), the pharmacist should spend a moment exchanging pleasantries. This should be brief, but should not be omitted, because it can help build an interpersonal relationship.

5. *State the Purpose of the Call*: The purpose of the call should be stated clearly, to signal that it is time for business. This will also help the health professional prepare mentally, as well as take the time to retrieve the patient chart or any other material necessary. The purpose should include the patient's name as well as any other identification generally used specific to the practice (e.g., chart number, clinic or office patient, or from hospital emergency visit). If it is anticipated that the purpose of the call might lead to a lengthy discussion, the pharmacist should state this and allow the health professional to arrange an alternate time if necessary.

6. *SOAP Format*: The SOAP format should be used as with any other written or verbal discussions regarding a particular patient.

7. *Show Respect for All Members of the Patient's Health Care Team*: Often the pharmacist has to speak with a nurse or receptionist before being allowed to speak with the physician. These people are part of the health care team, since they are usually familiar with the patient as well, and therefore should not be ignored or treated with a lack of respect. Building interpersonal relationships with all involved in the patient's care will ultimately improve the patient's care. Of course, care should be taken regarding confidentiality.

8. *Be Empathetic and Assertive*: Skills of empathy and assertiveness should be remembered when dealing on the telephone. For example, often when a pharmacist telephones a physician's office, the office is very busy, and the physician may even be with a patient when he or she takes the call. This may make it difficult for the physician to concentrate on the patient the pharmacist wishes to discuss. By using empathetic skills, the pharmacist can let the health professional know that he or she recognizes that this may be the case.

   The pharmacist may need to use assertive skills to make sure that the receptionist or nurse will allow the pharmacist to speak with the physician. Assertiveness may also be needed to ensure that the pharmacist's concerns or recommendations are considered by the physician.

9. *Summarize*: The telephone conversation should be summarized with a clear statement of what will be done, if anything.

10. *End on a Positive Note*: The pharmacist should try to end the conversation on a positive note, even if the situation was not resolved. Without being solicitous, the pharmacist should thank the health professional for his or her time.

Written Interaction

As discussed in Chapter 6, written information has become a mainstay of providing information to patients, although it should always be used together with verbal discussion, either before or after the patient has read the material. As discussed previously, this material should be prepared and used with consideration for appropriate content, readability, comprehension, and presentation format. Written communication is also used between pharmacy personnel and between pharmacists and other health professionals.

Written interaction in pharmacy includes notes, faxes, reports or documentation forms, e-mails, forms, and prescriptions. This kind of communication tends to be impersonal and often is poorly worded. As a result, the message is often interpreted negatively, for example, recommendations made in writing are perceived as demands for change, or reports of problems are perceived as accusations.

Since pharmacists often work opposite shifts so that there is little overlap or opportunity for face-to-face communication with other pharmacists or pharmacy staff, written notes are often used. Communication between pharmacists and other pharmacists or employees can be improved by using a dispensary communication book. Entries can be made at the end of each shift to raise issues that come up; keep track of special orders or circumstances; and share information about a patient, doctor, new drug, and so forth. Care should be taken, however, to address colleagues in a friendly rather than demanding manner and should preferably include social greetings and salutations.

Health Care Professional Communication Report

In order to communicate and share information with other members of the health care team, pharmacists need to document their interactions with shared patients. Pharmacists sometimes send recommendations to physicians following a medication review or pharmaceutical intervention using a form, but a more personal letter format is more likely to be well received. The format of the letter should follow the SOAP method used by physicians. An example of a letter is shown in Appendix B. This should be preceded or followed-up with verbal communication whenever possible.

Patient Consultation Report

When an assessment is made following a consultation with a patient such as a medication management consultation, nonprescription drug consultation, or a follow-up consultation in which medication-related problems are identified and actions recommended, it is useful to provide a written summary of this to the patient. This will provide similar information to that provided to the physician, but will be presented in more patient-friendly language and format. For efficiency, it can be a preprinted form with information filled in by the pharmacist, or it can take a personal letter format. An example of a patient consultation report is shown in Appendix B.

Making this report will serve as a confirmation to the patient that pharmacy services were provided. It can also be used in conjunction with an invoice to bill for services or as an introduction to additional pharmacy services for which the patient will be requested to pay. This will be discussed further in Chapter 9.

To avoid communication problems with written communication, pharmacists can observe the following suggestions:

1. Carefully organize and word written communication to avoid any suggestion that orders are being given, or blame is being placed for errors.
2. When developing forms such as intervention forms, incident reports, performance reviews, get input from all who will be using and receiving such forms.

3. Use a level of language appropriate for the audience, e.g., technical language for health professionals presented in SOAP format.

4. Add a personal note, in the form of a greeting or comments in hand writing by the sender, to help to soften the formality of forms and form letters.

5. Where possible, either precede or follow written forms or reports with a verbal message in person or by telephone to give the opportunity for more informal comment or discussion.

Electronic Communication

With the increasing utilization of computers and the Internet by both patients and health professionals, a new avenue of communication has become available. In a 2005 Internet survey, 46% of physicians reported using e-mail to communicate with patients, 27% using it more than weekly.[70] In 2003, 67% to 78% of adults in the US had Internet access, and 90% of those reportedly want to communicate with their physicians electronically.[71]

The advantage of e-mail communication is the speed, with most responses being sent within 8 business hours, so that 79% of patients and 61% of physicians prefer it to the telephone.[71] Total message volumes are decreased, less time is required for the interaction and with "telephone tag," and communication can be ongoing throughout the day.[71] There is, however, decreased satisfaction if more than 2 business days elapse for a response, so pharmacists using this method of communication must be sure to regularly receive and respond to messages. For the health professional, there is no payment mechanism for an e-mail consultation and privacy may be a concern.[71]

Computer networking is another form of electronic communication that is being used by health professionals. An electronic profile for a patient can be generated and shared between health professionals, with the ability to edit and comment on changes so that a discussion can occur regarding a patient intervention. It can enhance communication between health professionals, and has been found to be a benefit by allowing pharmacists to alert physicians to nonprescription medication use, and issues such as nonadherence.[72]

Videoconferencing and web messaging are further electronic communication techniques that allow for more frequent communication among patients and health professionals.[61,71] They have advantages of allowing for visual cues in the case of videoconferencing and providing better security of information with web messaging. In both cases, people need to be trained to use these technologies, and frustrations with technical glitches and cost can be barriers, but it is expected that these will gradually be reduced, making these forms of communication more widespread and useful.

SUMMARY

This chapter provided a review of communication and human interaction in pharmacy practice. Pharmacists should seek more in-depth understanding of these topics through readings and workshops when they are available. Practice is the most beneficial way to improve communication skills, and pharmacists should try to develop these skills over time.

Although this chapter discussed communication and interactions with patients in general, as well as with peers, there are specific kinds of communication difficulties that arise. These will be discussed in the next chapter with respect to tailoring counseling for the individual patient.

REFLECTIVE QUESTIONS

1. A father with two small children comes into your pharmacy with a prescription for an antibiotic suspension for the youngest child, Kevin, who is 2 years old. The man sighs as he hands you the prescription and asks how long it will be. You have several prescriptions for other clients waiting to be filled and when you inform Kevin's father that the wait time will be approximately 20 minutes, he appears angry and blurts out, "How could it possibly take that long?"

   Give a potential explanation for the father's reaction. How could you respond empathetically to his question?

2. Looking at the illustration earlier in this chapter of the pharmacist who spilled antibiotic liquid, what are the pharmacist's nonverbal messages? If you were the pharmacy manager, what would you say to the pharmacist in this situation?

3. Janet Brown is a 46-year-old woman who asks you for help recommending an over-the-counter sleep aid. Rephrase the following questions to make them more effective:

   Is this a recent problem?

   You're not drinking too much coffee, are you?

   Are you napping during the day or getting any exercise?

4. Bill is a pharmacist interested in providing a new service for diabetic patients in his pharmacy. He starts by advertising this to patients, and when he gets his first patient, he sends a written form to the physician with recommendations. What is the likely response of the physician to this? What stage of CWR is he at with physicians in his community? What actions should he take to develop a CWR?

REFERENCES

1. Kimberlin C. Communications. In: Wertheimer A, Smith MC, eds., Pharmacy Practice: Social and Behavioral Aspects, 3rd Edition. Williams & Wilkins, Baltimore, MD, 1989.
2. Ley P. Techniques for Increasing Patients' Recall and Understanding. In: Communicating with Patients: Improving Communication Satisfaction and Adherence. Croom Helm, New York, 1988.
3. Waitzkin H. Doctor-patient communication: Clinical implications of social scientific research. JAMA. 1984;252(17):2441–2446.
4. Hargie O, Morrow N, Woodman C. Pharmacists' evaluation of key communication skills in practice. Patient Educ Couns. 2000;39:61–70.
5. Worley M, Schommer J. Pharmacist-patient relationships: Factors influencing quality and commitment. J Soc Admin Pharm. 1999;16(3/4):157–172.
6. Gerrard B, Boniface W, Love B. Developing Facilitation Skills. In: Interpersonal Skills for Health Professionals. Reston Publishing, Reston, VA, 1980.
7. Bernstein L, Bernstein RS. An Overview of Interviewing Techniques. In: Interviewing: A Guide for Health Professionals, 4th Edition. Appleton-Century-Crofts, New York, 1985.
8. Gerrard B, Boniface W, Love B. Developing Skills in Understanding Interpersonal Behavior. In: Interpersonal Skills for Health Professionals. Reston Publishing, Reston, VA, 1980.
9. Funch, F. Transformational Dialogues: Facilitator Training Manual #1. An instruction manual of practical techniques for facilitating personal change. Available at: www.worldtrans.org/TP/TP1TP1TOP.HTML (accessed March 18, 2005).

10. Lively B. Communication as a transactional process—Basic tools of the community pharmacist. Contemp Pharm Pract. 1978;1(2):81–85.
11. Lawrence G. People Types and Tiger Stripes: A Practical Guide to Learning Styles, 2nd Edition. Center for Application of Psychological Type, Gainsville, FL, 1982, p. 13–25.
12. Nichol M, McCombs J, Johnson K, et al. The effects of consultation on over-the-counter medication purchasing decisions. Med Care. 1992;30(11):989–1003.
13. Dusay J, Dusay K, Transactional Analysis. In: Corsini R, eds., Current Psychotherapies, 3rd Edition. FE Peacock Publishers, Inc., Itasca, IL, 1984.
14. Elder J. Introduction to the Ego States. In: Transactional Analysis in Health Care. Addison–Wesley Publishing Co, Melno Park, CA, 1978, p. 2–7.
15. Samovar L, Porter R. The Challenge of Intercultural Communication. In: Communication Between Cultures, 4th Edition. Wadsworth, Belmont, CA, 2001, p. 3–20.
16. Samovar L, Porter R. Communication and Culture. In: Communication Between Cultures, 4th Edition. Wadsworth, Belmont, CA, 2001, p. 21–50.
17. Burroughs V, Maxey R, Crawley L, et al. Cultural and genetic diversity in America: The need for individualized pharmaceutical treatment. National Pharmaceutical Council, National Pharmaceutical Association. Available at: www.npcnow.org/issues_productlist/PDF/culturaldiversity.pdf (accessed November 3, 2003).
18. Samovar L, Porter R. Cultural Diversity in Perception. In: Communication Between Cultures, 4th Edition. Wadsworth, Belmont, CA, 2001, p. 52–80.
19. Samovar L, Porter R. Language and Culture. In: Communication Between Cultures, 4th Edition. Wadsworth, Belmont, CA, 2001, p. 136–160.
20. Samovar L, Porter R. Nonverbal Communication. In: Communication Between Cultures, 4th Edition. Wadsworth, Belmont, CA, 2001, p. 164–195.
21. Burroughs V, Maxey R, Levy R. Racial and ethnic differences in response to medicines: Towards individualized pharmaceutical treatment. J Natl Med Assoc. 2002;94(10)Suppl:S1–26. Available at: www.npcnow.org/issues_productlist/PDF/SupplementFINAL.pdf (accessed February 4, 2004).
22. Berger B. Building an effective therapeutic alliance: Competence, trustworthiness, and caring. Am J Health Syst Pharm. 1993;50:2399–2403.
23. Norris P, Rowsell B. Interactional issues in the provision of counselling to pharmacy customers. Int J Psychoanal Psychother. 2003;11:135–142.
24. Reiser D, Klein A. The Interview Process. In: Patient Interviewing—The Human Dimension. Waverly Press, Baltimore, MD, 1980.
25. West D, Wilkin N, Bentley J, et al. Understanding how patients form beliefs about pharmacists' trustworthiness using a model of belief processing. J Am Pharm Assoc. 2002;42(4):594–601.
26. Barnard D, Barr J, Schumacher G. Empathy. Person to Person. The AACP-Lilly Pharmacy Communications Skills Project. American Association of Colleges of Pharmacy, Bethesda, MD, 1982.
27. Meach B, Rogers C. Person-centred Therapy. In: Corsini R, eds., Current Psychotherapies, 3rd Edition. FE Peacock Publishers, Itasca, IL, 1984.
28. Bernstein L, Bernstein RS. The Understanding Response. In: Interviewing: A Guide for Health Professionals, 4th Edition. Appleton-Century-Crofts, New York, 1985.
29. Gardner M, Boyce R, Herrier R. Pharmacist-Patient Consultant Program. An Interactive Approach to Verify Patient Understanding. U.S. Public Health Service, Indian Health Service, 1991.
30. Knapp M. Nonverbal Communication: Basic Perspectives. In: Essentials of Nonverbal Communication. Holt, Rinehart and Winston, New York, 1980.
31. Samuelson K. Non-verbal messages can speak louder than words. Health Care. 1986;Apr: 12–13.

32. Knapp M. The Effects of Territory and Personal Space. In: Essentials of Nonverbal Communication. Holt, Rinehart and Winston, New York, 1980.
33. Lustig M, Koester J. Intercultural Competence: Interpersonal Communication Across Cultures, 3rd Edition. Addison Wesley, New York, 1999, p. 219.
34. DiMatteo MR, Taranta A, Friedman HS, et al. Predicting patient satisfaction from physicians' non-verbal communication skills. Med Care. 1980;18(4):376–387.
35. Gerrard BA, Boniface W, Love B. Developing Assertion Skills. In: Interpersonal Skills for Health Professionals. Reston Publishing, Reston, VA, 1980.
36. Anonymous. Privacy rule for health records. HIPAA Summary. Standards for the Privacy of Individually Identifiable Health Information. American Pharmacists Association, 2003. Available at: www.pharmacist.com/articles/h_hi_0001.cfm (accessed April 28, 2005).
37. Lau Carino J, Gulanick M. Using motivational interviewing to reduce diabetes risk. Prog Cardiovasc Nurs. 2004;19(4):149–154. Available at: www.medscape.com/viewarticle/496829 (accessed January 13, 2005).
38. Sandman P. Acknowledging uncertainty. Available at: www.psandman.com/col/uncertin.htm (accessed November 17, 2004).
39. Schillinger D, Piette J, Grumbach K, et al. Closing the loop: Physician communication with diabetic patients who have low health literacy. Arch Intern Med. 2003;163:83–90.
40. Bernstein L, Bernstein RS. The Probing Response. In: Interviewing: A Guide for Health Professionals, 4th Edition. Appleton-Century-Crofts, New York, 1985.
41. Morrow D, Leirer V, Altieri P, et al. Elders' schema for taking medication: Implications for instruction design. J Gerontol Psychol Sci. 1991;46(6):378–385.
42. Zimmerman G, Olsen C, Bosworth C. A Stages of change approach to helping patients change behavior. Am Fam Physician. 2000;61:1409–1416. Available at: www.aafp.org/afp/20000301/1409.html (accessed November 2, 2004).
43. McDonough R, Doucette W. Dynamics of pharmaceutical care: Developing collaborative working relationships between pharmacists and physicians. J Am Pharm Assoc. 41(5):682–692. Available at: www.medscape.com/viewarticle/406728 (accessed May 3, 2005).
44. Kassam R, Farris K, Buirback L, et al. Pharmaceutical care research and education project: Pharmacists' interventions. J Am Pharm Assoc. 2001;41(3):401–410.
45. Meade V. APhA survey look at patient counseling. Am Pharm. 1992;NS32(4):27–29.
46. Hepler C, Strand L. Opportunities and responsibilities in pharmaceutical care. Am J Hosp Pharm. 1990;47(3):533–543.
47. Ewen E, Triska O. What is the pharmacists' role in the community? Can Pharm J. 2001;134(6):33–39.
48. Rinelli P, Biss J. Physicians' perceptions of communication with and responsibilities of pharmacists. J Am Pharm Assoc (Wash). 2000;40(5):625–630.
49. Anonymous. 1999 Community Pharmacy Trends Report. Healthcare and Financial Publishing, Rogers Media, Toronto, Canada, 1999.
50. Halpin P. Reading the numbers. Interaction. Improving physician-pharmacist communication. Pharm Pract. 1997;Dec.(Suppl):26.
51. Anonymous. 1984 Schering Report explores pharmacist-physician relationships. Am Pharm. 1984;24(10):13–14.
52. Albro W. How to communicate with physicians. Am Pharm. 1993;NS33(4):59–61.
53. Ritchey F, Raney M. Effect of exposure on physicians' attitudes toward clinical pharmacists. Am J Hosp Pharm. 1981;38:1459–1463.
54. Brock K, Doucette W. Collaborative working relationships between pharmacists and physicians: An exploratory study. J Am Pharm Assoc. 2004;44(3):358–365.
55. Timmerman S. How to work with physicians. Am Pharm. 1992;NS32(2):39–40.
56. Welch P, Wright P, Harell A, et al. Development of a pharmacy/nursing orientation program. Abstract of Meeting Presentation. ASHP Midyear Clinical Meeting. 1991;26:127D.

57. Howard M, Trim K, Woodward C, et al. Collaboration between community pharmacists and family physicians: Lessons learned from the Seniors Medication Assessment Research Trial. J Am Pharm Assoc. 2003;43(5):566–572.

58. McDonough R. Interventions to improve patient pharmaceutical care outcomes. J Am Pharm Assoc. 1996;36(7):453–465.

59. Szeinbach S. Helpful ideas: Using interpersonal skills to resolve conflicts with prescribers. The Consulting Pharmacist. 1991;6(6):524,526.

60. Sepinwell S. Managing to communicate. The Leading Edge. 1992;2(3):8–9.

61. Phul S, Bessell T, Cantrill J. Alternative delivery methods for pharmacy services. Int J Psychoanal Psychother. 2004;12:53–63.

62. Anonymous. Telehealth Ontario. Ont Pharmacist. 2001;59(5):12.

63. Joeseph A, Franklin BD, James D. An evaluation of a hospital-based patient medicines information helpline. Pharm J. 2004;275:126–129.

64. Pinnock H, Bawden R, Proctor S, et al. Accessibility, acceptability, and effectiveness in primary care of routine telephone review of asthma: Pragmatic, randomised controlled trial. BMJ. 2003;326:477.

65. Gammaitoni A, Gallagher R, Welz M, et al. Palliative pharmaceutical care: A randomised, prospective study of telephone-based prescription and medication counselling services for treating chronic pain. Pain Med. 2000;1:317–331.

66. Clifford S, Barber N, Horne R, et al. Evaluation of pharmacist-delivered intervention to improve patients' adherence and reduce their problems with medicines. Presented at Health Services Research & Pharmacy Practice Conference, Belfast, 2003. Available at: www.hsrpp. org.uk/abstracts/2003_47.s html (accessed May 9, 2005).

67. Pal B. The doctor will text you now: Is there a role for the mobile telephone in health care? BMJ. 2003;326:607.

68. Smith D. Communicating with patients by telephone. Am Pharm. 1983;NS23(10):38.

69. Hunter R. Effective Telephone Communication. In: Tindall W, Beardsley R, Curtis F, eds., Communication in Pharmacy Practice. Lea & Febiger, Philadelphia, PA, 1984.

70. Medscape Instant Polling. How frequently do you use email to communicate with your patients? Available at: www.medscape.com/px/instantpllservlet/result?PollID=1283 (accessed January 4, 2005).

71. Liederman E, Lee J, Baquero V, et al. Patient-physician web messaging. J Gen Intern Med. 2005;20(1):52–57. Available at: www.medscape.com/viewarticle/500025_print (accessed March 10, 2005).

72. Sellors C, Sellors J, Levine M, et al. Computer networking to enhance pharmacist-physician communication: A pilot demonstration project in community settings. Can Pharm J. 2004;137(8):26–29.

Tailoring Counseling to Meet Individual Patient Needs and Overcome Challenges

CHAPTER 8

Objectives

After completing the chapter, the reader should be able to

1. describe the factors that may require the tailoring of counseling for individual patients.
2. be able to identify situations presenting special challenges in counseling.
3. list the variety of different challenges pharmacists face with patients with special needs.
4. describe techniques to use to improve counseling for the elderly, disabled, limited literacy, or critically ill patients.
5. describe techniques to handle difficult issues such as a medication incident, cultural issues, and non-drug-related patient concerns.
6. be prepared to deal with emotional situations and conflict during counseling.

The counseling protocols suggested in Chapter 5 and the educational and counseling techniques discussed in Chapters 6 and 7 do not necessarily apply to all patients and all situations. Patient needs vary and some situations present particular challenges. Pharmacists need to recognize these situations and understand the issues involved. Certain points in the counseling may need to be emphasized, and the various materials, methods, and techniques used in counseling may need to be altered. Tailoring counseling to meet individual patient needs in this way can assist the pharmacist in dealing with a variety of challenges while being efficient and effective in counseling.

It should be recognized at the outset of this discussion about various types of challenges that patients in no way form homogeneous groups and that each patient should be considered on an individual basis, i.e., not just as an elderly person or a disabled person. In addition, it must be emphasized that the patient himself or herself is not a problem, but the circumstances in relation to the pharmacist's concerns regarding patient counseling and the patient's individual health care needs are the challenge.

FACTORS TO BE CONSIDERED IN TAILORING COUNSELING

Pharmacists have reported that many factors contribute to challenges in patient counseling.[1] These factors include characteristics of the patient, the type of drug prescribed or condition being treated, and various aspects of the situation. In addition, there are factors involving the individual pharmacist that contribute to challenges. These are summarized in Table 8-1.

TABLE 8-1	Factors to Consider in Tailoring Counseling
Patient	Age
	Cultural background
	Abilities and preferences
	Disabilities
	Lifestyle and employment
	Gender, employment status, socio-economic status
Drug	Prescription or nonprescription
	Risk level and adverse effects
	Route of administration
	Time to effect
Condition	Seriousness
	Emotional arousal, e.g., fear, anger, and embarrassment
	Level of lifestyle modification needed
Situation	New or returning patient
	Conflict or emotional upset
	Pharmacy environment, e.g., interruption, limited time, and privacy
	Medication incident
	Nontherapeutic concerns, e.g., child abuse and threat of suicide
Pharmacist	Knowledge of patient
	Knowledge about drugs and conditions
	Communication skills
	Time
	Attitude
Pharmacy environment	Lack of privacy
	Poor patient accessibility
	Lack of time
	Isolation from health care team

Characteristics of the Patient

Certain patient characteristics will affect the emphasis that needs to be placed on certain aspects of counseling. The age of the patient may affect counseling in a number of ways. Elderly patients may use multiple drugs to treat several conditions and may experience unexpected reactions to medications resulting from the physiological changes of aging.[2] The pharmacist may therefore have to spend more time than he or she would with another patient in identifying problems, explaining directions, and helping the patient schedule dosing.[2] Similarly, pediatric patients require more attention regarding problem identification because of their physiological differences from adults. More time will also likely be required for providing detailed instructions to the caregiver about administration.[3]

The cultural background of the patient may also alter the emphasis in counseling. People with different cultural backgrounds may have different perceptions of their illnesses and of the purpose or effectiveness of medication.[4] For example, some Europeans are more accustomed to using herbal remedies, and they may have doubts about the effectiveness of prescribed medications. These patients may also require modifications to the information provided in terms of detail and selection of patient education materials as discussed in Chapter 6.

Some patients may also have various disabilities that may affect where counseling can take place, the patient education materials used, and the type of information that may be needed.[5]

A patient's type of employment and lifestyle may need to be considered. The dosage form, dosing schedule, and side effects may need to be modified, and special arrangements may need to be made. For example, a truck driver will have difficulty taking a medication that makes him drowsy.

The patient's gender, employment status, or socio-economic situation should not alter the type of counseling provided; however, these factors should be considered by the pharmacist during certain discussions in order to prevent embarrassing or offending the patient.

Characteristics of the Drug

As discussed earlier, the content of the counseling will vary depending on whether a prescription or a nonprescription drug is involved. Also, certain drugs are more likely than others to present problems with adherence, side effects, or precautions.

Where a drug is known to be associated with a high risk of interactions or adverse effects, this section in the protocol should be emphasized. Other medications, such as those administered by inhalation or injection, may require more emphasis on the method of use.

Another consideration with regard to the drug may be the length of time that it will take before a patient will recognize an effect, as with some antidepressants, or the lack of evident effect, as with antihypertensive medications. As discussed in Chapter 4, it is important in these situations to help the patient find ways to identify the medication effect in some way (e.g., through suggesting self-monitoring of blood pressure) to encourage adherence.

Characteristics of the Condition

Some conditions may arouse more emotion or concern for the patient than others.[4] For example, the diagnosis and prognosis of high blood pressure are often poorly understood. Similarly, a diagnosis of psychiatric illness may cause a patient embarrassment and worry about other people's reactions. In particular, where the illness may be fatal, such as cancer or AIDS, the patient will have a variety of concerns and emotions requiring special attention by the pharmacist.

In these situations, the pharmacist may need to spend more time in discussing the condition and the patient's feelings. It is also important to emphasize how the medication works in relation to controlling or reducing symptoms rather than curing the condition, and the consequences of missing a dose of the medication without, of course, resorting to scare tactics.

Some conditions require more lifestyle modification than others. For example, smoking, obesity, or diabetes require changes to habits and diet that can be extremely challenging. The pharmacist may need to spend a significant amount of counseling time discussing these issues, making referrals for further assistance as well as providing follow-up counseling to further support the patient.

Characteristics of the Situation

Certain situations can create challenges and call for different emphasis in counseling. As discussed in Chapter 5, the content of the counseling will vary, depending on whether the patient is new to the pharmacy or is a returning patient.

A situation in which a patient becomes angry, fearful, or emotionally upset can make counseling particularly difficult for the pharmacist. The pharmacist will need to deal with the patient's emotions before the counseling can proceed.

Difficult situations also arise when the patient's aims are in conflict with the pharmacist's, for example, when the patient is particularly in a hurry, or alternatively, wanting to talk more with the pharmacist than necessary.

Unfortunately, pharmacists are occasionally faced with situations involving medication incidents. Although we strive to prevent such incidents, patients occasionally receive the wrong medication or dose and may experience negative consequences as a result. The way such issues are handled can be critical to the outcome of the incident and to prevention of future incidents.

Finally, pharmacists are often consulted by patients with a range of nontherapeutic-related concerns from child abuse to threatened suicide. Although these situations do not require medication counseling, the pharmacist is required, because of his or her position as a public health resource in the community and as a caring human being, to respond to such situations.

Characteristics of the Pharmacist

There are always two sides to a story, and so in addition to patient factors that make counseling individual patients challenging, various pharmacist factors are also involved. Pharmacists are individuals also and they bring strengths and challenges to a situation. The pharmacist's level of knowledge about the patient (his or her concerns, family situation, conditions, and symptoms) can be important in understanding how to approach the patient, how much information to give, and how comfortable he or she is in dealing with the patient. The pharmacist's knowledge about the conditions and medications involved in counseling are also important, as the pharmacist must be able to anticipate issues that must be addressed and provide appropriate information. This is particularly important when dealing with patients who are critically ill. Some pharmacists find it helpful to acquire additional qualifications such as becoming a diabetes educator or specialist in geriatrics, gaining more knowledge and understanding of specific groups of patients and their conditions.

The pharmacist's ability to communicate with the patient and health professionals involved is also important. If the pharmacist is able to initiate conversations and gather pertinent information, he or she will be better able to assess individual patient's needs. The use of empathy is paramount in dealing with challenging situations, allowing the pharmacist to deal with the patient's emotions such as anger, embarrassment, fear, and confusion that generally exist in such situations.

Time is another factor for the pharmacist. If the pharmacist and patient feel rushed and pressured, with inadequate time to ask questions and discuss issues, then they will become frustrated and their needs will not be met.

Finally, the attitude of the pharmacist can be the overriding factor in creating, preventing, and dealing with all these various issues. The pharmacist must be tolerant, empathetic, and interested in the individual patient. This will be apparent to the patient and will allow for the development of a successful relationship.

Characteristics of the Environment

The pharmacy environment is often a source of difficulties in patient counseling. There is often lack of privacy, inadequate time, poor accessibility, and lack of specialized resources for dealing with a patient's individual needs. The isolated nature of the pharmacist can also be a difficulty, so that interaction with other health professionals in a team approach is infrequent and sometimes difficult, resulting in misunderstandings and poor information exchange.

Pharmacists should consider modifying various physical aspects of the pharmacy. This will be discussed further in Chapter 9. In order to allow the necessary time and modifications to counseling needed depending on the various needs discussed in this chapter, pharmacists should consider making appointments, home visits, and group sessions.[6] Arrangements that allow the pharmacist to interact frequently with other health care team members, such as shared physical facilities or virtual networks, can also assist the pharmacist in dealing with the individual patient's needs.

COUNSELING PATIENTS WITH SPECIAL NEEDS

As discussed briefly earlier, certain groups of patients have particular needs. This does not mean that patients in these groups are all the same, i.e., not just as an elderly person or a disabled person. They may even belong to several groups at once, e.g., an elderly, critically ill patient with limited literacy. Each patient should be considered on an individual basis, but the pharmacist can anticipate that patients with language comprehension and literacy difficulties, patients with disabilities, critically ill patients, and elderly patients will have certain needs in common, and require modifications to counseling to meet these needs.

Counseling Patients with Poor Comprehension

As discussed in Chapter 6, pharmacists are often confronted with comprehension difficulties of various sorts when counseling patients. Patients with difficulties in this area are at risk when dealing with medications in a number of ways. For one thing, they often lack knowledge of basic preventative health care and may be more likely to self-treat or borrow other people's medications. There is of course a greater potential for confusing medications at home and of misusing medication because of inability to comprehend the medication label and reluctance to ask questions. Difficulties can arise as a result of inability to read or comprehend dosing instructions, labeled warnings regarding expiration dates, and side effects, as well as confusion between look-alike brands.

Types of Comprehension Difficulties

Pharmacists often encounter challenges in counseling patients because a patient's first language is different from that of the pharmacist. Comprehension difficulties can include not only language comprehension, but also culturally different ways of expressing and perceiving things, which will be discussed later in this chapter.[7]

Even when the pharmacist and patient have the same mother tongue, pharmacists often find themselves using jargon, forgetting that many technical pharmaceutical terms are not readily understood by a large percentage of the population. Even well-educated people apparently have poor health literacy so that more than 90 million Americans cannot adequately understand basic health information.[8] For example, words such as "void" and "topical" have been reported to be intelligible to only one third of the population, and require a grade 12 to grade 13 education level to be understood, whereas the average comprehension level is considered to be grade 6.[9]

As discussed in Chapter 6, patients with low literacy levels have comprehension difficulties. Patients who speak English as a second language, are senior citizens, who have not completed high school, or who live in conditions of poverty are at greater risk for low literacy.[10] Forty million Americans are deemed to be functionally illiterate and 55 million are marginally literate.[8] They have problems with reading appointment slips and prescription labels and understanding terminology used by health professionals.[11–13]

A patient may also have comprehension difficulties because he or she has a developmental disability, previously referred to as being mentally retarded.[14] These individuals, with subaverage intellectual function (IQ of 70 to 75 or below), require more time to take in and interpret information, have flawed short-term memory, and have difficulty transferring problem-solving skills from one task to another.[14] As a result they require time and patience during medication counseling.

Detection of Poor Comprehension

The pharmacist must be tactful in detecting and inquiring about comprehension difficulties, as well as in dealing with those challenges. At no time should the patient be made to feel that this is a bother to the pharmacist, or that he or she is in any way inferior.

Sometimes pharmacists are unaware of patients' comprehension problems because people with comprehension difficulties are often skilled at concealing their difficulties.[15]

Pharmacists should be alert for patients at greater risk of low literacy as noted above (i.e., speaking English as a second language, being a senior citizen, not completing high school, and living in conditions of poverty).[10]

Patients with comprehension difficulties may not ask any questions, or they may ask a lot of questions. They may rely on a friend or relative to speak for them. They may be persistently nonadherent to medications, ignoring or misunderstanding even simple instructions.[16] Patients experiencing difficulty with written information may avoid filling out forms or questionnaires, never refer to written information received in the past, say that they left their glasses at home, or bring in a presigned checks.[15] Patients with low literacy may also show frustration or anxiety while reading.[17] Above all, patients may pretend to understand rather than risk embarrassment by revealing literacy or comprehension difficulties.[15]

The pharmacist can try to detect the presence and extent of comprehension difficulties by getting the patient to speak as much as possible during the opening and information-gathering phases of the counseling session. The pharmacist should try to gauge the patient's language level and vocabulary, and reflect this in his or her own speech. For example, if the patient says his or her medication is for "blackouts," then the pharmacist should use this term during counseling rather than terms such as "seizures" or "epilepsy."

Tailoring Counseling for Patients with Comprehension Difficulties

Pharmacists can improve counseling effectiveness with patients exhibiting comprehension difficulties by tailoring counseling in a number of ways.

1. *Simplify Explanations*: While avoiding any hint of condescension, the pharmacist should phrase explanations in the simplest terms possible, without sacrificing any necessary information. The patient can be invited to ask the pharmacist questions, and more information can then be provided at the patient's request. Oral communication may also need to be slower (but not louder) with repetition and summarizing.[14]

2. *Avoid Difficult Words*: Some alternate words for difficult or misunderstood words often used in patient counseling were suggested in Chapter 6 (Table 6-7). In addition, general phrases such as "plenty of water" and "on an empty stomach" have been found to lead to confusion and should be explained more precisely by the pharmacist.[18]

3. *Involve Family and Community Caregivers*: Where necessary (and where possible), a family member or other individual should be enlisted as an interpreter for those with a foreign language or as additional support for those with literacy needs. If this is done, the pharmacist should meet the patient and caregiver together and ask that the discussion be translated or explained in sections so that the patient can be involved and so that patient's queries can be responded to. This way the pharmacist can be sure that the information was actually transmitted to the patient and that any misunderstandings or concerns of the patient were dealt with. If the support worker for a patient with developmental disabilities does not accompany the

patient to the pharmacy, the pharmacist should ask the patient to have the worker call so that he or she can be briefed on the patient's medication needs.

4. *Use Various Counseling Methods and Aids*: Assisted labeling such as pictograms, charts, and clock diagrams, as discussed in Chapter 6, should be made available to clarify information. Adherence reminders, such as charts and dosettes, alarms, cue lights, and timing devices can also be used to clarify and remind patients about dosage regimens.[14]

   For patients with a foreign mother tongue, pharmacy computer software programs can make translations of prescription-label directions into other languages. However, the pharmacist or at least pharmacy personnel should be able to understand these instructions so that errors can be detected. Translations should also be made for information sheets of common medications and instructions on ophthalmic, vaginal, rectal, and inhaler use. Some organizations such as the Diabetes Association or local cultural groups may have literature available in a variety of languages.

   When low literacy is identified, print materials should either not be used or selected for easy reading (fifth grade level or lower) or availability in the patient's mother tongue.[19] Print materials may, however, be useful for patients to take home to read at their own pace and refer to as needed, or to give to caregivers who can help patients understand the information. Print material should be accompanied by verbal information and wherever possible be presented on several different occasions to reinforce understanding.[19]

   Multimedia computer-based educational programs can allow the patient to see or hear information about the condition.[19]

   For patients with developmental disabilities, training for problem solving is important so that they know what to do when various situations arise with medication use. This can be done by presenting scenarios or using role-playing games about such issues as what to do if medication runs out, if it is lost, or if it looks unfamiliar.[14] It can also be helpful to do task analysis, which involves dividing the task of self-medication into smaller steps such as hear the medication alarm ring, turn off the alarm, go to the medicine cupboard, take out the pill container, open the container, take out the correct number of pills, put the container back in the cupboard, and get a glass of water.[14] Reinforcement of correct behavior such as food or drink, other pleasant rewards, and praise and encouragement can help motivate the patient to adhere to instructions.[14] Written instructions should be limited to one or two only that state exactly what the patient needs to know, with complex instructions broken down into easy-to-understand parts.[14]

   The use of several different counseling methods is advisable so that a method that is most suited to the patient's needs is likely to be included.

5. *Obtain Feedback and Use the Teach-back Technique*: The pharmacist should solicit feedback from the patient at several points during the counseling session to ensure that the patient fully understands what he or she has heard. The teach-back technique discussed in Chapter 7 elucidates lack of knowledge or understanding and may reveal the nature of the misunderstanding, allowing a further communication by the pharmacist tailored to this.[20]

   In order to avoid embarrassment or reluctance on the part of the patient, this should be introduced in such a way as to place blame for any lack of understanding on the pharmacist rather than the patient, for example, "Just so I can be sure that I have made myself clear, could you show me how you are going to measure your blood sugar using the glucose meter."[20]

The pharmacist may also ask the patient, directly or through the translator, if the patient has any concerns or questions.

6. *Follow-up*: Follow-up contact with the patient or caregivers the next day and possibly regularly over the following weeks can be important to reinforce information and to detect any misunderstandings.

7. *Be Patient But Assertive and Allow Extra Time as Needed*: The pharmacist may need to make repeated efforts to make himself or herself understood, and may need to try a variety of counseling methods and education tools before being successful in gaining the patient's understanding. They should neither passively admit defeat nor aggressively persist with an unsuccessful method. Patients with comprehension difficulties require counseling to be slower, with repetition, and frequent praise for the patient's efforts. Patients with developmental disabilities have shorter attention spans and will benefit from frequent, short teaching sessions no longer than 15 to 20 minutes.[14]

8. *Respect the Individual Patient and His or Her Rights*: Above all, individual patients should be respected, regardless of their comprehension difficulties. They should never be talked down to or made fun of for their lack of comprehension.

Further suggestions for counseling patients with comprehension difficulties due to foreign language are made in the later section in this chapter about cultural issues.

Counseling Patients with Disabilities

Some patients have disabilities that can create challenges during patient counseling. One in five Americans reports having a disability, which may be a sensory disability such as hearing (deaf or hard of hearing) or sight (blind or visually impaired), a physical disability or mobility impairment, speech impairment or cognitive disability, or other self-care disability. In some jurisdictions, laws have been enacted to ensure that people with disabilities have accessibility to buildings, education, employment, and effective communication.[21,22] However, many health professionals are poorly trained to communicate appropriately and with sensitivity with patients with disabilities. Pharmacists and the pharmacy staff should be educated and prepared to interact with patients with disabilities with respect and understanding.

Tailoring Counseling for Patients with Disabilities

Recommendations have been made about etiquette for interacting with patients with disabilities and specifically issues involving communicating with and about people with disabilities. Pharmacists can improve counseling effectiveness with patients with disabilities by observing the following recommendations:

1. *Be Alert for Signs of Disabilities*: The pharmacist should note at the start of the encounter whether the patient has any apparent disabilities. Sometimes, however, disabilities may not be detectable at the beginning, but may become apparent during counseling. For example, a patient with hearing difficulties may respond inappropriately to questions; turn the head so that the ear faces the pharmacist; make

gestures to indicate that he or she is having difficulty hearing (cupping a hand behind an ear); make frequent requests for repetition; look around for the speaker; use loud speech; or omit word endings such as t, s, sh, f, and v.[23,24] The pharmacist must be tactful in detecting and inquiring about disabilities, and every effort should be made to make the patient feel comfortable and in no way inferior.

2. *Treat Patients with Disabilities with Dignity and Respect*: People often make inaccurate judgments about people with disabilities, particularly regarding their intellect and personalities.[1,21] In particular, it should be recognized that abilities vary with the individual patient and the type of disability so that, for example, patients with physical disabilities should not be considered to also have developmental disabilities. Actions such as addressing all patients with disabilities using slow speech, loud voice, or extravagant praise should be avoided.[25] However, neither the patient's disabilities nor the patient himself or herself should be ignored.

   Although the pharmacist may be interested or curious, he or she should not ask for details or the origin of a patient's disabilities as the patient may not want to discuss it.[22]

3. *Be Prepared for Feelings*: Pharmacists need to be prepared for the feelings that dealing with patients with disabilities may arouse in themselves and other staff such as embarrassment, aversion, pity, and dread.[25] In addition, the frustrations with their disabilities and irritation with others' attitudes can cause patients with disabilities to react aggressively or uncooperatively.[25] Pharmacists should try to make allowances for patients' feelings, and should perceive negative behavior as a result of these feelings rather than aimed personally at the pharmacist.

4. *Offer Assistance*: Assistance should be offered where the need is obvious or when the patient requests it, rather than automatically provided.[5,26] The patient should be asked what he or she would like done and how it can be accomplished, and the pharmacist should wait until the offer is accepted, then listen for instructions. For example, the patient should be asked how he or she prefers to be helped up the steps rather than just grabbing the patient's arms. One should never interfere with a person's control over assistive devices or move crutches or communication boards out of reach.[22]

5. *Allow Extra Time*: Extra time should be allowed for counseling patients with disabilities. Time may be needed for physical needs (e.g., maneuvering a wheelchair into a counseling area); the patient's slower speech; or the use of communication aids (e.g., pointing to words and letters on a communication board). Silence should be tolerated (for up to 20 to 30 seconds) to allow the patient to collect his or her thoughts and to prepare a response.[24] The pharmacist should simply wait quietly or cue the patient visually to indicate that the patient should continue. Of course, prolonged silence indicates communication breakdown.

6. *Communicate Appropriately*: Words and actions can be powerful, particularly when used inappropriately with and about people with disabilities. The focus should be on recognizing the patient as an individual rather than the disability; hence rather than speaking of "the disabled patient" we refer to "a patient with a disability."[26] Table 8-2 lists affirmative phrases to use as alternatives to negative phrases.[26]

   When first meeting a patient with a disability, if one would normally shake hands, then an offer should be made to shake hands even if the patient has limited hand use or wears an artificial limb, if necessary simply touching either the right or left hand or a prosthesis.

TABLE 8-2	Appropriate Words to Be Used When Communicating with and about People with Disabilities

Affirmative Phrases	Negative Phrases
Person with intellectual, cognitive, or developmental disability	Retarded, mentally defective
Person who is blind or person who is visually impaired	The blind
Person who is hard of hearing or person who is deaf	Suffers from hearing loss, deaf, deaf and dumb
Person with multiple sclerosis, cerebral palsy, muscular dystrophy, epilepsy, and so forth	Afflicted by . . . , victim of . . . , stricken by . . . Epileptic
Person who uses a wheelchair	Confined or restricted to a wheelchair
Person with a physical disability	Cripple, lame, deformed
Person unable to speak	Dumb, mute
Person with a psychiatric disability	Crazy, nuts

Adapted from Communicating with and about people with disabilities. U.S. Department of Labor. Office of Disability Employment Policy. Available online at www.dol.gov/odep/pubs/fact/comucate.htm (accessed June 2005)

7. *Involve the Patient and Solicit Feedback*: As discussed regarding patients with comprehension difficulties, efforts should be made to ensure that the patient is involved as much as possible in the discussion. The pharmacist should address the patient directly, rather than speaking to the caregiver. Direct vocal and eye contact should be made.[26]

   Every effort should be made to assess the patient's understanding and to respond to his or her concerns by soliciting feedback during patient counseling and using teach-back techniques. Follow-up contact should also be made to ensure patient understanding and to deal with any concerns or misunderstandings.

8. *Emphasize Nonverbal Communication*: Nonverbal communication is important when dealing with patients with disabilities such as facing the patient, inclining the body toward the patient, or holding the patient's hand. Such gestures can make the patient feel more comfortable and send the message that the pharmacist is interested in the patient. These nonverbal actions also cue the patient that the pharmacist is about to speak.[24] Although it is expected by people with disabilities that people may take a second look, staring for long periods is inappropriate, as is avoidance of eye contact altogether.

9. *Use Appropriate Counseling Methods and Aids*: The pharmacist should consider that printed or visual materials such as diagrams and videotape or computer-assisted programs may be more useful to patients with hearing disabilities, whereas patients with visual disabilities may prefer verbal counseling. Counseling aids such as braille labeling, various packaging methods, and calendars as described in Chapter 6 can assist patients to take medications and understand necessary information.

Where necessary, an interpreter or caregiver should be used as an intermediary, but the focus should continue to be on the patient.

10. *Attend to the Environment*: Preferably the counseling environment should be quiet and well lighted. The pharmacist should be positioned as close to the patient as possible for comfort, on the same level (e.g., the pharmacist should sit or squat down to the patient's eye level when speaking to a patient in a wheelchair). The pharmacy and counseling area should be accessible by wheelchairs and barriers such as boxes or extra furniture should be kept clear of walkways. Products and patient-information materials should be reachable from a wheelchair, and staff should be alerted to provide patients with assistance where it appears necessary. Decals and signs should be used in the pharmacy window to indicate that it is wheelchair accessible.[5] Some accommodations can be costly, but should be considered, such as telecommunication equipment or relay services (special operators who translate spoken into written words and vice versa).

    It should also be noted that automated telephone systems such as those often used in pharmacies for ordering prescription refills can pose difficulties for people with disabilities where comprehending instructions or pushing buttons can be a problem.[21]

11. *Learn More about People with Disabilities and How to Help Them*: Contact local chapters of organizations serving people with disabilities, such as the National Spinal Cord Injury Association, the Muscular Dystrophy Association, the Multiple Sclerosis Society, United Cerebral Palsy, and the Easter Seal Society.[5] Web sites such as the U.S. Department of Labor Office of Disability Employment Policy and National Organization on Disability, and Partnership for Clear Health Communication have many useful resources for dealing with people with various disabilities.

12. *Tailor Counseling to the Patient's Specific Disability*. Different disabilities require different modifications for counseling. Table 8-3 describes specific issues when dealing with patients who are deaf or hard of hearing, blind or have visual impairments, mobility impairments, speech impairments, or cognitive disabilities.[22,26]

Counseling Patients with Critical or Difficult Conditions

Although all patients have basic needs as human beings and as sufferers of illness, some patients have greater needs and require more specialized kinds of pharmacy services than others. Conditions where patients may have more intense needs and present particular difficulty in counseling include psychiatric illnesses and conditions that may be fatal, such as cancer and AIDS-related conditions. Other conditions such as diabetes, smoking, and obesity may be particularly difficult because they require significant lifestyle modification.

In these critical or difficult conditions, patients are faced with a variety of issues that significantly affect their emotions, their ability to cope and function in the community, and limit their quality of life. These all affect their pharmaceutical care needs and their ability to adhere to medication.

Pharmacists who practice in specialty clinics and hospital departments come to understand these issues and find ways to tailor counseling to best meet these patients' needs. With the advent of new technologies and treatment options, many of these special

TABLE 8-3	Tips for Communicating with Patients with Different Disabilities
Patients who are hard of hearing	Do not yell
	Enunciate clearly and face the person directly, with the light facing the pharmacist
	Avoid obscuring face with bowed head, beard, or masks
	Use simple sentences and familiar vocabulary to facilitate lip reading
	Supplement verbal explanations with written notes, print materials, or charts and diagrams
	In cases of total deafness, a family member or caregiver who knows sign language may be able to provide assistance
	Allow the patient to select preferred mode of communication, and supply it if at all possible, e.g., reading lips, writing notes, interpreter, teletypewriters (TTY), or telecommunications devices for the deaf (TDD)
Patients who are visually impaired	Identify yourself and any other people who are with him or her, using people's names to clarify to whom the conversation is being directed
	Vary the size of medication bottles and containers to help identification of different medications
	Use bright-colored stickers for patients with limited vision
	Use description when giving instructions, e.g., take the large, round pill in the tallest container
	If the patient uses a companion dog, do not pet the dog while he or she is working
	When offering a seat, gently place the individual's hand on the back or arm of the chair so he or she can locate the seat
Patients with mobility difficulties	Don't lean on a person's wheelchair
	Sit or squat down so that you will be at eye level
	When telephoning the patient, allow the phone to ring longer than usual to allow the patient time to reach the phone
Patients with speech difficulties	Concentrate on what the individual is saying
	Do not speak for the individual or attempt to finish sentences
	If you don't understand, do not pretend to understand, but rather ask the patient to repeat or ask the patient if writing is an alternative
Dealing with patients with cognitive disabilities	Move to a quiet or private area free of distractions
	Be prepared to repeat instructions
	Be patient and flexible
	See also previous section on patients with comprehension difficulties

Sources: Eigen B. Improving communication with the physically disabled. Am Pharm. 1982;NS22(10):37–40; Anon. Fact Sheet: The use of over-the-counter medicines. National Council on Patient Information and Education. Available online at www.bemedwise.org/press_room/sep_2003_fact_otc.pdf (accessed January 2005); Tabor PA, Lopez DA. Comply with us: improving medication adherence. J Pharmacy Pract, 2004;17:167–181; Disability etiquette tips. National Organization on Disability. Available on line at www.nod.org (accessed March 2005); Communicating with and about people with disabilities. U.S. Department of Labor. Office of Disability Employment Policy. Available online at www.dol.gov/odep/pubs/fact/comucate.htm (accessed June 2005).

and difficult conditions are being treated in the community and so community pharmacists need to understand and meet their needs.

Issues Faced by Patients with Critical or Difficult Conditions

Patients with critical or difficult conditions are faced with a number of issues including therapeutic, psychosocial, environmental, and communication challenges.[27] Understanding these issues will help pharmacists identify the increased pharmaceutical care needs of these patients, and ways that counseling needs to be tailored. Issues faced by specific patients with psychiatric illnesses, cancer, HIV/AIDS, and patients making behavior change such as quitting smoking or losing weight are presented in Table 8-4.[26]

Therapeutic Issues. Patients with critical or difficult conditions often have symptoms such as severe and/or chronic pain, extreme and disruptive moods, fatigue or physical disfigurement. At times this can be very debilitating, making it difficult for the patient to perform needed functions or attend counseling.

A variety of issues involving medication use result in a greater likelihood that patients with critical or difficult conditions will be nonadherent. They generally take a

TABLE 8-4	**Counseling Issues and Needs for Patients with Critical or Difficult Conditions**
Patients with psychiatric illnesses	May at times act "different," avoid eye contact, make bizarre statements, demand attention, have emotional outbursts
	May refuse to adhere to medications because of experiencing side effects, fear of side effects, perceptions of treatment ineffectiveness, length of time to experience effect, denial of need[31,32]
	Ability to communicate and focus on information may be affected by patient's mood, cognitive state
	Often experience social stigma and embarrassment because of condition
Patients with HIV/AIDS	On many different medications (up to 24 in some cases)
	Poor adherence to medication due to polypharmacy, forgetfulness, inconvenience, scheduling, occurrence or avoidance of side effects, uncertainty regarding drug efficacy[33]
	Often use alternative and unorthodox treatments without reporting use
	Access to costly medication can pose hardship
	Patient is often unable to work and therefore often in financial need
	Experience social stigma and isolation because of condition

(Continued)

TABLE 8-4 **(Continued)**	
Patients with cancer	Treatments provided at home and at intervals in hospital making continuity of treatment a problem due to lack of communication among health care providers
	Access to treatments may require travel to treatment center far from home, which is inconvenient and isolating from social support networks
	Treatments often cause severe adverse effects
	Nonadherence to pain medication results from fear of addiction
	May have poor control of pain because of poor pain management by health professionals
	Access to costly medications can pose financial hardship
	Often use alternative and unorthodox treatments without reporting use
	Must make decisions about multiple treatment options and digest complicated information about treatments and their risks
	Palliative care may involve many health professionals who may not communicate well
Patients making behavior change such as quitting smoking or losing weight	Need to understand the physical, social, environmental, and emotional aspects of the problem behavior
	Must be motivated to change
	Need support through various stages of change
	Consider medication and nonmedication approaches
	Must include behavioral management along with medication for success
	Patient should expect relapses and be encouraged to restart therapy
	Require ongoing support for 6 months to a year
	Consider social supports
	May require referral for additional help such as support groups, counseling, alternative therapies

Sources: Rantucci M. Counselling special patient groups. CE Compliance Centre National Continuing Education Program, 2004. Available at: www.pharmacyconnects.com/pdfs/2004/08/NovCE_Aug.pdf (accessed June 2005); Kelly GH, Scott JE. Medication compliance and health education among outpatients with chronic mental disease. Med Care. 1990;28(12):1181–1197; Hogan TP, Awad AG, Eastwood R. A self-report scale of drug compliance in schizophrenics: Reliability and discriminative validity. Psychol Med. 1983;(13):177–183; Foisy M. Pharmacists and HIV. Pharm Pract. 1995;11(5):56–58, 62–68.

variety of medications to manage their symptoms and the adverse effects of other medications. Multiple and varied administration schedules and administration routes may change frequently and can be confusing and uncomfortable as well as inconvenient, sometimes requiring the patient to be admitted to the hospital or attend an outpatient clinic to receive therapy. These medications are often potent and sometimes experimental, with a high risk of adverse events and side effects that are uncomfortable and often serious such as compromised kidney and liver function or decreased immunity to infections. There may also be embarrassing side effects such as hair loss, loss of libido, skin rashes, and diarrhea.

Patients with critical or difficult conditions may also seek out nontraditional treatments from a variety of alternative practitioners and substances. Some patients may ask the pharmacist about these treatments, but others may take them without consultation, possibly to avoid censure or ridicule. The results may be disastrous if these treatments counteract traditional medications or cause adverse effects or, worse yet, cause the patient to discontinue possibly effective treatments. It may also cause confusion since the efficacy of traditional treatments may not be accurately assessed.

Psychosocial Issues. As discussed in Chapter 3, patients faced with serious, chronic, or terminal illnesses may experience a range of feelings including frustration at the disruption in their lives and inability to perform usual activities and functions; fear and anxiety about symptoms and illness prognosis and the social consequences of their illnesses such as loss of job and status; feelings of damage or being "different" in some way as a result of physical changes as well as from just being ill and having to take medications. They may also experience anger, dependency, and guilt at not being able to be the person they were (parent, caregiver, lover, bread-winner). This may lead to feelings of loss of self-esteem and depression which may require treatment if it becomes severe.

Patients faced with terminal, chronic, or serious illnesses and their families may go through a series of emotional stages including denial, anger, bargaining, depression, and hopefully acceptance.[28] They may go through these stages in varying order or may continually cycle through these emotions as the disease progresses.

Although disease and public health organizations and the popular media have attempted to educate the public, patients with conditions such as HIV/AIDS and mental illness often face social stigmas. Pharmacists and other health care workers may also react with bias, fear, and discomfort causing them to minimize interaction with these patients, avoiding necessary information provision and monitoring. As a result patients may isolate themselves and resist communication.

As discussed in Chapter 3, patients may also have feelings surrounding medication use, such as embarrassment, resulting in nonadherence.[29] In addition, patients with critical and difficult conditions will have a large amount of information to process and assess about their prognosis, treatment choices, risk of side effects, and effectiveness of medications, and have difficult decisions to make. As discussed in Chapter 4, this is very difficult for most people to do, and can cause patients further distress and anxiety.

Finally, patients with critical or difficult conditions will have a diminished quality of life. Their perceptions of their abilities and satisfaction with those abilities will be changed; their physical, emotional, mental, and intellectual capacity may be diminished; and their ability to function at work, in social situations, and within the family may be seriously affected. Their motivation to make the necessary lifestyle changes and maintain them may also be limited.

Environmental Issues. Patients with critical or difficult conditions need a great deal of social support from family or friends including help with activities of daily living such as bathing, dressing, shopping, and transportation; help with medication administration and social contact. Unfortunately, some patients cannot get the needed support because they are isolated geographically or emotionally, causing them to deteriorate physically and mentally. They may also lose motivation to adhere to medication regimens.

Patients with critical or difficult conditions may also have difficulties accessing care. Waiting lists or geographical distance from health care facilities may make access to the necessary specialized physicians, physiotherapists, dieticians, psychologists, nurses, and pharmacists difficult. Treatments, diagnostic procedures, or medications may not be available or available only under specific, documented conditions as a result of hospital or drug-plan policies. As a result, necessary treatments may not be available, and monitoring of symptoms and therapeutic interventions may not occur. Adverse effects may go undetected or ineffective treatments may not be adjusted.

Communication Issues. Patients with critical or difficult conditions have a lot of information needs. However, the information provided is often very complicated, and may not include explanations or definition of terms, making it incomprehensible. In addition, because of their physical and mental states, these patients may find it difficult to read or hear information, or to concentrate or remember. They may require extra time as well as assurances.

Pharmacists may find patients with critical or difficult conditions demanding and difficult to communicate with. This may be a direct result of the condition, for example, psychiatric conditions can cause thought and mood disorders, or because of the various emotional, psychological, and environmental issues noted above. They may look to the pharmacist or others to fulfill some of their emotional needs.

Pharmacists may also find that they have to communicate with these patients through caregivers who may make inaccurate assessments of the patient's needs or miscommunicate information provided.

Tailoring Counseling for Patients with Critical or Difficult Conditions

Counseling in these situations can be most effective by tailoring counseling in a number of ways.

1. *Use Empathy and Tact*: It is particularly important for the pharmacist to be tactful in discussing the condition, being careful to use the patient's own terms. Be sure the patient is aware that his or her condition is serious or fatal before mentioning this.
2. *Deal with Personal Biases and Fears*: Pharmacists themselves may have biases and fears regarding the condition that may cause them to avoid discussion or to offer false reassurance.
3. *Identify the Patient's Needs*: The patient's understanding of the condition, as well as his or her attitudes toward treatment are important to ascertain, particularly concerning the patient's willingness to participate in the treatment.[30] Detailed questions should be asked in this regard, and an assessment form should be used to assist the pharmacist in asking specific questions related to the patient's condition.[30]

Documentation by the pharmacist of the patient's needs at the first counseling session and at follow-up sessions will help the pharmacist track particular concerns and take appropriate action. Needs specific to particular conditions are identified in Table 8-4.[27,31–33]

4. *Help the Patient Make Adjustments to Daily Life*: Since these conditions are long term and require many adjustments the patient's life, pharmacists should pay particular attention to helping patients integrate medication use into their daily lives. In addition, monitoring for effectiveness and side effects could be assisted through use of a log book for the patient to record daily occurrences, attentive follow-up by the pharmacist at repeat visits, and arranged follow-up telephone calls or home visits.

   Due to the complexity of regimens for many of these conditions, the pharmacist should assist the patient in organizing and remembering doses, as well as, where possible, making recommendations to the physician for simplifying regimens.[34]

   Referral to support groups will assist the patient in learning about others in similar conditions and provide self-help tools and social contact.

5. *Assist the Patient to Understand the Condition, Treatment Choices, and Risk Information*: Because of the large volume of information presented to the patient, he or she will need the pharmacist to help organize it and make sense of it. Providing educational materials in various forms (e.g., print, audiovisual, and computer Web sites) including information about risks and decision-making tools as discussed in Chapter 6 will help the patient make informed decisions. The pharmacist should review common terminology for the condition with the patient to assist the patient to comprehend information and to participate in discussions with other health professionals.

6. *Encourage Participation By the Patient in His or Her Treatment*: Participation by the patient is particularly important, since treatment will be ongoing. The patient should be taught how to monitor his or her condition, be encouraged to suggest changes according to his or her own needs, and take responsibility for his or her treatment as much as possible. This will increase the patient's feelings of self-worth and make him or her more psychologically able to deal with other aspects of the condition.

7. *Provide Additional Motivational Counseling*: Due to the long duration of treatment, the patient will need additional motivational counseling. More supervision, use of adherence aids, changes to reduce or eliminate side effects, goal-setting, and improvements in the patient–clinician relationship may be used to enhance the motivation of these patients.[30,34] The pharmacist should use the motivational counseling and behavior change techniques discussed in Chapter 7.

8. *Provide follow-up*: Ongoing reinforcement and support will be needed through follow-up. Appointments, home visits, and telephone follow-up can be used according to the patient's needs.

9. *Provide an Appropriate Counseling Environment*: Providing privacy is particularly important for counseling these patients, since discussions will likely involve the patient's feelings and concerns about his or her condition and treatment. They may also need somewhere to sit down as they will often be physically debilitated. If possible, the pharmacist should make home visits when patients are unable to come to the pharmacy.

10. *Provide Empathy and Emotional Support to Patients and Their Caregivers*: As discussed earlier, patients with critical or difficult conditions and their families experience a range of emotions and may go through various stages of emotions. Suggestions were made in Chapter 3 for ways that pharmacists can help patients with these emotions. The following suggestions are also helpful:[35,36]

   - Be as relaxed as possible.
   - Show genuine concern and care.
   - Use listening skills as well as nonverbal communication to let the patient know you are interested as well as to encourage the patient to express his or her own feelings.
   - Allow silence.
   - Be prepared to defer counseling to another time if the patient does not feel well enough.
   - Help the patient make choices.
   - Do not tell the patient how he or she should feel or that you know how he or she feels.
   - Do not try to talk the patient out of feeling angry, depressed, sad, and so forth.
   - Be as honest as possible.

   Support for patients and their caregivers can also be provided through referral to various community and disease-specific organizations such as the Cancer Society, which may provide a range of services such as transportation to appointments, education, respite for families, and counseling.

11. *Have a Nonbiased Approach to Patient's Treatment Choices*: Since patients with critical and difficult conditions may explore the use of alternative treatments, the pharmacist should be prepared to provide information in an unbiased way. Recommend reliable information sources such as the Cancer Society where up-to-date information on available treatments and tips on evaluating them may be provided. Patients should be counseled to follow the guidelines provided by the Cancer Society, including:[37]

   - Tell all involved health professionals about alternative treatments being used.
   - Use products for short periods and in moderation.
   - Do not use an alternative treatment in place of prescribed treatment and be aware of possible interactions.
   - Purchase products from reputable suppliers.
   - Be cautious when using highly concentrated oils and teas.
   - Do not give to children.

12. *Advocate for Patient's Right to Information, Access to Care, and Resources*: Because patients who are critically ill or have difficult conditions are preoccupied with their symptoms and the many issues discussed earlier, they may need assistance searching out information and finding the care and resources they need. Pharmacists can assist with this by keeping up-to-date lists of resources available in the community and be familiar with how the patient can access these; be aware of available treatment options; and when necessary make contacts for the patient and explain the patient's needs.

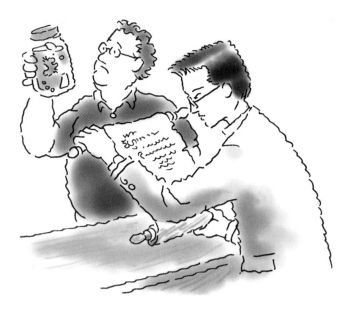

I haven't heard about Eye of Newt being helpful for
your condition, but I will try to find some information
for you.

13. *Become Part of the Patient's Care Team*: Because care for these patients is so involved, it is important for a team approach to be taken, with pharmacists involved in treatment decisions, monitoring and adjusting medications. Keeping the lines of communication open and preventing misunderstandings between the patient and other health professionals can be an important role for the pharmacist. This may require assertiveness as well as tact when dealing with other health professionals as discussed in Chapter 7.

Counseling Elderly Patients

Elderly patients comprise a growing segment of the pharmacist's clientele. As mentioned earlier, elderly patients in no way form a homogeneous group. They vary greatly, not only in their physical and mental capacities, but also in their financial circumstances and personal wants and needs. The number of illness conditions and medications used tends to increase with age, so that there may be great variations between 60-year-old and 90-year-old patients (all considered *elderly*), but there may also be great differences among individuals. As a result, each patient should be considered on an individual basis.

Issues in Counseling Elderly Patients

There are many issues that require special consideration of elderly patients in regard to medication counseling.

1. *High Drug Use*: Elderly patients use more prescriptions than any other group of patients. Although people over 65 years of age comprise 12% of the US population,

they use 30% of all prescription drugs and 40% of nonprescription drugs, so that two-thirds of persons 65 years and over take a prescription or nonprescription drug, on average four to five prescription drugs and two nonprescription drugs.[38,39]

2. *High Incidence of Illness*: Elderly patients experience an increased incidence of illness, particularly chronic illnesses; 80% of people over 65 years of age report at least one chronic ailment. On average, older persons have six diseases, more often chronic than acute, half of which their primary physician may be unaware.[40]

3. *Increased Risks of Drug-related Problems and Inappropriate Drug Use*: Since aging is accompanied by various changes in physiology, the pharmacokinetics of many drugs are different from expected, resulting in an increased risk of adverse reactions in elderly patients, nearly double that of younger adults.[19,24,41,42] Up to 75% of seniors have been found to have drug-related problems including drug interactions, adverse drug reactions, lack of effect or excess effects, and unnecessary use of medications.[43] A 2004 national US study found that 12.6% of elderly patients treated in emergency departments between 1992 and 2000 were administered an inappropriate medication.[41]

4. *Increased Limitations and Disabilities*: Forty-two percent of elderly Americans experience disabilities such as hearing loss (experienced by 60%) and vision impairment even with corrective lenses (experienced by 20%).[44] Other disabilities experienced by elderly people include physical, mental, dementia, language disorders often resulting from stroke (dysarthria, dysphasia), difficulties eating because of dental problems, altered pain threshold, transportation difficulties, diminished personal economic resources, loss of physical energy, and isolation.[24,45,46] As discussed earlier, these disabilities limit access to care as well as ability to adhere to medication, and require consideration when pharmacists interact with elderly patients.

5. *Decline in Cognitive Functioning*: Although cognitive functioning changes at varying rates with age, there is a general decline in short-term memory that may cause patients to forget or become confused about how and when to take medication, or the reason for taking it.[47] Elderly patients may also experience confusion as a result of sleep problems, changing drug regimes and drug-induced cognitive dysfunction.[48,49]

    Ability to learn also declines with age because of a decrease in general intelligence, information processing, problem solving, and approach to learning.[50,51]

6. *Difficulties Adhering to Medication Regimens*: Studies of elderly patients find that nonadherence (intentional and nonintentional) ranges from 26% to 59%, which is not significantly different from other age groups, but may have different causes.[47] Misunderstanding the purpose, forgetfulness, difficulty seeing or hearing instructions, intolerable adverse effects, inability to take medication (difficulty opening vial, trouble swallowing), belief that drug is not needed, fear of side effects, perceived lack of efficacy, and cost have been reported as reasons for elderly patients' nonadherence.[47] In addition, elderly patients have been found to have more difficulty than younger patients in distinguishing between tablets of similar size, shape, and color.[18]

7. *Attitudinal Barriers to Communication*: Apart from the barriers of disabilities and cognitive decline as discussed earlier, elderly patients experience attitudinal barriers to communication. Pharmacists may view elderly patients in a stereotypical

way, as frail, confused, slow, hard of hearing, and needy. Younger pharmacists in particular may have difficulty in understanding an elderly patient's point of view, the effects of history and experiences on their attitudes, and ways of behaving that have become rigid over time and experience. Pharmacists may experience fear of aging such as anxiety about changing appearance, infirmity, dependence, and death and this may cause stress in the relationship.[50]

Elderly patients may also have attitudes that can inhibit communication as they may adhere to beliefs, values, and perceptions from their younger years such as the need to hoard medications, embarrassment about their body functions, keeping health matters private, and suffering in silence.[52]

8. *Literacy and Cultural Issues*: Elderly patients may be more likely than other age groups to have a low level of education such that educational materials may pose difficulties. Elderly patients in many countries such as the United States may be from a wide variety of cultures, and although acclimatized to a large degree, may have language difficulties or beliefs and health practices that may interfere with communication and medication use.

9. *Access and Affordability to Health Care Services*: Most elderly people are on fixed and diminished incomes such that the increasing costs of drugs, if not privately or publicly funded, can cause hardship or lack of adherence.

Tailoring Counseling for Elderly Patients

A survey of elderly patients found that they tend to be quite loyal customers (three out of five said they use only one pharmacy regularly) and are generally satisfied with their pharmacies.[53] Although low costs were at the top of their wish lists, the elderly also reported wanting quality of care, information from the pharmacist, and friendliness. In another survey, elderly patients were more willing than other age groups to pay for information services from the pharmacist.[54]

Pharmacists should tailor counseling for elderly patients in the following ways:

1. *Recognize Feelings and Attitudes toward Aging*: Pharmacists should remember that the elderly patient has not always been old.[45] The pharmacist should ask himself or herself, "What was this person like when he or she was my age? When was that? What was going on in the world then? What has happened in the intervening years?"[45] In this way, the pharmacist might better understand what the patient's difficulties are today, particularly if he or she spends a few minutes actually discussing some of these questions with the patient before getting down to the details of the medication counseling.[45]

2. *Conduct Regular Medications Reviews and Be Alert for Drug-related Problems*: As a result of the greater risks of elderly patients experiencing drug use problems, patient counseling for elderly patients should involve regular, detailed discussion of medication use, particularly for patients whose clinical conditions have changed. This should include regular monitoring for adverse reactions. Psychoactive drugs should be aggressively monitored and signs of extrapyramidal, cognitive effects, and constipation should be particularly noted. The dosing of new drugs should be assessed for appropriateness, preferably starting low and slowly increasing. Drugs with high risk of cognitive effects such as hypnotics, narcotics, and those with anticholinergic effects should be avoided if possible.[49,55,56]

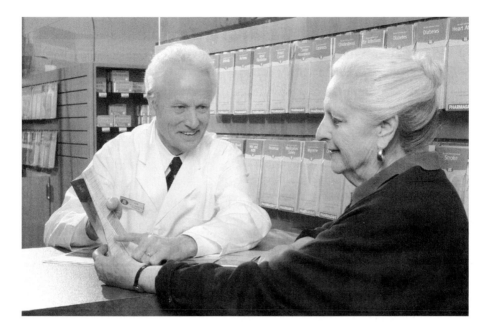

Figure 8-1   Elderly Patients Should Be Educated about How to Monitor Medication Effectiveness (Courtesy of Pharmasave Drugs National Ltd.)

3. *Educate Elderly Patients about Self-monitoring*: Patients should be given information regarding the purpose of all medications and ways to detect effectiveness. They should also be told ways to identify adverse effects, ways to reduce the chance of occurrence, what to do if they occur, how to modify the effects, and when to report to the physician immediately (Figure 8-1).

4. *Allow Time*: In the initial phase of the counseling session, pharmacists should spend time making the patient comfortable, discussing general topics as desired by the patient. This not only helps the pharmacist–patient relationship (particularly for lonely, isolated patients), but also allows the pharmacist to evaluate difficulties that may potentially interfere with medication use as mentioned above.

5. *Allow for Disabilities*: If disabilities are identified, the pharmacist should make sure that the techniques discussed earlier for counseling patients with disabilities are used. If memory problems or dementia of any type is suspected, the pharmacist may consider administering a mental status assessment such as the Short Mental Status questionnaire.[57] If this indicates a concern, then the patient should be asked if other family members or caregivers can be contacted to reinforce medication information. The pharmacist should also ask permission to discuss concerns with the patient's physician, as this may be the first indication of problems.

6. *Provide Follow-up*: For patients who live alone, careful monitoring is important, and follow-up contact arrangements should be made.

7. *Provide Privacy*: Privacy should also be considered, since the elderly often become embarrassed at sharing personal information.[54]

8. *Emphasize Adherence*: In a review of studies of drug use by elderly patients, Green et al. found that, in spite of all the difficulties faced by the elderly, there is no evidence to conclude that the elderly are more nonadherent than younger patients.[58] However, since the need of the elderly to adhere to medication is particularly critical given the seriousness of many of their conditions, the pharmacist should tailor counseling to put some emphasis on ensuring adherence. Attention should be made in particular to the causes of nonadherence more specific to the elderly as discussed earlier.

9. *Select Appropriate Counseling Methods and Aids*: When selecting the method of information provision to elderly patients, pharmacists should consider patients' disabilities as well as their learning style and provide material that they can easily use and understand (e.g., large print labels). Compliance packaging and referral to home care for assistance with medication use will assist the patient with adherence.

   Studies of different education strategies used for the elderly have concluded that drug knowledge is most likely to be improved by providing small amounts of specific information, and by a combination of reminder aids with oral reinforcement.[59,60] Since registering new information and retrieving information tend to be impaired in the elderly, simple formats such as short lists and uncomplicated content and frequent review of material should be used.[51] Well-organized materials, related where possible to previously learned material, will assist patients' problem-solving ability.[51] It may be helpful to schedule several sessions to cover information about large numbers of new medications (e.g., when a patient is discharged from the hospital) so that the patient does not become overwhelmed.

   Studies of the elderly have found that they like information grouped into categories: General information, how to take medication, and outcomes. When counseling is organized in this way, it is more likely to be remembered.[61] Written materials should also be organized in this way, and be in readable form (i.e., large print if necessary). In addition, elderly patients reportedly like having written information to take home and peruse at their own pace, or possibly to review with another caregiver.

10. *Involve Caregivers and Community Supports*: If caregivers are available, they should be informed about the potential risks for drug-related problems and, wherever possible, included in counseling. If the elderly patient is without supports at home, he or she should be referred to available community resources for assessment and if necessary to supply help with activities of daily living and medication use. Where possible, pharmacists should occasionally make home visits to elderly patients in order to assess medication use habits such as storage and organization.

DEALING WITH DIFFICULT ISSUES

As noted at the beginning of this chapter, regardless of the patient's characteristics or conditions, issues arise in pharmacy practice that present challenges and require modification of counseling or special approaches to handle the situation. These issues include cultural issues, medication incidents, and a variety of nontherapeutic issues that do not involve a particular drug or therapy but require appropriate handling such as on patients' questions and suspected child abuse, unwanted pregnancy, drug abuse, or threatened suicide. It should be noted here that the pharmacist should view the issue, not the patient, as the problem.

Cultural Issues

As discussed in Chapter 7, communication and counseling can be challenging in a multicultural society. Pharmacists and their patients often come from diverse cultural backgrounds that can affect their perceptions of health and medication use and how they communicate.

Culture is multidimensional and involves language, nonverbal behavior, and how one relates to others. It helps determine beliefs, values, and world view.[62] All individuals belong to a culture, although they may adhere to a set of cultural patterns in varying degrees. People tend to be ethnocentric, seeing other cultures from their own culture's perspective. This leads to poor intercultural communication and lack of sensitivity.

Pharmacists need to understand, acknowledge, and respect cultural diversity in order to communicate and counsel patients and meet their needs. It should be noted here, however, that ethnicity does not necessarily predict individual behavior.[63] All humans share feelings of need, fear, mistrust, and lack of control and hope, in spite of cultural diversity.[63]

Culturally based issues may affect treatment choice (from the patient's and health professional's clinical and personal perspectives), reaction to illness and treatment, and patient–health professional communication. As a result it can affect counseling in many ways. It may affect rapport with the pharmacist because of biases by the pharmacist or patient (e.g., the patient does not want to speak with a male or female pharmacist) or communication barriers; ability to gather information, assess patient's needs, or identify drug-related problems; and ability to provide information and resolve drug-related problems.[61]

Effect of Culture on an Individual Patient's Health Care

A patient's culture can affect his or her health care in many ways including health beliefs, treatment choices and prevention strategies, religion, family roles, personal health disclosure, language barriers, nonverbal communication, health literacy, and attitude toward health care workers. Communication and health literacy aspects were discussed in detail in Chapters 6 and 7.

Health Beliefs. A patient's understanding of the cause, treatment, and prevention of illness and how he or she perceives his or her health problems and treatments are all affected by the patient's health beliefs. People have beliefs about how one becomes sick or injured, the words to use to describe body parts and symptoms, how to behave when one is ill or injured, what one needs (or is allowed) to say or do to feel better.[65]

It is important for the pharmacist to recognize health beliefs so that treatments can be matched accordingly. Patients may not seek treatment or will wait until conditions are at a late stage, due to culturally based attitudes that illnesses should be kept private or illness is simply fate resulting in misdiagnosis, unnecessary procedures and treatments, and failure to treat.[58]

It can be difficult, however, to recognize patients' health beliefs since patients may not be aware that they need to discuss them, or may be reluctant to reveal that they are being treated by a nontraditional healer, or that they are using folk remedies.[64]

Three general systems of health beliefs are held by various cultures around the world: Biomedical, personalistic, and naturalistic.[66] Table 8-5 illustrates the

TABLE 8-5	Cultural Health Belief Systems and Effect on Health Care

Belief System	Health Beliefs	Effect on Health Care
Biomedical system	Dominant health belief system in North America Focuses on an objective diagnosis and scientific explanation for disease Illness is believed to result from abnormality in body functioning or structure through agents such as bacteria, viruses, or physical conditions such as injury or aging Disease is diagnosed when the body is clearly deviating from the norm The focus of the biomedical belief system is on the body, not the mind	Believe the goals of treatment are to return the body to normal by destroying or removing the causative agent, repair affected body parts, control the affected body system, and return the body to normal with medication, surgery, or nutrition Preventing illness involves avoiding the causes of illness
Personalistic system	Held by some Asians, Vietnamese, and Laotians Believe that disease or illness is caused by a supernatural or nonhuman being (deity, ghost, or evil spirit), or a human witch or sorcerer as a form of punishment	Aim to create a positive relationship with the entities causing the illness by shocking or scaring the spirit into leaving the body Prefer treatments that physically ward off evil spirits, consulting with folk healers and conducting ceremonial exorcisms
Naturalistic system	Belief that disease is an imbalance among elements in the body, mind, or environment Asians believe the balance is between yin and yang Mexicans and Puerto Ricans believe in the need to balance 4 body humors: Blood (hot and wet), yellow bile (hot and dry), phlegm (cold and wet), and black bile (cold and dry) African, Haitian, Jamaican, and Native Americans believe that illness is caused by disharmony with nature Native Americans view illness as a fate to be accepted like birth or death	Treatment involves restoring balance, often with a remedy that is opposite in nature Foods and herbs restore balance by treating cold illnesses with hot remedies, and hot illnesses with cold remedies Folk remedies involve looking beyond the symptoms of the illness for imbalances in relationship with the environment, emotions, social, spiritual, and physical factors Prevention involves maintaining the balance of forces

Based on information presented in Samovar L, Porter R. Cultural Influences on Context: The Health Care Setting. In: Communication Between Cultures, 4th Edition. Wadsworth, Belmont CA, 2001. p. 241–258.

various cultural health beliefs and the effects on treatment choices and preventive measures.

Religion. Spirituality may have an impact on prevention and treatment of illness. Positive effects of religious commitment such as diet and social practices and mental attitude generally far outweigh the negative effects.[66] However, specific religious teachings may cause refusal of treatment (e.g., Jehovah's Witnesses) and fatalistic beliefs can lead people to deny responsibility for health or illness.

Family. Some cultural groups have close-knit extended families, church, and community organizations that provide support and can play an important role in response to treatment and recovery. Conversely, treatment can be difficult when culture causes families to react negatively to such conditions as mental illness or unwanted pregnancy.

Fairly rigid family roles in some cultures result in male dominance, modesty and female purity, and specific rituals involving pregnancy and childbirth.[66] In Middle Eastern, Asian, Latin American, Mexican, and African cultures, men will generally answer questions, make decisions about a family member's health care, and sometimes refuse to deal with female health care workers. In other cultures, such as Hispanic, the mother or grandmother may make health care decisions.[63]

Cultural beliefs about modesty may prevent women from seeking care or medical advice. A girl may be punished for immodesty in order to preserve family honor and may refuse to undress for a medical examination.

Attitudes, practices, and behaviors surrounding childbirth and pregnancy are specific to most cultures. For example, the expression of emotion or pain during childbirth may be considered shameful (Asian cultures) or welcomed (Middle Eastern, Mexican, and Italian cultures).

Personal Disclosure. The ability or willingness of a patient to discuss personal information with health care providers may also be influenced by culture. There may be a lack of trust of medicine or health care providers.[63]

Some high-context cultures view talk about personal matters in poor taste and some may not wish to discuss "female problems." Since family members or others may need to translate, the patient may feel inhibited about discussing certain issues.

Communication. As discussed in Chapter 7, language and different meanings of words for symptoms and so forth can affect communication between cultures. Certain symptoms or feelings may be difficult to articulate and health jargon may be nontranslatable. Low literacy resulting in lack of health knowledge causes poor self-management skills and nonadherence.[63]

Cultural issues affecting nonverbal messages such as eye contact, facial expression, space, and touch can also make the patient–health care provider relationship difficult.

Attitude toward Health Care Workers and Health Care. Health care providers may be perceived as less credible because of casual dress or informal forms of address. Alternatively, white-coated health professionals may represent authority figures, causing reluctance or distress for immigrants who have suffered from torture or abuse. Misunderstandings due to language and communication issues and dissatisfaction with health care professionals can also result in poor response to medications.[67]

Western treatments may also be viewed with disbelief or caution, causing patients to take smaller doses or stop taking medications altogether. Views of treatment as symptom removal may make it difficult to treat patients with a chronic illness because they see no need to continue once symptoms are gone.[63]

Finally, confusion and dangerous side effects may occur because patients may access medications from their home country where fewer drug regulations make drugs that are available only by prescription in their new country available for self-treatment without the knowledge of current health care providers.[63]

Disease and Treatments. Some people have increased susceptibility for some illnesses and varying effects of treatments as a result of cultural environment, health beliefs, and behavior and genetic differences.[63,65] Culture may also affect the types of treatments patients expect, accept, or adhere to.

Poor metabolism and increased side effects can occur as a result of genetic variation in drug metabolism enzymes and proteins involved in drug response or disease progression.[63,65] These gene variations have a higher likelihood of occurring in some racial groups, most clinically significant in cardiovascular and central nervous system agents.

Some ethnic groups are also more susceptible to certain disease conditions. Most notably, people of African descent in North America have higher prevalence of hypertension, retaining more salt.[63] They are also more likely to suffer from death and disease from smoking because of higher rates of smoking and slower metabolism of nicotine.

Diet and lifestyle may contribute to ethnic differences in disease and drug effects. For example, aboriginal people in Canada suffer from a higher rate of rheumatism and arthritis, high blood pressure, and diabetes as a result of genetic predisposition to fat storage combined with a less-active lifestyle and a high-fat diet.[68]

Mental and emotional health problems due to loss of personal and cultural identity, depression, and post-traumatic stress disorder can be a major problem for refugees in their new countries.[69,70]

Techniques to Address Multicultural Issues

Pharmacists can provide pharmaceutical care and counseling to multicultural patients and improve intercultural communication by addressing personal attitudes and biases, and by using techniques to address language differences and cultural sensitivities.[71,64]

1. *Be Aware of Personal Attitudes and Perceptions and Multicultural Issues*: Pharmacists must recognize the complexity of the situation and cultural issues and be willing to address them. They must recognize their own cultural biases and stereotyping of other cultures. They must examine their beliefs and note how they influence attitudes toward individual patients and how they tend to communicate with people who are different. They should consider their levels of tolerance of strong accents or different modes of dress. Above all they should try to view things from the patient's point of view, i.e., although the idea of a male family member speaking for the female may seem wrong to a North American female, the pharmacist should consider that a woman from a different culture is probably comfortable with it.

2. *Make Concessions to Cultural Preferences and Customs Where Possible*: Pharmacists should get to know the various cultural groups that are predominant in their practice community. They should attempt to learn some of the important customs, forms of communication, and health beliefs by attending cultural events or studying the culture. These issues should then be addressed during interactions with multicultural patients. All pharmacy staff should be educated on cultural issues of groups in the community.

3. *As Much as Possible Communicate in an Understandable Language*: The pharmacy staff should match the cultural mix in the community as much as possible so there is always someone who can translate or clear up misunderstandings resulting from

cultural issues. Although it is not always possible for pharmacists to learn new languages, they can learn how to pronounce common names and proper ways of addressing people (last names are not always used and family names can be confusing). Key phrases, greetings, ways of referring to symptoms, and common medication instructions can also be learned. As discussed earlier, various counseling methods and counseling aids should be used to assist in language comprehension.

4. *Be Aware of Nonverbal Language*: As discussed in Chapter 7, pharmacists should be aware that nonverbal language, such as gestures, eye contact, speaking distance, pointing, and touching, mean different things in different cultures. Pharmacists should use universal symbols such as those found on auxiliary labels or used at airports.

5. *Be Empathetic*: Pharmacists must recognize or anticipate emotions caused by health conditions, medications, and interactions in unfamiliar health care settings. In particular, they might anticipate anger, frustration, fear, confusion, and embarrassment. The use of empathy will let the patient know that the pharmacist is caring and at least trying to understand.

6. *Be Assertive*: The pharmacist should let the patient know that he or she wants to understand. Rather than giving up in frustration, or ignoring the patient's comments, the pharmacist should tell the client that he or she cannot understand and ask the patient to repeat what was said more slowly or state it in another way. The pharmacist should accept the onus for lack of understanding, apologize, and ask the patient to help him or her understand the patient's needs and concerns. The patient will appreciate the attempt.

7. *Encourage Feedback and Use Teach-back*. The pharmacist should offer ample opportunity and time during counseling for patients to acknowledge that they understand and ask questions. The patient should be asked at intervals if the pharmacist is making himself clear, putting the onus on the pharmacist rather than on the patient for any misunderstandings.

8. *Recognize Poor Literacy/Health Literacy Skills*: As discussed earlier in this chapter and in Chapter 6, poor health literacy is frequently found in people of different cultures and mother tongues. The pharmacist must be sensitive to the embarrassment that poor literacy can cause by not making an issue of it. Techniques discussed earlier to overcome comprehension difficulties should be used.

9. *Treat Each Patient as an Individual*: Pharmacists and pharmacy staff must avoid stereotyping based on skin color, accent, clothing, or other visible differences. Each patient has individual needs, and these needs should be identified and addressed.

10. *Be Alert to Atypical Drug Responses or Poor Response to Treatment*: A patient's report of unusual drug ineffectiveness or adverse effects should not be discounted until cultural reasons have been ruled out. Reasons may include genetics, misunderstanding directions, nonadherence for cultural reasons, or misdiagnosis due to misunderstandings during initial diagnosing.

11. *Involve Family as Needed But Focus on the Patient*: In situations where no translator is present and English is poorly spoken or nonexistent, the pharmacist should ask if there is a family member who speaks English. Indicate to the family member to translate what is being said and wait for him or her to do this after speaking, signaling this with nonverbal language. Often a child can be enlisted. If so, this should be accepted, but counseling should be adjusted to avoid embarrassment to the child or

parent. Even if another family member is the spokesperson or translating, the pharmacist should make it clear that the conversation is with the patient not the translator by looking at the patient as well as the family member when speaking.

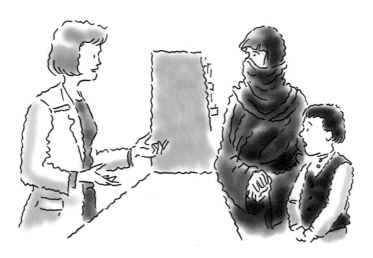

If a child is enlisted as a translator, counseling should be adjusted to avoid embarrassment.

Medication Incidents

The issue of medical errors and patient safety is one that hits close to home for pharmacists and technicians, since few can say they have never been involved in a medication error at some point in their careers. In recent years, a greater awareness and openness regarding all types of medical errors has evolved among health professionals and the public alike. The U.S. Institute of Medicine report, "To Err is Human, Building a Safer Health System," focusing on the quality of health care in America, estimated in 1999 that as many as 100,000 Americans die in hospitals annually from adverse events (more than from car accidents, breast cancer, or AIDS).[72] Reports such as this in the United States, Australia, and Canada have noted that great personal and financial costs to both patients and the system result from a wide range of adverse events that can and do occur when patients enter the health care system. A large percentage of these adverse events, many of which are preventable, involve medications.[73]

Rates for medication incidents vary considerably depending on how they are measured, gathered (e.g., anonymously, through chart reviews and observations, self-reported, or through incident reports), and what is included (e.g., whether they include missed doses, near misses, and wrong time). Estimates range from one error per patient per day in hospital, to 0.04% to 2.9% of doses dispensed during the hospital cart-filling processes, to 1.5% to 4% of prescriptions filled for ambulatory patients.[74]

When medication incidents occur, it is important that a process be followed so that the patient is appropriately treated and the incident is properly reported. In addition, the incident should be investigated through a root cause analysis to identify system and immediate causes, and to develop strategies to prevent future incidents from happening.

Handling Medication Incidents in Community Pharmacy

When a medication incident occurs, it is important that action be taken to deal with the outcome with the patient. In addition, an investigation should be undertaken to discover what happened, and why, and action taken to prevent future incidents. It is most helpful if a prearranged protocol is followed so that all involved know what needs to be done. This will reduce confusion and ensure that all appropriate steps are taken.

A protocol for handling medication incidents in a community pharmacy is suggested in Figure 8-2. If the discrepancy is identified in the pharmacy, then the pharmacist

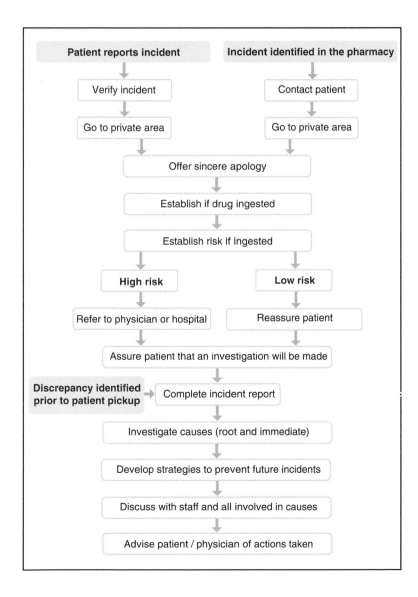

Figure 8-2 Protocol for Handling Medication Incidents

should inform the patient of the incident and offer a sincere apology. If the patient identifies the discrepancy, then the pharmacist should speak with the patient in a private area of the pharmacy. The incident should be verified to ensure that any discrepancy was not the result of intentional changes to the prescription.

If the pharmacist handling the incident was not the one who dispensed the medication, he or she should assure the patient that the other pharmacist will be informed, without making negative remarks or blaming the other pharmacist. The other pharmacist should be contacted so that he or she can also speak with the patient and apologize as soon as possible.

The pharmacist should establish if the drug was ingested and if there is a risk to the patient. If so, the patient should be referred to the hospital or his or her physician and appropriate measures taken. Otherwise the patient should be reassured there is no risk, without trivializing the incident. If necessary, the physician should be contacted at this point and communicated with appropriately (to be discussed later). The pharmacist also needs to reassure the patient that the pharmacist is genuinely concerned, that the situation will be handled appropriately, and that such an incident is not a usual occurrence.

An incident report should be completed and the patient should be told the incident will be investigated. A root cause analysis should be undertaken to identify causes and develop strategies to prevent future similar incidents. At the end, the patient, all staff, and any other parties in the system that may have contributed to the cause of the incident (e.g., manufacturer and physician) should be informed of the outcome.

Communication Issues When Handling a Medication Incident

Appropriate communication is a critical part of handling an incident, including communication with the patient, the physician if necessary, staff, and with any others involved. When medication incidents are mishandled they are more likely to result in a complaint to a pharmacy regulatory body or legal action. How things are said—the tone of voice, the words used, the attitude and approach of the pharmacist—are all important to an outcome that is satisfying to the patient and the pharmacist.[75,76]

The following are recommendations and techniques for handling a medication incident with an ambulatory patient:[76–79]

1. *All Involved Should Be Honest and Open*: Patients involved in incident investigations have stated, "If the pharmacist had been upfront instead of trying to cover up his or her mistakes, I would never have complained."[76] The pharmacist should be open and honest with the patient and with any investigating bodies so that an investigation can be conducted to protect the public and hopefully prevent further similar incidents.[76] The pharmacist should be assured, however, that the intent is not to determine guilt or innocence but to investigate in an unbiased manner. Only a no blame system can result in open and honest reporting.

2. *The Pharmacist Should Deal with the Situation*: The pharmacist rather than technicians or clerks should deal with the patient. If necessary, the pharmacy manager may offer further apologies and help to calm the situation. It may be difficult for the pharmacist to remember full details of the incident when confronted, so he or she should be allowed time to think about what happened (for a brief time only) in order to avoid self-contradiction later.

3. *The Pharmacist Should Communicate Directly with the Patient*: A relationship exists already between the pharmacist and patient, and hopefully this is a trusting and respectful one. An intermediary such as a family member may not have a full understanding of the circumstances and may be less forgiving or emotional than the patient.

4. *The Pharmacist and Anyone Else Involved Should Give a Sincere Apology*: Whether or not harm resulted or a cause was found, the pharmacist should apologize. This is not an admission of guilt or blame but an apology for any inconvenience or upset resulting for the patient. The patient should also be thanked for being understanding and patient, for bringing this issue to light, and for continued patronage of the pharmacy.

5. *The Welfare of the Patient Should Be Assured*: It should be determined whether the patient ingested the wrong medication. If so, the pharmacist should provide appropriate information about the potential outcome. If the effect is negligible, the pharmacist should not belittle the patient for his or her concern, or trivialize the incident.

6. *The Patient Should Be Assured That an Investigation Will Be Conducted*: The pharmacist should explain that everything possible will be done to determine what went wrong and to ensure that it will not happen again.

7. *Discussion Should Take Place in a Private Area*: A private area should be used so that other patients do not overhear and become concerned.

8. *The Pharmacist Should Be Properly Prepared*: Many pharmacy owners have a policy or procedure to follow. It should be thought through ahead of time so that a protocol for handling medication incidents and for communicating with the patient is clear to the pharmacist at the time of the incident. This reduces the stress as well as the chance that the incident will be mishandled. Pharmacists should also make sure that they are properly insured for individual liability (not just for the pharmacy) and know what their insurance clause requires. Some may have a recommended procedure and require immediate notification.

9. *The Pharmacist Needs to Deal with Personal Emotions*: The pharmacist may first experience panic, particularly if the seriousness of the outcome is not yet known. Every effort should be made to stay calm by breathing deeply and not letting the imagination run away with thoughts of tragedy. It may help to engage in self-talk such as "stay calm," "just take one step at a time," "find out what happened before panicking."

10. *Words Should Be Chosen Carefully*: Particular attention should be paid to avoid trigger words and questions that tend to raise emotions or lead to further questions or concerns. Table 8-6 lists some recommended words and phrases to be used when discussing a medication incident with a patient.[80]

11. *The Focus Should Be on the Patient's Issues*: Although the pharmacist's instinct may be for self-protection, concern with his or her own plight, or the repercussions on the pharmacy, personal concerns should be secondary. As the patient is the injured party, the pharmacist should focus on the patient as an individual.

12. *The Pharmacist Should Show Empathy for the Patient*: The patient may be experiencing a variety of emotions such as fear, anger, frustration, indignation (this shouldn't happen or why me), loss of trust, and inconvenience. Before asking questions and verifying that an incident has occurred, the pharmacist should acknowledge

TABLE 8-6   Communication about a Medication Incident

1. Use the word "incident" rather than "mistake" or "error," which are blaming and emotional words
2. Use the words "and" or "however" rather than "but" since this word negates what was just said, e.g., "I'm sorry about this, *and (rather than but)* I'll check into it"
3. Use the phrase, "is there a reason" rather than "why," which tends to make people defensive
4. Use the words "issue," "question," or "situation" rather than "problem," which has a negative connotation
5. Use words of agreement and helping as much as possible such as "You're right, this shouldn't have happened"; "That may be, and . . ."; "It may seem that way, and . . . ."; "I'm as concerned as you."
6. Use one of the following phrases to notify the patient that an incident has occurred: "There has been a medication incident/adverse medication event"; "There appears to have been a medication incident/adverse medication event"; "A medication incident/adverse medication event has occurred."
7. Nonverbal language should portray confidence and caring. Stand erect, with chin up, nodding when listening
8. Take deep breaths and try to keep the voice low since one's voice tends to raise in pitch when one is nervous
9. Show empathy by using one of the following phrases: e.g., "I can see that you're very worried about this"; "I understand why you would feel angry about this"; "This may be frightening for you"; "You have every reason to be concerned and upset about this situation and we are too."
10. Avoid leading questions or blaming. For example, say, "In order for me to help you I need to find out . . ." rather than "Didn't you check it was your name on the label before you took it?"

Sources: Quiring, V. How to respond when medication errors occur. Presented at APhA 2001—14th Annual Meeting and Exposition, San Francisco, U.S.A. March, 2001; Rantucci M, Stewart C, Stewart I. Safe medication practices- A pharmacist's guide to preventing and managing medication incidents. Pharmacy Practice. Rogers Publishing Ltd. Toronto. 2004.

and empathize with the patient's feelings. This will demonstrate caring and a willingness to listen. If the patient expresses anger, the pharmacist should not take this personally and let him or her vent (see the later section on dealing with conflict).

13. *There Should Never Be Blaming or Making Excuses*: Blame must not be ascribed to the patient, the physician, or another pharmacist. Although contributing reasons for the incident should be sought, the pharmacist should not offer excuses such as "We're only human"; "We were busy"; "These things happen"; "No big deal"; "It's not really dangerous."

14. *The Physician Should Be Informed If Necessary*: If the outcome of the incident could in any way be negative such as the patient is missing critical dosing such as diabetic medication or chemotherapy, or a high-risk or high-dose medication has been ingested, then the physician should be informed. As discussed earlier in regard to patient communication, honesty and calm are the best approaches. The pharmacist

should speak directly to the physician, never a third person, and explain as clearly as possible what the patient received and when. An explanation about why it happened or who did it is not necessary at this point, just the assurance that it is being investigated and that this is not a regular occurrence. The suggestions for wording shown in Table 8-6 also apply here, such as avoiding the word "error."

15. *The Pharmacist Should Follow-up with All Involved*: An explanation for the incident and actions being taken to prevent future similar occurrences should be provided to the patient, physician, and anyone else involved when the investigation is complete. A further apology and thanks for their patience should be included, preferably in a formal letter from the pharmacist and pharmacy manager.

Issues Involving Primary Care and Nontherapeutic Situations

Although pharmacists deal with patients primarily in the area of medication counseling, they are also generally considered to be the most available health professionals in the community. It has been estimated that a number of people equivalent to the total population of the United States visits one of the many pharmacies in the country every 3.5 weeks.[81] The pharmacist may, therefore, be the first person that a patient will turn to in order to discuss a variety of concerns. Not only is no appointment generally needed with the pharmacist, but the patient may also feel more comfortable discussing personal matters with the pharmacist than with a more formal caregiver—especially if a helping and trusting relationship has developed between the patient and the pharmacist. Pharmacists are in a unique position, and therefore have a responsibility to become involved in many situations not directly related to therapy, but rather primary care and prevention.

Involvement in primary care and prevention involves promoting health maintenance in individual patients by providing counseling and education on topics such as smoking, alcohol use, nutrition, and exercise.[81] Pharmacists actively pursue this role by inquiring about these issues during medication counseling or by holding group education programs or clinics, either in the pharmacy or elsewhere in the community. Pharmacists are also approached by patients to answer questions about these issues and, in some cases, about social problems.

Handling Patients' Questions

It is a good idea to provide a patient-information section in the pharmacy that holds pamphlets and patient-oriented reference books regarding not only medications but also various illness conditions. Patients should be encouraged to discuss this information with the pharmacist at any time. In addition, pharmacists should become involved in national health observances such as National Mental Health Month and National Arthritis Month, or hold store promotions related to a particular condition, thus inviting questions from the public. Pharmacists involved in screening for hypertension, diabetes, or colorectal cancer also need to be prepared to answer questions and discuss the condition with the patient.

In dealing with general questions about drugs or illness, it is best to gather some information about the request before responding. The pharmacist should find out why the patient wants to know, what specifically he or she wants to know, where he or she heard about the drug or illness in question, and what he or she already knows. This will allow the pharmacist to determine the nature of the patient's needs.

Sometimes the patient making the request is new to the pharmacy. Some pharmacists prefer not to answer questions in this situation, preferring instead to refer the patient to his or her "regular" pharmacy where there may be a more complete record of medications and conditions. However, many patients use more than one pharmacy so that there is no one place that has all their information. In addition, the opportunity may be lost to assist the patient in a critical decision, as the patient may become discouraged from being rebuffed. It is also an opportunity to gain the trust and future patronage of a new patient. As long as the patient's full history is obtained prior to answering the patient's questions, it is appropriate to consult with a previously unknown patient in this way. The pharmacist may wish to ask the patient to pay a consultation fee since there is no professional fee being charged for medication. The pharmacist can also impress upon the patient the importance of patronizing one pharmacy offering a full range of consultation services.

If a patient requests a reference book, it is preferable to provide prepared information pamphlets or books designed specifically for patients, as discussed in Chapter 6. It is not advisable to simply hand the patient a pharmacists' reference text, which is too detailed and technical for most patients to understand, and may indeed be mystifying, alarming, or misleading. If the patient is familiar with and requests to see a particular pharmacists' reference text, the pharmacist should not appear to be withholding information. In cases where it would be awkward to refuse to show the book to the patient, the pharmacist should stay with the patient and ask questions as suggested above to determine the patient's needs or concerns. The pharmacist can then help to clarify the information in the reference in terms that the patient can more easily understand, and put the information into perspective. It would be advisable following this discussion to suggest that the patient make an appointment with the pharmacist and perhaps the physician for a more complete discussion of the patient's issues.

If the question involves an issue requiring behavior change such as weight loss or smoking cessation, the pharmacist should compliment the patient for his or her concern and offer to help. The pharmacist may choose to provide information about the issue, then refer the patient to another health professional providing in-depth counseling or arrange an appointment to provide more in-depth counseling himself or herself. Counseling involving behavior change and motivation can require significant time and skill as discussed earlier in this chapter and in Chapter 4.

Dealing with Patients' Social Issues

Patients may also approach the pharmacist with a range of social issues, or alternatively, the pharmacist may become aware of these issues through discussion or observation. These issues may include alcoholism, legal or illegal drug abuse, family planning, unwanted pregnancy, child abuse or family violence, and suicidal thoughts.

Patients may not know where to get help for such issues, or they may not be quite ready to seek more formal care. Patients in these situations need assistance in finding out where they can get more specialized help. They may need confirmation that the issue can and should be dealt with. They may need encouragement to seek help.

They may also need reassurance about the source of referred help regarding confidentiality and the nature of the encounter with that caregiver. Finally, they may need some help in the practical aspects of accessing or contacting that source.

Pharmacists are not usually trained to counsel in these social counseling situations, which often require more specialized professional counselors. Since pharmacists are approached, however, they have a responsibility to deal with the patient rather than turning him or her away. Regarding child abuse, pharmacists are professionally, and in some jurisdictions, legally responsible to report suspected cases to the proper authorities.[82]

When confronted with social issues, although not prepared to provide specialized counseling, pharmacists can deal with the patient compassionately and appropriately as follows:

1. *Listen to the Patient in an Unbiased and Nonjudgmental Manner*: As with other counseling situations, the pharmacist should begin by allowing the patient to express his or her feelings or concerns, empathizing with the patient. Some gentle probing may be needed for the pharmacist to get a full understanding of the patient's needs.

2. *Provide Privacy*: Because these situations are of a very personal nature, the pharmacist should be sensitive to the need for privacy. If a private area is not available for the discussion, a time might be arranged to speak with the patient when there will be privacy in the pharmacy. Alternatively, the pharmacist might arrange to speak with the patient on the telephone.

3. *Ensure Confidentiality*: The pharmacist should keep in mind the need to maintain confidentiality. If, in the pharmacist's opinion, someone else should be informed about the situation—a physician, parent, family member, or social-service worker—he or she must first discuss it with the patient and get his or her consent. Patients should be encouraged to first speak with these people themselves. If a patient feels unable to do this, the pharmacist may offer to intervene, but only with the patient's consent. The only exception to this rule may be in the cases where the pharmacist is legally (in some jurisdictions) or ethically responsible for reporting, such as child abuse, or where the patient may harm himself or herself or another individual.[82] In any of these cases, discussion of the patient's situation with other pharmacy staff or with acquaintances must also be restricted.

    Throughout any discussion with the patient, confidentiality should be emphasized to encourage and comfort the patient.

4. *Encourage Patients to Seek Their Own Solutions*: The pharmacist should avoid giving advice, even if asked directly—instead, he or she should stress that such decisions are up to the patient. The pharmacist should, however, help the patient explore appropriate options.

5. *Refer Patients to Appropriate Resources*: In order to handle these situations properly, the pharmacist must be familiar with resources in the community to which the patient can be referred. These may include physicians; specialized clinics (e.g., family planning clinics); religious leaders; school counselors; specialized treatment centers (e.g., addiction treatment centers); self-help organizations (e.g., Alcoholics Anonymous); crisis-intervention services (e.g., suicide hotlines); and social-service agencies.

It is useful to keep a list of community resources, with phone numbers and the name of a contact person, if available. When making up such a list, it may also be helpful for the pharmacist to contact the resources personally to find out about their referral procedures and the sort of treatment the patient can expect to receive from them. This way, the pharmacist will feel more confident in making referrals and be able to reassure patients by explaining what will happen when they reach the particular helper.

6. *Provide Follow-up*: The pharmacist should ensure that the patient was able to contact the referred resource and offer any further assistance as needed. It is best to inform the patient in advance that he or she will do so. This will encourage and reassure the patient that the recommended help is indeed necessary and that he or she can rely on the support of a concerned individual.

Emotional Situations and Conflict

Pharmacists must sometimes deal with patient-counseling situations that are particularly difficult, because there is a strong emotional element or an element of conflict. The source of the conflict is usually a difference in opinion between the pharmacist and patient, such as a patient's complaint about a particular product. A patient's strong emotions may be a result of the pharmacist's actions or for a reason unrelated to the pharmacist, such as extreme worry about illness or medication use, or emotional upset for any number of personal reasons. In addition, pharmacists should realize that patients are often in physical discomfort. When people have these kinds of feelings, they often react with strong emotions like anger, or appear distraught and depressed, sometimes tearful.

Conflict may also occur between the pharmacist and other health professionals, pharmacy peers, or staff. Strong emotions may be at the root of these conflicts also since such people are often under stress in the health care system. Consider Counseling Situation 8.1.

COUNSELING SITUATION 8.1: The Angry Patient

Mr. Williams is a middle-aged executive who has been waiting in the pharmacy for a refill of his prescription for bupropion 150 mg for smoking cessation. It is now ready and the pharmacist calls him to the pharmacy counter.

Pharmacist: Hello, Mr. Williams. Your prescription is ready for you now. I'll just spend a few minutes to discuss it with you to make sure you're getting the most benefit from it.

Patient: *(looking and sounding aggravated)* It's about time! I've been waiting here half my lunch hour, and I think it's ridiculous! I'm a busy person, and I simply don't have the time.

Pharmacist: *(ignoring the patient's comments and cutting in)* Well, it's ready now. I see you've been taking this for a few months now. How have you been taking it?

Patient: *(still fuming)* Twice a day, just as it says on the label.

Pharmacist: *(ignoring the patient's obvious anger)* Good. And how's it been going?

Patient: *(raising his voice more)* Just fine, until I had to come in here and get the run around. I think . . .

Pharmacist: *(cutting in)* Well, we've been very busy today. If you'd phoned 24 hours ahead as it says on the label . . .

Patient: *(cutting in, almost yelling)* I phoned ahead like it says on the label, and it still wasn't ready.

Pharmacist: *(sounding a little unsure)* Oh, well, I wasn't here yesterday. They probably had to call the doctor.

Patient: *(still sounding angry)* Why do they have to do that? She knows I need this stuff.

Pharmacist: *(more sure of herself now, authoritative tone)* Legally we need to contact the doctor to refill prescriptions.

Patient: *(yelling, attracting the attention of other waiting patients)* I don't care about your laws. I'm supposed to be on this all the time, and the doctor said I could get it whenever I wanted.

Pharmacist: Oh, well, I don't know anything about that. I just came on duty a few minutes ago. The other pharmacist must have handled it.

Patient: Sure, just pass the buck. That's always the way with you people. You just put in your time and don't give a hoot about what's going on.

Pharmacist: *(angry now, raising her voice)* What do you mean "you people?" I'm a very responsible pharmacist. You have no right to say that about me!

Patient: *(giving up, still yelling)* Just give me my prescription and let me get out of here! And I won't be back, that's for sure!

Pharmacist: *(practically throwing the prescription at the patient)* Fine! Here! *(Patient walks away, angrily commenting to other waiting patients as he passes about the inefficiency of this pharmacy)*

This patient probably won't come back to the pharmacy. More importantly, the pharmacist was not able to discuss the medication, and therefore, didn't have a chance to discover that the patient was experiencing some dizziness, causing him to skip doses on days when he has important meetings. In addition, the patient didn't have the opportunity to ask whether he could have a drink at a party he planned to attend that evening. Even more importantly, the pharmacist did not get the opportunity to discuss the patient's success in quitting smoking, and provide support as needed. Finally, both the patient and the pharmacist left the situation feeling stressed.

In such situations, the pharmacist's first instinct may be to avoid the issue, for his or her sake or the patient's comfort. If the counseling is to proceed, however, the patient's emotions or the source of conflict must be dealt with first. Strong emotions will distract the patient from participating, making it difficult for the pharmacist to gather information and for the patient, in a turbulent state of mind, to learn anything about the medication. By trying to resolve the situation, the pharmacist might even discover important information pertaining to medication use.

Counseling Patients in Emotional Situations and Conflict

The techniques for dealing with these difficult situations involve using many of the communication techniques discussed in Chapter 7. The most important elements in handling such situations are to recognize the patient's feelings and concerns and, if at all possible, to discuss them. The emphasis during the counseling session should be placed on resolving the patient's concerns and calming strong emotions. Specific suggestions for tailoring counseling to deal with difficult situations are as follows:

1. *Remain in Control of Personal Emotions*: When presented with an emotional patient or a conflict, the pharmacist must deal with his or her own emotions as well as the patient's, resulting in interpersonal stress.[83] The most common causes of interpersonal stress for pharmacists include commands given by others, anger directed toward the pharmacist, criticism, inattentiveness by another individual (not listening, ignoring, avoiding eye contact), impulsive behavior by another, and making mistakes.[83] The resulting emotions may be anger, frustration, embarrassment, disgust, or general discomfort about the topic under discussion.

   To deal with difficult situations, the pharmacist should be prepared for such feelings. By recognizing and accepting these feelings (rather than trying to deny them), the pharmacist will be better able to control such emotions and maintain a detached and nonjudgmental attitude with the patient. This by no means implies that pharmacists should remain cold or unfeeling; on the contrary, it suggests that by becoming familiar with his or her own responses, the pharmacist will be better equipped to maintain a professional demeanor and help the patient deal with emotions. Responding with an emotional outburst is invariably counterproductive.

   One technique for dealing with interpersonal stress is desensitization.[83] This is a technique whereby the pharmacist gradually makes himself or herself "less sensitive" to a stressor. It involves being exposed to the stressor for increasing lengths of time until the pharmacist "learns to put up with it." This often occurs over time as pharmacists gain experience in dealing with patients. However, a more painless and quicker way is to actively pursue desensitization through a relaxation exercise in which the pharmacist imagines the stressful situation in detail for 5 seconds at a time, then imagines a peaceful, relaxing scene.[83] This is repeated several times, increasing the length of time of imagining the stressor by 10 seconds each time. This whole process is repeated several times a day for several days until the pharmacist feels comfortable with the situation.

   Another technique involves the pharmacist saying positive coping statements to himself or herself, while the situation is occurring. Such statements may be: "I can handle this"; "I can cope with this"; "It's not so terrible"; "I can stand it"; "Everything's going to be all right."[83] These can also be more specific to the situation, for example, "Stay calm"; "He doesn't really mean it personally"; and "He isn't feeling well."

   A third technique is covert rehearsal, whereby the pharmacist imagines himself or herself successfully coping with the stressor.[83] As with desensitization, the pharmacist imagines a situation that he or she generally finds difficult. Then, the pharmacist imagines going through the situation, what he or she might say, perhaps imagining the surroundings and how the patient is behaving, but imagining that things work out and that the patient responds to his or her statements More details about these technique and practice exercises are provided by Gerrard et al.[83]

Other techniques useful for coping in such situations include visualizing that the situation is over, distracting oneself with activities such as doodling (as long as it is out of sight of the patient), and simply not responding to personal criticism or insults from the patient, since they are often designed simply to put the pharmacist at a disadvantage.

2. *Provide Privacy*: Because most of these situations are quite sensitive, the pharmacist should provide privacy, as early in the discussion as possible. If necessary, the discussion should be continued later, by telephone. This allows both the pharmacist and the patient to be more comfortable in the discussion, as well as preventing others from becoming involved (e.g., another nearby customer entering into a disagreement about pricing).

3. *Let the Patient Vent His or Her Feelings*: The scientific training that pharmacists have received will have taught them to be analytical in their problem-solving approaches. As a result, they may tend to focus on the problem rather than on the patient. As discussed in the previous chapter, pharmacists often tend to deal with situations by asking questions and making judgments or giving advice. This, however, removes the focus from the patient and may result in an angry response. It is more effective, particularly in difficult situations, for the pharmacist to focus on the patient.

   The pharmacist should start by giving the patient an opportunity to vent his or her feelings. By passively listening, the pharmacist will allow the patient to get his or her concerns, or any emotions, out in the open and possibly to calm down a little.[84] If the patient is very distraught, and possibly even in tears, he or she should be allowed to sit quietly, preferably in privacy, to regain control. If the patient is extremely upset and unable to regain self-control, it may be necessary to defer medication counseling to a later time, to be conducted either on the telephone or in person.

4. *Express Empathy for the Patient*: As discussed in Chapter 7, expressing empathy is an important part of patient counseling, and this is particularly true in difficult situations.[85] After the patient has had his or her say, the pharmacist should empathize with his or her situation. Rather than arguing, becoming defensive, or jumping to give advice, the pharmacist can encourage the patient to discuss any problems and complaints through active listening. This allows the patient to clarify what is bothering him or her, and it helps the pharmacist to better understand the situation (e.g., the patient isn't actually angry at the pharmacist but frustrated with the doctor).

5. *Probe to Clarify the Issue*: At this point it is useful to try to make clear more details about the issue. As discussed in the previous chapter, probing requires a certain degree of skill to avoid causing the patient to become defensive or impatient. Again, this not only helps the pharmacist get a better grasp of the issue at the root of the conflict or emotions, but also helps focus and calm the patient.

6. *Provide Explanations and Suggestions*: Once the pharmacist has a grasp of the issue, he or she may need to offer the patient an explanation or simply provide some information. The patient's point of view, not the pharmacist's, should always direct the pharmacist's explanations. For example, when explaining that a prescription cannot be refilled without the doctor's authorization, rather than simply stating pharmacy law, the pharmacist should explain that it is in the patient's interest that the physician be apprised of the situation.

   Where possible, suggestions should also be offered to help deal with the issue. Several alternatives should be offered where possible, so that the patient can maintain a feeling of choice, and hence, can feel more in control of the situation. Recall from Chapter 3 that patients often feel a lack of control because of their condition and treatment in the health care process, which often results in frustration, anger, or feelings of hopelessness. By allowing the patient to make some decisions, the pharmacist can improve the patient's feelings of self-worth and control.

If the reason for the patient's distress involves a medication incident, then the procedure discussed in the earlier section of this chapter should be followed.

Even if the pharmacist dealing with the situation is not personally involved in the issue (e.g., if another pharmacist originally dealt with the patient), he or she should still accept the responsibility of dealing with it. It's best to avoid making excuses or "passing the buck." If, however, the patient demands to speak with someone else, this should be politely arranged.

7. *Be Assertive*; Assertiveness on the pharmacist's part can help resolve the situation in such a way that neither party ends up as the "loser."[85] If the situation cannot be resolved because outside input is necessary or because the patient is too upset to continue, assertiveness is critical. The pharmacist may simply have to stand his or her ground and end the situation.

   Although the patient's point of view should be considered first, the pharmacist can ask the patient to consider the pharmacist's own point of view later in the discussion. The pharmacist may also state his or her feelings, for example, "I feel very embarrassed about this."

8. *Provide Positive Messages to the Patient*: Positive messages, both verbal and nonverbal, will help calm a situation and improve the interaction. Such things as using the patient's name, smiling, giving the patient full attention and honest recognition, and apologizing for any inconvenience caused by the pharmacist or pharmacy, all help to provide a positive message. In addition, comments should be phrased in a positive light. For example, rather than "I can't help you," the pharmacist should say, "I'd like to help you. I just need a little more information."

9. *End the Situation on a Positive Note*: Attempt to end on a positive note perhaps by recapping a positive solution, or by reiterating what has been tried to resolve the situation. The pharmacist might also suggest some sort of follow-up, such as asking the patient to telephone to discuss the outcome of suggested measures, or offering to call the patient.

   Sometimes situations involving distressed or upset patients cannot be resolved at the time. It may be necessary for the pharmacist to end the encounter if the patient is unable to regain control, or if the session threatens to become too lengthy. Assertiveness on the pharmacist's part may be needed here to summarize the situation, and bring it to a close. Arrangements might be made for further discussion or for the patient to seek other help. A statement might be made to curtail the situation, such as "I'm sorry I'm not able to help you any further today. I've tried to explain the situation to you and offered some suggestions. Perhaps we can discuss this further when you're feeling calmer." The pharmacist can then use nonverbal language to indicate that the discussion is over (e.g., turning his or her body to begin walking away, making eye contact with the next patient, and stapling the prescription bag).

If the pharmacist had used these techniques, the counseling situation with Mr. Williams would have ended differently.

Pharmacist: Hello, Mr. Williams. Your prescription is ready for you now. I'll just spend a few minutes to discuss it with you to make sure you're getting the most benefit from it.

Patient: *(looking and sounding aggravated)* It's about time! I've been waiting here half my lunch hour, and I think that's ridiculous! I'm a busy person, and I simply don't have the time to stand around and wait in this pharmacy.

Pharmacist: *(listens and waits for patient to finish speaking, empathetic tone)* I can see that you're upset about having to wait, and I can understand why that would annoy you. Let's step over to the counseling area to talk. *(leads the way to the counseling booth)* I'm sorry if you were inconvenienced.

Patient: *(calmer but still fuming)* Well, why wasn't it ready?

Pharmacist: *(empathetic tone)* I know it may seem like a long time to get your prescription ready, but we did need to contact the doctor, to . . .

Patient: *(cutting in angrily)* Why did you have to do that? She knows I need this stuff.

Pharmacist: *(calmly)* Yes, and she also likes to be kept informed of how often you need your medication, so she can know how your condition is and whether the medication is helping.

Patient: *(calmer)* Oh, I guess that's true, but I thought I had refills on this prescription.

Pharmacist: *(sounding confident)* I'll check on that for you. I wasn't here at the time it was processed but I'll find out what happened.

Patient: *(still a little angry)* Sure, just pass the buck.

Pharmacist: *(controlling her own anger and speaking in a calm voice)* It may seem like that, but I'm just trying to explain why I wasn't sure about the refill order. Again, I'm sorry if you're upset.

Patient: *(calming down and feeling sorry for insulting the pharmacist)* OK. I shouldn't have become so worked up. I sure wish I could have a smoke, but I'm trying to quit with the help of these pills. I've got a big case I'm working on, and I guess I'm on edge.

Pharmacist: *(smiling, empathetic tone)* That's OK. It sounds like you're really under stress. Let's just slow down for a few minutes, and I'll go over your pre-scription to make sure you're getting the most benefit from it. It'll just take a few minutes and then you'll have some time left to relax before heading back to your work. Maybe we can talk later about other things to help you quit smoking.

Patient: *(smiling back)* OK. I could use some fresh ideas on that. I also wanted to ask you about drinking with this medication . . . *(Patient and pharmacist proceed to discuss the medication. The pharmacist identifies the patient's medica-tion-related problems, then counsels him regarding alcohol use, and arranges a time to talk about smoking cessation.)* (She also checks the patient file and confirms that there were no authorized refills and explains to the patient that his prescription will be ready for him next time if he allows a full 24 to 48 hours for the pharmacist to contact the physician.)

This time the pharmacist responded right away to the patient's anger. She listened passively until he finished speaking, then suggested they move to a more private area to avoid other patients overhearing. She responded empathetically and then tried to explain what had happened. Her explanation did not cite the law, but used optimal control of therapy as the reason for having to call the doctor. She did not let herself get angry, even when the patient made personal comments, but remained assertive, letting the patient see her point of view. Her smile, calm voice, and empathy for the patient allowed the counseling to maintain a positive note. Having dealt with the patient's anger first, she was then able to proceed with counseling the patient effectively, identifying and resolving drug-related problems, and providing further help with smoking cessation.

SUMMARY

Much has been written in the previous chapters about what pharmacists should do regarding patient counseling; however, the question arises as to how the average pharmacist in everyday practice is able to accomplish this. This chapter in particular highlights some of the challenges for pharmacists with respect to performing this important duty. The following chapter will further discuss challenges facing pharmacists in patient counseling and will offer some practical suggestions for pharmacists to overcome some of these challenges and develop optimal counseling involvement.

REFLECTIVE QUESTIONS

1. An elderly Asian lady accompanied by a younger man comes into your pharmacy with a prescription for an antianxiety agent. What types of difficult issues can you anticipate might arise?
2. When you speak to the Asian lady mentioned in the previous question she appears unable to speak or understand your English language very well. What techniques might you use to provide counseling?
3. An elderly gentleman comes to the pharmacy to ask for a cane. Just by looking at him, you suspect that he may also have hearing or cognitive impairment. What type of bias would you be exhibiting?
4. How would you determine if the gentleman in the previous question has these disabilities? How would you tailor counseling to allow for this and his need for a cane when counseling him for his medications?
4. Bill is a patient who is complaining about receiving the wrong dose of medication. The prescription was prepared by another pharmacist. What would you say to the patient about this?
5. If Bill becomes very angry and accuses you of incompetence, how would you deal with this?

REFERENCES

1. Morrow N, Hargie O. An investigation of critical incidents in interpersonal communication in pharmacy practice. J Soc Admin Pharm. 1987;4(3):112–118.
2. Klein L, German P, Levine D, et al. Medication problems among outpatients: A study with emphasis on the elderly. Arch Intern Med.1984;144(6):1185–1188.

3. Schoepp G. For kids only. Drug Merch. 1990;71(1):26–31.

4. Mechanic D. Illness Behavior. In: Medical Sociology, 2nd Edition. Free Press, New York, 1978.

5. Eigen B. Improving communication with the physically disabled. Am Pharm. 1982;NS22(10):37–40.

6. Penna R. Pharmacists should make appointments to serve patients with chronic diseases. Am Pharm. 1991;NS31(7):57–59.

7. Myerscough P. Aspects of Transcultural Communication. In: Talking With Patients: A Basic Clinical Skill, 2nd Edition. Oxford University Press, Oxford, 1992.

8. Kirsch I, Jungeblit A, Jenkins L, et al. Adult literacy in America. A first look at the results of the National Adult Literacy Survey. U.S. Department of Education. National Center for Educational Statistics. Educational Testing Service, Princeton, NJ, 1993.

9. Wilson J, Hogan L. Readability testing of auxiliary labels. Drug Intell Clin Pharm. 1983;17(1):54–55.

10. Gillis DE. Beyond words. The health literacy connection. Canadian Health Network, Public Health Agency of Canada, 2005. Available at: www.canadian-health-network.ca/servlet/ContentServer?cid=105968393879&pagename=CH-RCS%2FCHNResource%2FCHNResourcePageTemplate&c=CHNResource (accessed March 2005).

11. Williams MV, Parker RM, Baker DW, et al. Inadequate functional health literacy among patients at two public hospitals. JAMA. 1995;274(21):1677–1682.

12. Anonymous. Fact sheet: The use of over-the-counter medicines. National Council on Patient Information and Education. Available at: www.bemedwise.org/press_room/sep_2003_fact_otc.pdf (accessed January 2005).

13. Tabor PA, Lopez DA. Comply with us: Improving medication adherence. J Pharm Pract. 2004;17:167–181.

14. Bennison C. Step into the picture. Pharm Pract. 2004;21(4):27, 29–32, 34–35.

15. Work D. We've come a long way . . . or have we? Am Pharm. 1987;NS27(7):48–50.

16. Weygman L. Managing conflict. On Cont Pract. 1988;15(1):19–20.

17. Baker DW, Williams MV, Parker RM, et al. Development of a brief test to measure functional health literacy. Patient Educ Couns. 1999;38:33–42.

18. Hurd P, Butkovich S. Adherence problems and the older patient: Assessing functional limitations. Drug Intell Clin Pharm. 1986;20(3):228–230.

19. Nichols-English G, Poirier S. Optimizing adherence to pharmaceutical care plans. J Am Pharm Assoc. 2000;40(4):475–485.

20. Schillinger D, Piette J, Grumbach K, et al. Closing the loop: Physician communication with diabetic patients who have low health literacy. Arch Intern Med. 2003;163:83–90.

21. Iezzoni L, O'Day B, Killeen M, et al. Communicating about health care: Observations from persons who are deaf or hard of hearing. Ann Intern Med. 2004;140:356–362.

22. Disability etiquette tips. National Organization on Disability. Available at: www.nod.org (accessed March 2005).

23. Miller B. Break the sound barrier with the deaf person in your pharmacy. Drug Merch. 1984;65(10):44.

24. Chermak G, Jinks M. Counseling the hearing-impaired older adult. Drug Intell Clin Pharm. 1981;15(5):377–382.

25. Myerscough P. Other Aspects of Doctor-patient Communication. In: Talking with Patients—A Basic Clinical Skill, 2nd Edition. Oxford University Press, Oxford, 1992.

26. Communicating with and about people with disabilities. U.S. Department of Labor. Office of Disability Employment Policy. Available at: www.dol.gov/odep/pubs/fact/comucate.htm (accessed June 2005).

27. Rantucci M. Counselling special patient groups. CE Compliance Centre National Continuing Education Program, 2004. Available at: www.pharmacyconnects.com/pdfs/2004/08/NovCE_Aug.pdf (accessed June 2005).

28. Kübler-Ross E. What is it like to be dying? Am J Nurs. 1971;71(1):55–60.

29. Conrad P. The meaning of medication: Another look at compliance. Soc Sci Med. 1985;20(1):19–37.

30. Torre M, Sause R. Counseling the diabetic patient. Am Pharm. 1982;NS22(10):45–46.

31. Kelly GH, Scott JE. Medication compliance and health education among outpatients with chronic mental disease. Med Care. 1990;28(12):1181–1197.

32. Hogan TP, Awad AG, Eastwood R. A self-report scale of drug compliance in schizophrenics: Reliability and discriminative validity. Psychol Med. 1983;(13):177–183.

33. Foisy M. Pharmacists and HIV. Pharm Pract. 1995;11(5):56–58, 62–68.

34. Raleigh F. Counseling the patient with psychiatric conditions. Cal Pharm. 1990; Feb:33–35.

35. Okolo N, McReynolds J. Counseling the terminally ill. Am Pharm. 1987;NS27(9):37–40.

36. Buckman R. I Don't Know What to Say. Key Porter Books Ltd., Toronto, 1988.

37. Health professional info—Unconventional therapies. BC Cancer Agency. Available at: www.bccancer.bc.ca/HPI/Unconventional Therapies/default.htm (accessed June 2, 2004).

38. Health Care Delivery. In: The Merck Manual of Diagnosis and Therapy, Chapter 293. Geriatric Medicine. Available at: www.merck.com/mrkshared/mmanual/section21/chapter293/293b.jsp (accessed June 2005).

39. General. In: The Merck Manual of Diagnosis and Therapy, Chapter 304. Drug Therapy in the Elderly. Available at: www.merck.com/mrkshared/mmanual/section22/chapter304/304a.jsp (accessed June 2005).

40. Disorders Common in the Elderly. In: The Merck Manual of Diagnosis and Therapy, Chapter 293. Geriatric Medicine. Available at: www.merck.com/mrkshared/mmanual/section21/chapter293/293c.jsp (accessed June 2005).

41. Caterino J, Emond J, Camargo C. Inappropriate medication administration to the acutely ill elderly: A nationwide emergency department study, 1992–2000. J Am Geriatr Soc. 2004;52(11):1847–1855.

42. Billow J, Mort J, Vreugdenhil D, et al. Tips on communicating with the elderly. Am Pharm. 1991;NS31(4):51–54.

43. Howard M, Dolovich L, Kaczorowski J, et al. Prescribing of potentially inappropriate prescription medications for community dwelling seniors. Presented at the CPhA Conference, Vancouver, 2003.

44. Disability status: 2000—Census 2000 brief. U.S. Census Bureau, Census 2000, Summary File. Available at: www.census.gov/hhes/www/disable/disabstat2k/table1.html (accessed March 2005).

45. Currie CT. Talking to the Elderly. In: Talking with Patients—A Basic Clinical Skill, 2nd Edition. Oxford University Press, Oxford, 1992.

46. Galizia V, Sause R. Communicating with the geriatric patient. Am Pharm. 1982;NS22(10):35–36.

47. Pavlakovic R. Geriatrics: Special pharmacotherapy considerations. CE Lesson. Pharm Pract. 2004;20(2).

48. Coambs R, Jensen P, Her M, et al. Review of the scientific literature on the prevalence, consequences, and health costs of noncompliance and inappropriate use of prescription medication in Canada, Health Promotion Research, Toronto, 1995, p. 46–54.

49. Virani A. Drugdaze—How to prevent or manage drug-induced cognitive impairment. Pharm Pract. 2003;19(10):35–43, 47.

50. Peterson DA. Facilitating Education for Older Learners. Jossey-Bass, San Francisco, CA, 1983.

51. Moore SR. Cognitive variants in the elderly: An integral part of medication counseling. Drug Intell Clin Pharm. 1983;17(Nov):840–842.

52. McKim W, Mishara B. Compliance in the Elderly. In: Drugs and Aging. Butterworths, Toronto, 1987, p. 26–31.

53. Epstein D. What older patients want from you. Drug Topics. 1991;135(5):50–52, 55.

54. Culbertson V, Arthur T, Rhodes P, et al. Consumer preferences for verbal and written medication information. Drug Intell Clin Pharm. 1988;22(5):390–396.

55. MacKinnon N. Early warning system—How vigilant pharmacists can prevent drug-related morbidity in seniors. Pharm Pract 2002;18(8):40–44.

56. Recommendations on drug use in the elderly. 13th Annual Report of the Geriatric and Long-Term Review Committee to the Chief Coroner for the Province of Ontario, 2002. Pharm Connect. 2004;11(2):30–31.

57. Robertson D, Rockwood K, Stolee P. A short mental status questionnaire. Can J Aging. 1982;1(1/2):16–20.

58. Green L, Mullen P, Stainbrook G. Programs to reduce drug errors in the elderly: Direct and indirect evidence from patient education. J Geriatr Drug Ther. 1986;1(1):3–18.

59. Ascione F, Shimp L. The effectiveness of four educational strategies in the elderly. Drug Intell Clin Pharm. 1984;18(11):926–931.

60. Tett S, Higgins G, Armour C. Impact of pharmacist interventions on medication management by the elderly. A review of the literature. Am Pharmacother. 1993;27(1):80–86.

61. Morrow D, Leirer V, Altieri P, et al. Elders' schema for taking medication: Implications for instruction design. J Gerontol Psychol Sci. 1991;46(6):378–385.

62. Samovar L, Porter R. The Challenge of Intercultural Communication. In: Communication Between Cultures, 4th Edition. Wadsworth, Belmont, CA, 2001, p. 3–20.

63. Burroughs V, Maxey R, Crawley L, et al. Cultural and genetic diversity in America: The need for individualized pharmaceutical treatment. National Pharmaceutical Council, National Pharmaceutical Association. Available at: www.npcnow.org/issues_productlist/PDF/culturaldiversity.pdf (accessed November 3, 2003).

64. Rantucci M. Counselling in a multicultural society. CE Compliance Centre National Continuing Education Program, 2004. Available at: www.pharmacyconnects.com/pdfs/2004/06/NovCE June.pdf (accessed June 2005).

65. Burroughs V, Maxey R, Levy R. Racial and ethnic differences in response to medicines: Towards individualized pharmaceutical treatment. J Natl Med Assoc. 2002;94(10)Suppl. Available at: www.npcnow.org/issues_productlist/PDF/SupplementFINAL.pdf (accessed February 4, 2004).

66. Samovar L, Porter R. Cultural Influences on Context: The Health Care Setting. In: Communication Between Cultures, 4th Edition. Wadsworth, Belmont, CA, 2001, p. 241–258.

67. Lustig M, Koester J. Intercultural Competence—Interpersonal Communication Across Cultures, 3rd Edition. Addison Wesley, New York, 1999, p. 219.

68. A second diagnostic at the health of First Nations and Inuit people in Canada. Health Canada. Available at: www.hc-sc.gc.ca/fnihb/cp/publications/second_diagnostic_fni.pdf (accessed November 3, 2003).

69. Samovar L, Porter R. Nonverbal Communication. In: Communication Between Cultures, 4th Edition. Wadsworth, Belmont, CA, 2001, p. 164–195.

70. Fowler N. Providing primary health care to immigrants and refugees: The North Hamilton experience. CMAJ. 1998;159:388–391.

71. Samovar L, Porter R. Accepting and Appreciating Similarities. In: Communication Between Cultures, 4th Edition. Wadsworth, Belmont, CA, 2001, p. 262–296.

72. Kohn LT, Corrigan JM, Donaldson MS, eds. To Err Is Human: Building a Safer Health System. National Academy Press, Institute of Medicine, Washington, DC, 1999. Available at: www.nap.edu/html/to_err_ is_ human/ (accessed May 2, 2004).

73. Brennan T, Leape LL, Laird NM, et al. Nature of adverse events in hospitalized patients. Results of the Harvard Medical Practice Study II. N Engl J Med. 1991;324(6):377–384.

74. Flynn E, Barker K. Medication Errors Research. In: Cohen M, ed., Medication Errors—Causes, Prevention and Risk Management. APhA. Jones and Bartlett, Boston, MA, 2000, p. 6.1–6.30.

75. Quiring V. How to respond when medication errors occur. Presented at APhA 2001—14th Annual Meeting and Exposition, San Francisco, CA, 2001.

76. Vieira-Conti C. Close-up on complaints. Pharm Connect. 1997;4(4):12–13.

77. Murphy Enright S, Smith K, Abel S, et al. Preventing medication errors. U.S. Pharmacist Continuing Education. ACPE Program No. 430-000-00-031-H01. Available at: http://www.uspharmacist.com/ce/mederrors/default.cfm (accessed June 3, 2002).

78. Anonymous. Practical tips for errors and omissions prevention. Ont Pharm. 2002:60(1):32.

79. Anonymous. What to do in case of a dispensing error/incident. Ont Pharmacist. 2001;59(4):35–37.

80. Rantucci M, Stewart C, Stewart I. Safe Medication Practices: A Pharmacist's Guide to Preventing and Managing Medication Incidents. Pharmacy Practice. Rogers Publishing Ltd., Toronto, 2004.

81. Jinks M, Cornely P, Mayer F. The pharmacist's role in individual preventive health care. Am Pharm. 1983;NS23(7):10–17.

82. Mangione R. The pharmacist's role in child abuse prevention. Am J Pharm Educ. 1988;52(3):161–163.

83. Gerrard BA, Boniface W, Love B. Developing Skills for Coping with Interpersonal Stress. In: Interpersonal Skills for Health Professionals. Reston Publishing, Reston, VA, 1980.

84. Steptoe A. Psychophysiological Processes in Disease. In: Steptoe A, Mathews A, eds., Health Care and Human Behaviour. Academic Press, London, 1984.

85. Albro W. Dealing with difficult patients. Pharm Student. 1992;Feb:13–15.

9 Implementing Patient Counseling as a Pharmacy Service

Objectives

After completing this chapter, the reader should be able to

1. identify different opportunities for providing patient-counseling services.
2. be aware of challenges in providing patient-counseling services and ways to overcome them.
3. be prepared to take the necessary steps to select and implement patient-counseling services.

So far, this book has provided pharmacists with some theory and background information about patient counseling in order to provide an appropriate perspective for counseling. In addition, some practical aspects of counseling have been discussed concerning the content of counseling, materials and techniques, and skills required. Having understood this material, many pharmacists still find it difficult to become involved in patient counseling to the extent required today by professional and regulatory standards. Pharmacists need to recognize that patient counseling is a pharmacy service and therefore involvement in patient counseling means more than having the ability to interact with a patient; it means being able to identify what pharmacy services will be provided and implementing them.

This chapter will make suggestions to assist pharmacists in implementing patient counseling as a pharmacy service.

ENVISIONING PATIENT COUNSELING AS A PHARMACY SERVICE

Patient counseling in pharmacy does not stand alone. It is part of an array of activities that pharmacists can become involved in, over and above the traditional product-oriented dispensing functions. As discussed in Chapter 1, pharmacists need to counsel in order to meet patient care needs and demands of the health care system in which we practice, as well as to meet professional and business demands. When we view patient counseling as a pharmacy service we can envision a range of services as shown in Table 9-1. Some patient-counseling services are related to the act of dispensing; some are related to patient needs at the time of dispensing; pharmaceutical care services can be provided apart from dispensing; and some services are more specialized services.

TABLE 9-1	Range of Pharmacist Counseling Services
Services related to dispensing	Special needs labeling
	Adherence aids
	Refill reminders
	Management of prescription interpretation issues
	Management of third-party issues
Counseling services involving patient needs at the time of dispensing	Training for device, home health products, or nonprescription drugs
	Resolution of more complex drug-related problems
	Training for self-monitoring, e.g., blood glucose levels and blood pressure
Non-dispensing-related pharmaceutical care services	Medication management consultation
	Self-care consultation
	Disease-specific consultations, e.g., smoking cessation, emergency contraception, travel consultation, and menopause management
	Health care team consultations, e.g., palliative care team, home health care worker, social worker, and hospital discharge pharmacist
Specialized consultation services	Diabetes educator
	Drug abuse program
	Smoking cessation program
	Drug/poison information
	Collaborative prescribing
	Consult on a wide variety of medication-related issues for various organizations (e.g., health care organizations, governments, or education systems)

Counseling Services Related to Dispensing

When pharmacists are supervising the dispensing process, issues arise that require consultation with the patient or others involved with the patient. These services often require an investment of time and effort by the pharmacist, beyond being simply involved with supervising that the correct patient gets the correct drug at the correct time as required by most regulations. It may come to the pharmacist's attention that the patient needs modified labeling (e.g., large print and different language) or modified packaging (e.g., easy-open vials and pictographs for instructions) to deal with disabilities; or aids to adherence (e.g., refill reminders and unit of use packaging). The pharmacist will need to discuss this with the patient and/or caregivers; explain how it will help; and arrange for this to be done.

The pharmacist may also identify the need to contact the prescriber to clarify the interpretation of the prescription (e.g., clarify drug, dosage form, dose, duplicate drug or class, and availability). There may also be issues involving eligibility for third-party reimbursement that the pharmacist may have to communicate with the third party, the physician, and the patient.

Counseling Services Involving Patient Needs at the Time of Dispensing

At the time of dispensing, the pharmacist will need to counsel the patient about his or her medication, but the pharmacist may also need to provide training for a device (e.g., inhaler and blood glucose monitor), a home health product (e.g., ostomy aid and mobility aid), or discuss self-monitoring (e.g., blood glucose level and blood pressure). During the standard medication consultation, the pharmacist may identify complex drug-related problems that cannot be handled simply. For example, actual or potential drug-related problems may be identified (e.g., need different drug or dose, too late, or too early). The pharmacist may also identify a change in the patient's health status, a lack of desired outcome by a drug, or an adverse effect. This will require intervention by the pharmacist and additional communication with the patient and the prescriber. These services require additional time by the pharmacist.

Nondispensing-related Pharmaceutical Care Services

Although pharmacy services have generally been provided at the time of dispensing, there are many services that are not related to a particular drug, and are more amenable to an arranged appointment time with the patient or others involved. They require more time than can be provided at the time of dispensing and cannot usually be provided unless time is purposely set aside.

Providing services such as conducting a medication management consultation requires from 30 minutes to several hours and may also require additional time for the pharmacist to consult references, formulate recommendations, and write necessary reports and communicate verbally with physician and others as necessary.[1]

Although pharmacists often provide counseling for nonprescription drugs in a few minutes in the aisle near the product, a more complete self-care consultation would be more beneficial, although it requires additional time. Patients with chronic conditions such as allergies, constipation, or eczema could benefit from a better understanding of their conditions and nondrug treatments, in addition to nonprescription drug information.

Patients with specific condition-related needs also require a more in-depth consultation, e.g., smoking cessation, emergency contraception, travel medicine consultation, and menopause management.

As discussed in Chapter 8, pharmacists can also play an important role on health care teams managing care for patients with more complex and critical needs. Pharmacists can provide services consulting with, for example, palliative care teams, home health care workers, social workers, and hospital discharge pharmacists, as well as patients and their caregivers.

Specialized Consultation Services

Patient needs in regard to disease management may be met by a variety of health care providers in different settings in the health care system, but for various reasons such as limited funding, resources, or local availability, pharmacists find themselves ideally positioned to fill a care gap. Pharmacists generally need additional training to better understand the therapeutic area and ways to meet patient needs, and to add credibility in their ability to provide these services. Pharmacists may take certificate programs to become diabetes educators, drug abuse counselors, and drug or poison information pharmacists. They may provide smoking cessation programs for individuals or groups, and they may enter into agreements with physicians to do collaborative prescribing for patients in certain agreed-upon circumstances such as emergency contraception. Pharmacists providing these services may practice in a variety of settings in addition to a community pharmacy including a hospital or community clinic, a residential care facility, a physician's practice, or a health center. They often provide services through referral and may be funded by another organization (e.g., government, hospital, clinic, and health maintenance organization), third-party insurer, or directly by the patients.

Pharmacists may also consult on a wide variety of medication-related issues for various organizations including health care organizations, governments, or education systems. This generally requires the pharmacist to have specific knowledge and experience, often gained through advanced education and training.

CHALLENGES TO PROVIDING COUNSELING SERVICES

Gaps and trends in patient care have created a need for the wide range of pharmacy services described here. The role of pharmacists in patient care and counseling has become entrenched in standards of practice and pharmacist education in the United States and most industrialized countries (e.g., Canada, Australia, New Zealand, Britain, and Sweden). The majority of pharmacists report that they would like to spend more time counseling patients and that counseling is their most preferred activity.[2–4]

In spite of this, the quantity and quality of pharmacist–patient communication has apparently improved little over the last 25 years.[4] Between 33% and 42% of patients in various surveys have reported receiving counseling from a pharmacist, although observational studies of pharmacists report a higher figure of 54% to 74%.[5] A 2003 observational study of 306 pharmacies in eight US states found that pharmacists provided written information to 89% of the study shoppers but verbally interacted with only 75% and provided on average 2.3 items of drug information during that interaction with 53%.[5] Pharmacy services that involve patient counseling such as clinic days, disease management programs, or drug reviews are being provided to some degree (about half of pharmacies in Canada in a 1999 survey, a third to a half in a 2002 Australian study).[6,7]

What prevents pharmacists from maximal involvement in counseling services? When it comes to the practice of counseling patients, pharmacists in one survey offered more than 50 "excuses" for not communicating with patients.[8] Pharmacists are apparently confronted by many challenges to making patient counseling part of their regular activities and in implementing pharmacy services.[7–10] Pharmacy researchers have added their views as have pharmacy leaders.[1,4,11–14] More importantly, the perspectives of patients have been considered as it has been recognized that once the pharmacist overcomes barriers to initiating counseling, the patient may be a limiting factor in the length and depth of what occurs.[15]

Table 9-2 lists the major challenges that face pharmacists in providing patient-counseling services. These include challenges embedded in the system, the environment

TABLE 9-2	Challenges to Providing Patient-counseling Services
System challenges	Lack of time (appropriate support staff)
	Lack of incentives—economic, regulatory
	Workforce dynamics
	Lack of quality measures and processes
	Lack of culture of quality improvement and accountability for patient outcomes
	Lack of policy change (corporate, health care)
	Regulations
	Lack of acceptance by physician
Pharmacy environment	Lack of privacy
	Physical barriers
	Inaccessibility of the pharmacist
	Atmosphere conducive to communication (color, light, sound)
Patient challenges	Patient's poor perception of the pharmacist
	Lack of awareness on the part of the patient of the need for counseling and of its availability
	Comprehension difficulties
	Lack of time
	Lack of choice
Pharmacist challenges	Lack of knowledge (about drugs and the patient's history)
	Lack of confidence
	Lack of skills (problem solving, interpersonal, counseling, self-assessment)
	Busyness and poor prioritization and time management
	Business skills
	Lack of resources (software, designated space)
	Perception of the importance of the patient's need for the information
	Inability to disengage old practice model
	Lack of ability/knowledge to change
The challenge of change	Global practice reorientation
	Internal and external changes needed
	Structural changes
	Procedural changes
	Role orientation
	Change in organizational culture

in which pharmacists practice, challenges presented by pharmacists themselves and by their patients, and finally the challenge of change itself.

System Challenges to Providing Patient-counseling Services

An Australian study found that industry-wide change as well as individual pharmacy change was needed in order for pharmacists to implement patient-counseling services.[7] One example of this is the time challenge. Everyone agrees that providing patient-counseling services requires more time than traditional dispensing services. It has been estimated that patients can provide pharmaceutical care services to 40 to 45 patients in a 9-hour day with at least an additional hour at the end of the day to complete documentation.[1] Not surprisingly, the most commonly cited factor preventing pharmacists from becoming involved in patient counseling is lack of time.[8–10,16,17] Pharmacists report that it is the greatest source of stress in their jobs (being interrupted, not having enough staff to provide necessary services, having so much work that everything cannot be done well).[18] Part of the difficulty seems to be the type of activities that pharmacists engage in. Pharmacists report that 30% of their time is spent in nonpharmaceutical activities, and acknowledge that this is too much.[19]

The time challenge is related to a number of system issues. One is the need for sufficient and adequately trained support staff to take on many of the administrative tasks and, where possible, dispensing tasks.[13,20] When pharmacists attempt to take on additional patient care tasks involved in expanded pharmacy services they also find it helpful to use additional support staff or other health care workers working together with the pharmacist, e.g., nurses.[21] Because of the additional time required for counseling services, more pharmacists are needed. However, human resource shortages as well as corporate pharmacy policies (some requiring pharmacists to dispense a set number of prescriptions or keep staffing to within limits) make it very difficult for pharmacists to provide much beyond minimal counseling.

A further system issue related to the time and human resource issue is that of incentives and policy change.[11,14,22,23] Many pharmacists and industry managers say that reimbursement for pharmacy services must occur before they can be implemented. Yet when pharmacists implement pharmaceutical care services, they often find that revenue is not forthcoming.[21] Most existing payment models allow for payment related to dispensing only, and that allows for minimal counseling without expanded pharmaceutical care services that are best provided apart from dispensing. Health care policies must recognize the value of pharmacy services and incorporate them into funding and delivery models.

Policies regarding pharmacist education and human resources as well as pharmacy laws and regulations must be aligned to fund, reward, and provide frameworks for pharmacists to provide patient-counseling services.

A culture of quality improvement and accountability for patient outcomes is also needed to encourage pharmacists and systems in which they work to do what is necessary to assist pharmacists in providing services.[1,14] Quality measures and processes to use the measures need to be put into place so that pharmacists can know what is expected of them and get feedback on how they are progressing.[14]

Corporate policies need to recognize pharmacists' changing roles and the need for quality accountability and measures. Health care organizations and pharmacy owners who maintain standard dispensing-oriented facilities, organizational policies, and administration make it almost impossible in many cases for pharmacists to implement counseling services.

It has been suggested that the degree of state regulation seems to be one of the most important factors in determining the degree that pharmacists talk to patients, provide risk information, assess patient understanding, and provide oral information.[5] Regulators need to recognize this and put such regulations in place.

As part of the system, physicians can present a challenge to pharmacists. They are part of policy making and part of everyday practice. Their attitudes and policies to encourage pharmacists' expanded roles, teamwork, and funding must become a positive force for pharmacists to provide services.[14,24]

Challenges in the Practice Environment

The environment in which pharmacists practice presents a further challenge to pharmacists' patient-counseling activities.[1,4,7–13,25] Traditionally, pharmacists have been confined to the dispensing area of the community or hospital pharmacy with significant physical barriers between the pharmacist and patient. Raised platform dispensaries, high counters, and more importantly, lack of privacy make the patient inaccessible to the pharmacist and create an atmosphere that is not conducive to therapeutic interaction. Such physical challenges have been shown to create a negative attitude in the patient toward the pharmacist.[26] The patient's perception of the pharmacist's expertise and frequency of contact are important to developing a high quality patient–pharmacist relationship.[25]

It has been suggested that having a completely separate and private area away from the dispensary for the pharmacist to meet with the patient emphasizes to the patient the pharmacist's expertise and encourages the patient to communicate freely, allowing the pharmacist to provide appropriate pharmaceutical care services.[1] Most patients report that they want privacy, preferably in the form of a private consulting area in the pharmacy.[27,28] Studies have found mixed results about the effect of having a private counseling area, overall indicating that it does not dramatically change pharmacists' or patients' communication practices during the encounter, but does tend to increase the time spent interacting.[4,29,30]

A study comparing pharmacists providing high versus low levels of pharmaceutical care services in Canada found significant differences between groups in regard to the pharmacy environment. A higher proportion of pharmacies with high levels of services had a policy of sit-down counseling for new prescriptions, unelevated pharmacist workstation, accommodation for needs of the disabled, a patient waiting area, and AV patient education equipment.[11]

Other physical factors, such as the decor of the area—the use of color and the arrangement of furnishings—as well as lighting and noise levels, may also affect patient–pharmacist communication.[31,32] Pharmacies designed for dispensing, emphasizing factory-like efficiency and sterility, are not adequate or appropriate for pharmacists to provide counseling services, particularly services that are not provided as a part of dispensing.

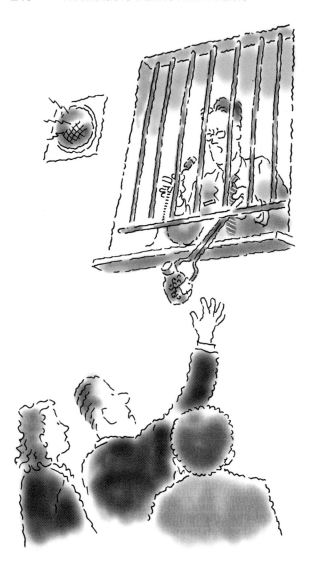

*The environment in which pharmacists practice
presents a further challenge to pharmacists'
patient-counseling activities.*

The need for extra staff, equipment, and changes to the environment increase the pharmacy department's overhead, adding to the economic challenges. Early estimates of the cost of counseling were $1 to $2 per prescription (not including the cost of the pharmacist's time).[31] A pharmaceutical implementation project conducted in North Carolina in 1997 calculated that the average cost of conversion was $36,207 (including personnel, education, remodeling, equipment, education materials, consultants, and marketing).[21]

Patient Challenges to Counseling Services

Although pharmacists may be willing to provide counseling services to patients, they often find it difficult to proceed past the initial interaction.[15] It has been found that once counseling is initiated, patient expectation for counseling and perceived importance of information determined the length and the content of counseling.[15] Patient expectations were affected by their need for cognition, experience with counseling, and self-perceived knowledge. Another study found that 1% of patients did not have time for counseling.[1] But most patients are cooperative with receiving pharmaceutical care services and understand the purpose, coming to expect it.[1] In fact, 81% of patients in another study reported expecting to receive information, but only 33% received it.[10] Many other studies have found that patients want more in-depth information than pharmacists generally give.[33–36]

Patients may be unable to access pharmacy counseling services because they subscribe to health care plans that limit their choice of pharmacy (36.8% of patients in a 1995 US study).[25] Health care programs must be made to recognize that pharmacy services can be beneficial and cost-effective.

A more significant challenge to pharmacists providing patient-counseling services is the variety of patient comprehension difficulties that pharmacists face during patient counseling. As discussed in the previous chapters, comprehension difficulties may include not only the patient's difficulties in speaking the English language because of foreign origin, but also difficulties in comprehension owing to the patient's low literacy level. The pharmacist's technical jargon and various patients' disabilities can also inhibit patient comprehension.

Pharmacist Challenges to Providing Patient-counseling Services

Pharmacists are sometimes reluctant to become involved in patient counseling because of lack of confidence in their abilities in patient counseling and in their pharmaceutical knowledge.[10] They may fear that the patient will ask a question that they cannot answer. They are often unsure of their knowledge base and worry about not being able to provide all the information that might be required. Because new drugs are continually being developed, it can be difficult for the pharmacist to keep abreast of current information. Pharmacists involved in pharmaceutical care implementation projects have found that lack of confidence was one of the challenges they faced and that participation in the implementation projects helped to overcome this, ultimately making interactions with physicians and patients easier.[37,38]

Pharmacists report that education and training are very important to providing counseling services.[6,37] It has been recognized by pharmacy educators that pharmacists require training within the undergraduate curriculum as well as continuing education (CE).[14] Pharmacists in many jurisdictions are required to participate in CE, but it may be necessary for pharmacists to do more than the minimum required, particularly for specialized counseling services. A study of pharmacies providing high and low level pharmacy services found that formal training of pharmacists was significantly higher in high service pharmacies.[29]

Lack of knowledge about the patient's medical and medication history has also been recognized as a challenge to counseling.[6,14] Fifty-one percent of pharmacists report that an up-to-date and accurate patient profile is very important to counseling.[6] Pharmacists can gather much of the information they need directly from the patient, provided that they use appropriate interviewing skills as discussed in Chapter 7. However, additional information may be needed from the physician or from hospital records and this is often not accessible by the pharmacist. Pharmacists practicing within a physician clinic setting have reported that having access to patients' records was extremely important and useful.[38]

That leads to another challenge to patient counseling, the pharmacist–physician relationship.[8,9] As discussed in Chapter 7, physician–pharmacist relationships need to be developed and nurtured for pharmacists to fulfill their roles in pharmaceutical care. Studies of the pharmacist–physician relationship indicate that physicians are not wholly accepting of pharmacists recommendations regarding drug-related problems identified in pharmaceutical care (76% of the time in a recent survey).[2,22] Concerns of physicians seem to be on the expansion of pharmacists' roles and concern about whether pharmacists have the required knowledge and skills to offer many of the proposed services.[6,24] They are also concerned that pharmacists sometimes will provide inappropriate information, or that pharmacist counseling may conflict with their advice or scare patients.[39,40] They are often unwilling to share patients' medical information that pharmacists need in order to provide pharmaceutical care services.[24] Studies indicate that, although there are areas of tension between physicians and pharmacists, physicians agree with the need for increased physician–pharmacist interaction, communication, and collaboration.[7,24,38]

Another recognized challenge that pharmacists themselves present to providing patient-counseling services is their lack of communication and interpersonal skills when interacting with physicians and with patients.[1,6,14] The importance of communication skills for pharmacists was discussed at length in Chapter 7, and problems of pharmacists in this area have been identified.[4,5,10] Lack of problem solving skills has also been recognized as a difficulty for pharmacists in providing pharmaceutical care.[1]

Pharmacists are aware of the many skills they need, but it is a challenge for pharmacists to consistently use those skills.[41] It has been found that the busyness of the pharmacy is a factor in determining the degree that pharmacists talk to patients, provide risk information, assess patient understanding, and provide oral information.[5] Prioritization and time management skills are also needed in order to deal with the demands of new roles.[1]

Because patient-counseling services require different policies and environments, pharmacists also need resources such as computer software and hardware and space. They need to have business skills to design and deliver pharmacy services and find new revenues that can provide a return on investment.[14] In addition, pharmacists need to be able to assess their progress in providing services and making the necessary changes.[14]

Along with the challenge of knowledge and skills, the pharmacist's perception of the importance of the patient's need for the information has been found to affect the degree of pharmacists' interaction with patients.[15]

Finally, pharmacists need the ability and knowledge to make necessary changes. They must disengage old practice models and be prepared to take on the challenge of change.

The Challenge of Change

It has been recognized that health care as a whole in many countries is struggling with change.[14,23] We welcome technological and program innovation but resist systematic change so that "2000s technologies are embedded in 1940s structures."[23]

Some pharmacy researchers suggest that pharmacists' involvement in counseling services require internal and external changes. Pharmacists who have implemented pharmacy services have found that they cannot just add on more patient care responsibilities but rather "global practice reorientation" is needed.[42] Pharmacists must have a role orientation for counseling as well as structures, procedures, and policies that allow them to practice in this role.[7,15]

The changes required involve many phases beginning with improving the efficiency and effectiveness of current practice, then gradual expansion of services along with strengthening stakeholder relationships before implementing the services.[20]

Structural changes are needed that involve acquiring resources such as education materials, computer hardware and software instruments, as well as social changes.[22] Procedural changes involve changes in the way people work and interact within the pharmacy as well as interaction between the pharmacist, the patient, and the physician.[22]

It has been noted that a change in organizational culture or "how we do things around here" must also change. The most important part of this is change in the management of human resources (team work, performance management, and training).[23] There must be effective teamwork within the pharmacy and within the health care system so that pharmacists, technicians, and clerks as well as pharmacists, nurses, physicians, and other health care professionals function with the patient as the most important member and the focus of the team.[23] This means that the hierarchies that exist among health care workers must be removed, and that is a huge challenge.

Performance management is also needed with members of the team, managers sharing decision making and goals, and performance appraisals that measure and reward the team rather than individual performance.[23] Training needs to be sophisticated and ongoing, not only to keep up to date on clinical issues, but also to change the way people think and work. In many organizations, pharmacists are expected to obtain their own CE in their own time and at their own expense, presenting a challenge to many.[23]

The change of the role orientation is perhaps the most challenging, and takes time and considerable effort.[20,37,38]

Many implementation projects have been undertaken to assist pharmacists with the challenge of change. They assist pharmacists to make cultural as well as structural and procedural changes. Pharmacists who participated in a project conducted in Alberta, Canada reported that they changed their perceptions of pharmaceutical care versus traditional pharmacy.[37] They found key differences, in particular in the continuity and longevity of the pharmacist–patient relationship. They derived a sense of pride and job satisfaction, increased their knowledge base and confidence level, changed their relationship with physicians, and came to take on the responsibility of ensuring a positive outcome for the patient and of decision making.[37]

However, once the projects are over, pharmacists still have the challenge of continuing on the programs and maintaining instituted changes.[38]

OVERCOMING THE CHALLENGES AND IMPLEMENTING PATIENT-COUNSELING SERVICES

The major challenges to patient counseling have now been discussed, and it can be seen that there is much that needs to be done for pharmacists to overcome these challenges and implement patient-counseling services. The challenges to implementing patient-counseling services may vary for each pharmacist and with each practice setting. Pharmacists must therefore analyze their own situations to see where challenges exist and how they may be overcome. Although this is a difficult task, we are coming to understand what is involved and that it can be approached in a logical fashion. The first task is to prepare for the change. The next is to plan the change through development of a business plan. Perceptions and goals must be changed and developed; help and resources must be accessed and allocated. A protocol for the planned services should be developed. Everyone involved must be ready to provide the planned services through motivation and management of resistance. Finally, continual evaluation should be planned.[7,20] This is summarized in Table 9-3.

Preparing for Change

Studies have been done to investigate pharmacists' readiness to change their practices so that they can offer counseling services. Change readiness is an organization's plan for change and its ability to execute that change.[7] It takes into account perception of benefits, the risk of failing to change, and demands of imposed changes.

Whether the cultural and personal changes come first or the structural and external changes is a "chicken and egg" puzzle that may never be solved. In an industry-wide report prepared by the Pharmacy Guild of Australia, pharmacists and the pharmacy industry were studied to discover their readiness to provide a range of expanded pharmacy services.[7] It was found that overall, although the majority of pharmacists were open to new ideas and to providing a range of proposed expanded services, over half

---

TABLE 9-3   **Steps to Implement Patient-counseling Services**

1. Prepare for the change
2. Select appropriate services to be offered
3. Plan the change through development of a business plan
4. Develop goals and change perceptions
5. Develop a protocol for the planned services
6. Access and allocate help and resources
7. Promote the services
8. Provide the planned services
9. Motivate and manage resistance
10. Evaluate

Sources: Dunphy D, Palmer I, Benrimoj S, et al. The Shape of our Futue-Change management and community pharmacy project. Pharmacy Guild of Australia, 2003. Available online at www.guild.org.au/public/researchdocs/2003–06_change_finalreport.pdf (accessed June 2005); Janke K, Tobin C. Getting ready for pharmaceutical care. Pharm Pract, 1997:13(10):39–42, 44–46.

TABLE 9-4   **Issues to be Considered in Preparing for Change**

- Desired level of remuneration
- Experience and approach to change
- Threats and rewards and assessment of risk
- Assess knowledge and skills
- Availability of resources and time

Source: Dunphy D, Palmer I, Benrimoj S, et al. The Shape of our Future-Change management and community pharmacy project. Pharmacy Guild of Australia, 2003. Available online at www.guild.org.au/public/researchdocs/2003–06_change_finalreport.pdf (accessed June 2005)

would not change unless they perceived a threat. The project studied pharmacists who had implemented changes in practice toward provision of pharmacy services and concluded that pharmacists needed to be ready for change.[7] They envisioned this as a progressive process that they called "the pharmacy readiness to change wheel" in which the pharmacist must consider a series of issues. Some of these issues are addressed here and summarized in Table 9-4.

Desired Level of Remuneration

Although some pharmacists are prepared to change the way they practice for the benefit of the patient and for the personal and professional satisfaction that they derive, many pharmacists will not make significant change without knowing that they will ultimately be paid. Some want to be paid from the start, others will start with the expectation that shown the benefit of the service, patients, third parties, or governments will eventually pay.[7] State programs are coming into effect in many jurisdictions, and private insurers and individual patients or their families are recognizing the value of paying for extended, individualized pharmacy services (U.S. Medicaid, Australian Community Pharmacy Agreement, British INH).[7,13,14]

Pharmacists need to identify their own level of acceptability of profit, and do a cost/benefit analysis of providing various services. Some services may be more profitable than others, whereas others may be more professionally desirable for the pharmacist.

Experience and Approach to Change

Some pharmacists are innovators, always looking for ways to do things better or differently, while others prefer the comfort of doing the same thing continually. If experience has shown that either of these perspectives works for the individual pharmacy, then pharmacists will be unlikely to change. If there has been a past negative or positive experience with providing new services, the perspective will also change accordingly.[7]

Because implementing change in counseling services can require an expenditure of time and money, involving some major changes, pharmacists must be convinced that it is important and worthwhile, and must be committed to the concept.

Pharmacists should review the benefits that counseling can bring to them and to their patients as discussed in Chapter 1. If these benefits correspond to the pharmacist's values, he or she will be prepared to embark on the necessary personal and professional development.

Threats and Rewards of Change and Assessment of Risk

As noted earlier, only threats may force change for some pharmacists.[5,7] Threats may involve loss of income due to loss of customers, regulatory enforcement of government programs, or pharmacy regulatory body standards of practice. A pharmacy banner may also have standards requiring involvement in pharmacy service programs, and the pressure of professional bodies may be felt. On the other hand, there may be rewards of personal satisfaction in helping patients, practicing professionally, or improved customer loyalty.

Pharmacists need to weigh these out and determine the risks of change or, alternatively, of not changing.

Assessing Knowledge and Skills

When preparing for change in providing counseling services, pharmacists must consider the knowledge required to provide the services and what skills they and their staff possess. Pharmacists are trained to provide most counseling services, but some may require additional knowledge about the condition or about patient needs. As discussed earlier, lacking skills in regard to communication, business management, time management, and change management can be barriers to providing counseling services. The pharmacist must consider whether they are prepared to get the additional training needed.

Availability of Resources

Providing new pharmacy services may require additional space, staff, and equipment (computers and software), as well as working capital to make necessary changes. Time and funding may be needed to train staff and for educational materials (books, journals). Promotional materials as well as counseling aids may be needed. Pharmacists must determine what is needed and if it is available.

Having the time not only to plan and implement the service, but ultimately to perform the services must also be considered. As discussed earlier, this is often a limiting factor, particularly if human resources are in short supply and demands of providing current pharmacy services are too great.

Selecting Appropriate Services to Offer

When and if pharmacists are ready to change their practices, and embark on providing counseling services, they must select what services would be most appropriate. As discussed at the beginning of this chapter, there are a range of counseling services that pharmacists can offer, from services provided at the time of dispensing to specialty services that can be offered outside the pharmacy. This should be determined according to the pharmacy clientele's needs and the pharmacist's interests. For example, the clientele may be predominantly elderly, needing frequent medication reviews and monitoring; young families with children with asthma needing education and monitoring for asthma treatment; middle-aged men and women needing menopause and hypertension management; or young community needing contraceptive counseling and travel consultations. There may also be opportunities related to a nearby medical specialty clinic such as smoking cessation, cancer, or pain management.

It is helpful to do a patient survey to identify patient needs and wants, and to discuss the communities' needs with local health care workers, public health authorities, and local physicians. Common interests may be identified as a result of this, and collaboration and teamwork may be initiated.

Planning the Change

Once a decision has been made to proceed with implementing new patient-counseling services, and the services have been decided upon, planning is critical. Development of a business plan is the best way to do this.[43] The first part of this is defining the scope of the services. One service or a range of related services may be offered locally or on a larger scale, e.g., outside the community.[7] Goals and objectives of implementing the services should be identified, including how many services would be provided over what period of time.

A list of resources needed should be made including consultants, education and training, technology, equipment, redesigning of space, additional staffing, marketing, and promotion. Organizational issues should also be considered, including the need for reorganizing work schedules and job descriptions.

A timeline for implementation should be identified.[43] This should be realistic, allowing for preparation and implementation of services and time to become profitable. In a study of US pharmacies implementing services, an average of 5 months were needed to complete the modifications, and a further 2 months after marketing services were needed before any revenue was gained.[21]

Financial implications should be estimated accounting for costs of resources and potential income, and a fee for the services should be identified based on this and the number of services identified in the goal setting.[43] A marketing plan should be developed along with a budget for it.

Changing Perceptions and Goals

Although the pharmacist planning the services may be convinced of the need, others may have negative perceptions. Pharmacy staff should be involved as much as possible in any planning and reorganization. If other pharmacists are involved, they should be encouraged in their commitment to the patient and patient counseling. The benefits may not become apparent until pharmacists begin to become engaged in providing the service, begin to develop relationships with patients and physicians, and overcome fear at giving advice and discussing patient therapy with physicians.[37] However, they can be reassured that training and practice will be provided and that benefits will become apparent.

Nonpharmacist staff members should be made aware of the purpose of the planned changes, and made party to some of the planning. A front store clerk with many years of experience, for example, may be asked to take on new roles in administration and record keeping. This requires tact and assertiveness and, if ignored or mishandled, can lead to disgruntled staff. New roles should be presented as advancements and staff should be complimented for their abilities and encouraged to be open-minded and enthusiastic about new opportunities.

As discussed earlier, physicians may feel threatened by pharmacists providing expanded patient services. To avoid problems in this area, local physicians should be

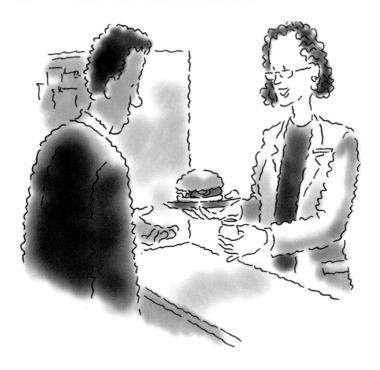

Would you like fries with your pharmaceutical care?

contacted and the nature and purpose of the new patient-counseling service should be explained. Samples of any patient education material supplied to patients can be provided for the physician's perusal. The pharmacist should be careful to present this as a service the pharmacist is providing to complement the physician's efforts in this area, and for the ultimate benefit of the patient.

Patients, too, may wonder about the changes associated with a new patient-counseling service, such as a new pharmacy layout and staffing changes. They may also be wary of the pharmacist's increased interest in them. As discussed in Chapter 5, the counseling protocol should always include an explanation of the pharmacist's purpose in the counseling, in order to prepare the patient for the potentially personal nature of the discussion, and to get the patient's agreement to continue. Patients must also be prepared that counseling services require time. As a pharmacist once said, "The patient has to understand that pharmaceutical care is going to take a little bit more of their time. I can put together a prescription as quickly as you can put together a 'Big Mac,' but that's not really providing patient care."[44]

It may be advisable to send a form letter to the pharmacy's regular clientele and provide brochures about available services and what is involved to introduce the new services. This would not only prepare patients for the change in the nature of their interaction with the pharmacist, but also promote the pharmacy and its services.

Pharmacists must also adjust their perceptions about their work environment and their priorities to cope with time challenges in providing new services, as this is one of the biggest barriers to implementing services as discussed earlier. This requires an honest and in-depth evaluation and, if overlooked at this point, attempts at patient-counseling services are destined to become frustrating. Pharmacists should consider their professional duties and rank them in order of priority within their professional role, from "immediate" to "mid-range," "low," and "complete waste of time."[45] This exercise described in Table 9-5 will help discover where time can be reallocated and change perception that there is not enough time.

As discussed earlier, pharmacists must also recognize that it will take time to make the necessary changes and implement the service.[21]

TABLE 9-5	**Assessing and Reallocating Time for Counseling Services**
Immediate priority	Duties that the pharmacist considers critical to his or her role or to the health of the patient. (The pharmacist committed to providing patient counseling would consider patient counseling an immediate priority.)
Midrange	Duties that are important to the role of the pharmacist, but have a lesser urgency in terms of time—they can more easily be rescheduled or reorganized (e.g., calling physicians and checking prescriptions)
Low priority	Routine duties necessary for the operation of the prescription department or of the whole pharmacy or the pharmacy department
	Critical to the day-to-day running of the pharmacy
	To a certain degree amenable to scheduling at the pharmacist's convenience
	Include placing orders, seeing sales representatives, doing administrative paperwork, and organizing staffing
	Some need not be performed by the pharmacist alone
	Staff retraining might allow them to be undertaken, in full or in part, by nonpharmacist staff, e.g., a nonprofessional staff member might be assigned to meet with sales representatives, with the pharmacist making the final approval of purchase orders
Complete waste of time	Interruptions during a day that pharmacists endure, sometimes out of politeness, other times out of a lack of control
	Includes telephone calls that are unrelated to pharmacy, inventory functions (stocking, unpacking, ordering), answering the delivery door, and day-to-day staffing functions
	Delegate and reorganize to minimize such interruptions

Source: Weygman L. Time management. On Cont Pract.1988:15(3):27–28.

Accessing and Allocating Help and Resources

Becoming involved in patient counseling may mean getting consulting assistance, a change in the pharmacy's physical layout, an investment in personal development and training for the pharmacists and others, accessing equipment, and obtaining counseling aids.[21] A study of pharmacies where services had been implemented found that pharmacies that gained revenue from the new services invested more in resources (on average two and a half times).[21]

Obtaining Assistance

It has been found that gaining the assistance of a consultant, a pharmacy banner, or franchise organization can be most beneficial to pharmacists implementing pharmacy service changes. A study also found that 56% of the pharmacies who had implemented services used such assistance and that those using it were significantly more successful in terms of revenue ($7283 vs. $861).[21]

Considering the Pharmacy Design and Decor

Access to the pharmacist and the atmosphere of the pharmacy are very important to providing pharmacy services. Remodeling the pharmacy may be necessary in order to provide privacy, space for new activities, and an appealing atmosphere. In a study of US pharmacies implementing new services, 84% remodeled the pharmacy, and one third remodeled a second time as they came to better understand their needs.[21]

Pharmacies should be designed to remove physical challenges and provide privacy for counseling. The pharmacist must be visible in order for patients to see that there is a pharmacist available. Sometimes pharmacists forget that the nature of a patient's illness and medication use is very personal. An atmosphere is needed in which a patient can feel comfortable asking the pharmacist's advice and discussing his or her prescription and illness.

A low prescription counter without barriers or stacked products along the divider will allow the patient to see the pharmacist. In addition, the pharmacist should be identifiable and in some way distinct from the other pharmacy staff, by wearing a nametag and a distinctive lab coat or uniform.

Even if the pharmacist is visible, the patient may not be prepared to talk particularly about personal matters. Reducing physical challenges such as removing the raised platform of the dispensary or at least providing a step down at the counter can allow the pharmacist to get physically closer to the patient, lessening the feeling of intimidation for the patient, and increasing the feeling of intimacy. The pharmacist might also lead the patient away from the counter, possibly into a quieter aisle, and position himself or herself so that the patient is between the pharmacist and the wall, thus creating a private corner.

An atmosphere of privacy can also be achieved through the use of a semiprivate counseling area. Signs or partial dividers can be used to indicate to other waiting patients that an area is designated for private counseling, discouraging them from crowding the patient being counseled (Figure 9-1). A waiting area that is out of earshot of the counseling area can also help create a greater degree of privacy.

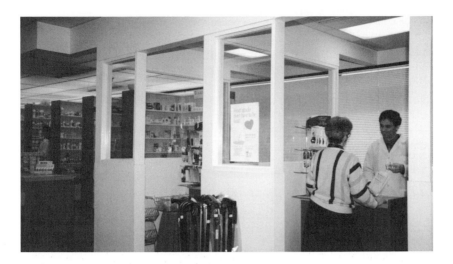

Figure 9-1   Semiprivate Counseling Booth (Courtesy of King Medical Arts Pharmacy and Home Health Care in Mississauga, Ontario, Canada)

Although pharmacies often provide counseling areas, these are often not well designed and are inconvenient or unappealing for the pharmacist to use.[46] The pharmacy layout should ideally provide a number of counseling areas, including a semiprivate and a private area (Figure 9-2). For the majority of pharmacy services provided at the time of dispensing, a semiprivate area can be incorporated adjacent to the dispensing area so that the flow of work is efficient. Some pharmacists find this is best located so that the pharmacist receives the patient at the beginning of the process, evaluating the prescription and counseling the patient prior to dispensing (known as *forward pharmacy* in Australia).[47] Alternatively, it can be located where the prescription is given to the patient.

Situations that require more privacy, such as those that involve an embarrassed or upset patient, or that call for a more detailed discussion, should be conducted in a private area. For pharmacy services provided apart from dispensing, a private area for the pharmacist to meet with the patient and prepare documentation can be away from the dispensing area or away from the pharmacy entirely. It has been suggested that this separation of the pharmacist from the dispensing area helps designate the different role the pharmacist is taking on.[1]

The pharmacy layout behind the prescription counter must also be evaluated to determine how well it provides a workflow that allows optimum efficiency and accuracy and allows the pharmacist to be available to patients. The pharmacy layout must allow for easy access by the pharmacist to the counseling areas and the nonprescription drug area.[31,48]

The general atmosphere of the pharmacy can also contribute to effective counseling. By removing clutter from the counter area and reducing noise levels (such as loud music or loud telephone bells), the pharmacist can make the environment even more

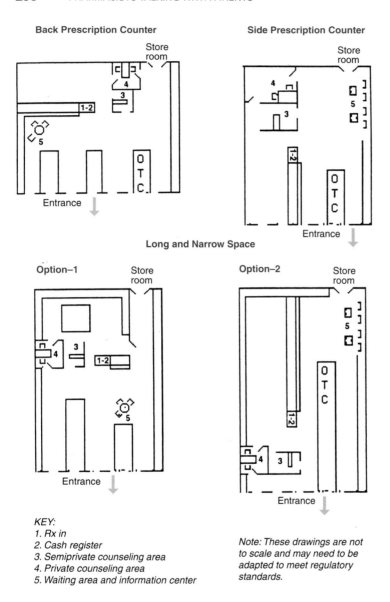

Figure 9-2 Suggested Pharmacy Layouts for Effective and Efficient Patient Counseling

conducive to conversation.[31] Some background music, however, is desirable since it reduces the ability of waiting patients to overhear the pharmacist's conversations with other patients. Lighting, color, sound, temperature, and aesthetics should all be considered.[32] Table 9-6 provides some information about these design aspects.

Figure 9-2 shows some suggested pharmacy layouts to allow maximum availability of the pharmacist. Some examples of private and semiprivate counseling areas and of a waiting area are shown in Figures 9-3–9-5.

TABLE 9-6 Pharmacy Decor Considerations	
Design Element	**Design Considerations**
Lighting	Has a physiologic, psychologic, and aesthetic effect on individual
	More intense light needed in dispensing area (30% decrease in error when significant increase in lighting)
	More natural light is more comfortable and increases satisfaction
Color	Soft colors promote calmness and would best suit a patient waiting and consulting area—blue, green, purple
	Bright colors are stimulating—red, yellow, orange
Sound	Loud ambient noise has been found to have a negative impact on patients' outcomes in hospitals
	Music and pleasing sounds (wind, water, bird song) decrease anxiety and pain and are more conducive to following instructions and cooperating
Temperature and humidity	Different people have different comfort zones
Aesthetics	Well-groomed and well-dressed staff reflect respect for patients
	Color-coded uniforms differentiate staff
	Artwork can inspire and nurture the human spirit

Source: Seifert P, Hickman D. Enhancing patient safety in a healing environment. Topics in Advanced Practice Nursing eJournal, 2005;5(1):1–11. Available online at www.medscape.com/viewarticle/499690.htm (accessed 4/1/2005).

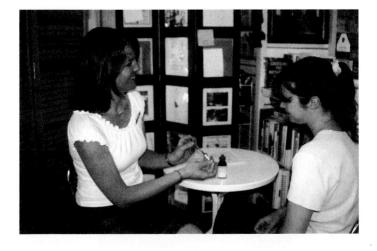

Figure 9-3   Counseling Area Built Using Room Dividers (Courtesy of Victoria Compounding Pharmacy, Victoria, BC, Canada)

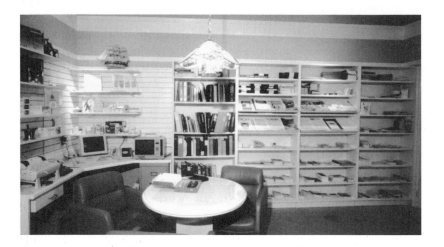

Figure 9-4   Private Counseling Room (Courtesy of Brant Arts Pharmacy, Burlington, Ontario, Canada)

Redesigning and reorganizing the pharmacy may be costly or require significant amounts of time but is well worthwhile. Pharmacies in a Canadian study which provided significantly more pharmaceutical care activities were more likely to have accommodation for needs of the disabled, an unelevated workstation, patient waiting area, patient education materials, and equipment.[11] Pharmacies that generated revenue from providing pharmaceutical care services in a US study spent on average $30,000 more on pharmacy renovation.[21] In other words, investing sufficiently in pharmacy design pays off! There may also be some financial assistance available through tax credits for modification that would accommodate disabled persons.[46]

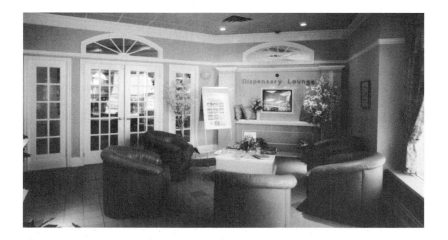

Figure 9-5   Waiting Area (Courtesy of Brant Arts Pharmacy, Burlington, Ontario, Canada)

Obtaining Counseling Aids and Documentation

As discussed previously in Chapter 6, a variety of counseling aids can be used to assist the pharmacist. The pharmacist should arrange for the convenient storage of counseling aids so that they are available at the time of counseling. In addition, a display area may be provided in the waiting area for patient-information materials, and possibly equipment for audiovisual resources made available.

Documentation is an important part of providing services, and resources must be accessed or developed for this with the input of pharmacists who will be using it. Computers and software programs and/or paper-based forms should be made available and, if necessary, training to use them.

Get Sufficient and Appropriately Trained Personnel and Manage Workflow

One of the most important and costly resources needed to implement counseling services is the human resource. It may be necessary to reallocate nonpharmacist staff as well as retrain them. In a study of Canadian pharmacies implementing services, those that provided a greater level of services had decreased involvement of pharmacists in technical functions and greater involvement of the technicians.[29]

Pharmacists need assistance with the dispensing function in order to allow them to interact more with patients. Different states have different regulations regarding what pharmacy technicians (also termed *ancillary*, *supportive*, or *nonlicensed* personnel) can do, if indeed they are recognized at all.[49] Where allowed by regulation, the pharmacy technician should perform the necessary clerical and administrative functions (e.g., stock control), technical tasks (e.g., picking, counting, and packaging), preparing the prescription, entering the necessary information into the computer, and checking the prescription through a "tech-check-tech" process, allowing the pharmacist the freedom to talk to patients. Technology is also available to do many of the technical tasks. Computer software programs are available to assist in identifying problems such as adverse drug reactions, duplication, interactions, and allergies.[50] As a result, the pharmacy technician should be able to perform most of the dispensing functions, alerting the pharmacist when problems are indicated through the computer program.

Ideally, the pharmacist should greet the patient and receive the prescription so that he or she can check any initial details with the patient, and arrange to conduct a medication management consultation interview if necessary. The pharmacist should then check the patient's medication profile to identify any drug-related problems that may show up there (e.g., duplicate drug, over- or underuse, and drug interactions). There are a few options on how to proceed from here. The pharmacist can proceed to counsel the patient at this point (known as forward pharmacy in Australia), or wait until after the medication has been dispensed.

If two computer terminals are not available, the patient's most recent drug history could be printed out with the prescription label, allowing the pharmacist to review it when checking the prescription and refer to it when talking to the patient.

Although pharmacy technicians play an essential role in the pharmacy, neither they nor the store clerks should act as intermediaries between the patient and the pharmacist. The pharmacist should be free to interact personally with the patient for prescription and nonprescription drugs, and should be the only person who counsels the patient.

The workflow and roles should be assessed and prioritized so that staffing decisions can be made.[51] One way to do this is to list the major tasks arranged in terms of priority for the pharmacist and for technicians and clerks. Asking the question "What is the value of the pharmacist completing this activity?" can help determine responsibilities.[52]

In order for a pharmacist to be available to each patient, it may be necessary to increase pharmacy staff, with either additional pharmacy technicians or an additional pharmacist, particularly during peak times. In a US study of 25 pharmacies implementing services, only 4 out of 25 needed to hire additional pharmacists, 11 hired additional technicians, and 6 hired clerks or other personnel.[21]

Getting Appropriate Training and Education

Pharmacists will likely also require additional education to improve their knowledge, skills, and confidence, particularly if specialized services will be provided such as diabetes education or palliative care. Training in communication skills, critical thinking, drug and disease knowledge, and understanding of the pharmaceutical care process (e.g., identifying drug-related problems and developing patient care plans) may be needed. This may be accomplished by books, computerized and Internet learning, and attendance at workshops, and may require travel to programs.[21] Keeping up with new information can also be assisted by subscribing to journals and by joining a professional journal club.

Developing a Protocol and Practice Guidelines for Services

A protocol for each service should be developed, specifying exactly what the service is. It should include the name of the service, e.g., Medication Review. This should be a simple but descriptive name that is helpful when it comes to marketing the service. The protocol should also describe the goals of the service in terms of the patient outcomes and benefits, e.g., improve understanding of the condition and identify adverse effects. It should list the steps included, e.g., review all medications, explain purpose, consult with the physician, document, provide a report to the patient, and follow-up. The approximate time that it should take or range of time, e.g., 30 minutes to 1 hour, should be estimated and the price of the service should be suggested. This could be per unit of time, per service, or a capitation fee per patient per year.[21] A price can be determined by considering the service in comparison to those provided by other groups (e.g., physiotherapists and physicians); comparison to dispensing services; required training, expertise and materials (e.g., blood glucose tracking software); and time required. Some pharmacists waive the fee in order to get the service established, but it is still advisable to put a price on the service and let the patient know what it would be if and when the pharmacy begins to charge.

In addition to this detailed description of services, pharmacists also need to develop guidelines and policies detailing expectations for the quality of work and new ways of working.[14,20] This may include things such as to whom the services will be offered, how the offer would be made, where the service will be offered, how many services will be performed, and requirements for documentation. This helps guide the change in the way pharmacists practice. In a study of Canadian pharmacies implementing services, those with higher levels of pharmaceutical care activities were more likely to have a policy requiring sit-down counseling for all new and refill prescriptions.[11]

Promoting Counseling Services

Pharmacists need to promote their services through a variety of means. All products benefit from marketing, and this is no different for pharmacy services. The public is generally unaware of the role of pharmacists in health care today, what services pharmacists offer, and why they need those services. Consumer expectations are low and there is a lack of demand.[14] In addition, potential payers of services such as third-party insurers, governments, and employers need to be made aware of pharmacy services available and the benefits, in terms of health outcomes, increased worker productivity, and dollars saved to drug plans and health care costs. Pharmacies who gained revenue from pharmacy services spent twice as much on marketing as those who made no revenue in a study of US pharmacies.[21]

There are many different marketing methods including brochures (in the pharmacy and placed in offices of other health care providers), signage in the pharmacy, newspaper and media advertisements.[21,43] Reputation and word of mouth can be very powerful and so it is important to maintain a maximal level of quality so that satisfied patients will spread the word.

Other health care providers should be contacted and asked to promote the pharmacists' services and refer patients. Personal "detailing" of physicians by pharmacists is important in gaining their support. This involves arranging appointments with physicians to describe the services the pharmacists will offer and invite them to participate. Physician "detailing" and use of brochures have been found to be related to greater revenue from services.[21] As discussed earlier, this should also be accompanied by maximizing opportunities to develop relationships with physicians through a variety of social, educational, and patient-centered activities. This will take time and effort to develop, so pharmacists should not become frustrated with this.

Pharmacists can further enhance the public's awareness of their availability by reaching out to their communities through speaking to community groups and schools as discussed in Chapter 6.[53]

Providing the Service

When preparations have been made ready to provide patient-counseling services the tasks involved with providing the service begin. It may need a period of time to work into full services and all involved should be patient.

Ensuring Basic Services Are Operating Efficiently

It has been suggested that pharmacists need to make sure the basic pharmacy services are operating at optimal efficiency, that current services are assessed and improved where needed, and that workflow be assessed and optimized before new services are implemented.[20] Changes in staffing and responsibilities as well as pharmacy redesign will cause changes in the way people work and this must be well thought out and run smoothly.

Working into Full Service Gradually

If pharmacists are new to providing counseling services they may find it helpful to use a series of steps. These steps are as follows:

1. *Personally Interact with Each Patient*: Receive prescription orders from patients and give out the completed prescriptions. The pharmacist will become accustomed to introducing herself or himself to patients, explaining counseling, and discussing basic prescription information (e.g., name of drug, purpose, directions, and adverse effects), answering any questions that might arise.

2. *Provide Complete Counseling in Steps*: Once the pharmacist is comfortable speaking to patients in this manner, the pharmacist can embark on complete counseling sessions for the most common classes of drugs, for example, antibiotics, anxiolytics, antihypertensives, and analgesics. To prepare for this, he or she can review the relevant pharmacology and therapeutics to provide appropriate information about the drugs in these categories. The pharmacist can also practice expressing such information in a language that most patients would comprehend and following the complete counseling protocols, incorporating pharmaceutical care suggested in Chapter 5. The pharmacist can then gradually add other more complicated issues, gaining further training in patient and therapeutic issues in order to tailor counseling as discussed in Chapter 8.

3. *Provide Community Outreach*: The pharmacist may want to develop his or her communication and counseling skills further by giving presentations to community groups about the safe use of medications or by taking part in clinics, such as "brown-bag clinics" for the elderly, in which patients' drug use is reviewed.

Identifying Patients Appropriate for Services

When all is ready to provide the complete counseling services, pharmacists should identify patients who may need or want the services, e.g., elderly patients, those on more than four drugs, and first-time users of asthma drugs. Pharmacists should be alert to patient needs when answering questions or providing medications, e.g., a patient asking about immunizations for a trip may be a candidate for a travel consultation and a mother worried about her child's increasing need for asthma medication is a candidate for an asthma consult.

Being Prepared to Offer Services

The pharmacist should plan and rehearse the "offer" of the service and be prepared to describe the service and its benefits. Brochures describing the service are particularly helpful here as the patient can use this to assist in the offer. Table 9-7 shows some phrases that can be used to offer the service and ask for commitment.[54]

Preparing for Each Counseling Session

Before meeting with individual patients, the pharmacist should take a moment to prepare for the encounter in the following ways:

1. *Review Patient Record*: For a new patient, conduct a medication management consultation, then review it for any problems that need to be discussed. For a returning patient, review the patient record for any problems.

TABLE 9-7	**Suggested Phrases to Offer Counseling Services**

Offer the service:

    "Our pharmacy offers a special service to help people with . . . and there is a fee"

    "There are additional services we provide for a fee to help people with . . ."

    "I can arrange for a *name of service* for you to discuss . . ."

Ask for commitment:

    "Do you agree that this would help you manage your *name of condition* better?"

    "Do you see how participating in this program will make it easier/help you with . . . ."

    "When would be a good time for an appointment to get started?"

Reprinted with permission from Quiring V. Above and Beyond Dispensing: How to Explain the Value of the Services and Request Payment. Live CE presentation, American Pharmacists Association Annual Meeting 1998.

2. *Organize*: Organize in your mind all the information that you must provide to the patient. If necessary, consult reference sources.

3. *Select Materials*: Select any patient-counseling aids and educational materials to be used in the counseling session.

4. *Have the Medication Available*: If the counseling session is conducted as part of the dispensing process, instruct pharmacy technicians to leave the bag unsealed, allowing the pharmacist and the patient to look at the medication bottles at the time of counseling. If the counseling session is part of a non-dispensing-related service, ask the patient to bring medications so that they can be reviewed and referred to during the consultation.

5. *Remember the Counseling Protocol*: Have the appropriate counseling protocol in mind and follow the process (Chapter 5 and Appendix A). However, remember that this should be a two-way conversation, allowing for patient questions and feedback. Also remember that individual patient's needs must be met and the session should be tailored for this as discussed in Chapter 8.

6. *Have Patient Information Available*: During counseling, the pharmacist should have access to the patient's information in the form of a computer printout of the patient record or immediate access to the patient record via a computer terminal.

Conducting the Session Efficiently and Effectively

Requirements for pharmacists to provide patient-counseling services in an effective and efficient manner can be summarized in four words: Availability, atmosphere, attitude, and approach. A summary of the methods for pharmacists to improve each of these when conducting the counseling session is shown in Table 9-8.

Availability. The pharmacist must make himself or herself available to the patient. Through time management, prioritizing, and reallocating responsibilities, pharmacists should be able to dedicate necessary time to each patient. If providing counseling at the time of dispensing, time will be limited.

TABLE 9-8	Conducting the Counseling Session
Availability	Be visible by attending to design, workflow, and human resource issues
	Manage time
	Make appointments
Atmosphere	Provide a private and semiprivate counseling area
	Use nonverbal language to create a sense of personal conversation
	Improve the general atmosphere
Approach	Use an organized approach and protocol
	Tailor counseling
	Adopt a helping approach
	Use good communication skills
	Use appropriate educational methods and counseling aids
Attitude	Attend to nonverbal messages
	Be assertive
	Be persuasive
	Be confident
	Be a lifelong learner
	Take advantage of new technologies
	Be a believer

If more time is needed, arrangement should be made for a further appointment with the patient in the pharmacy, on the telephone, or at the patient's home.

Atmosphere. Along with the design and decor of the pharmacy, the pharmacist can also enhance the atmosphere of intimacy through the use of nonverbal language.[26] To create the sense of a personal conversation rather than of a lecture, the pharmacist should position himself or herself within 2 to 4 ft of the patient. Using a quieter tone of voice, maintaining eye contact, and slightly inclining the body forward will help create a more personal and intimate atmosphere. As discussed earlier, privacy should be achieved through a semiprivate or private counseling area, and the pharmacist must decide when the situation demands this.

Approach. In order to be effective and efficient, the pharmacist should have a systematic and organized approach to any situation that a patient presents, at all times taking into consideration the specific patient and the specific situation.

Since the pharmacist has quite a lot to think about when counseling a patient (in addition to medication information), it is best to have a specific plan, or protocol, to follow. Following an organized protocol, as suggested in Chapter 5, will allow the pharmacist to grasp the situation and identify the facts involved quickly. Having an idea of specific words, actions, and sequences to use can take some of the guesswork out of counseling, allowing the pharmacist to cover the necessary information in a minimum amount of time (for suggested dialogues for counseling refer to Appendix A).

As described in Chapter 8, by considering the specific characteristics of the patient, the drug, and the situation, the pharmacist can tailor his or her counseling time in the areas most critical to optimal medication use by the patient.

The most important aspect of the pharmacist's approach to patient counseling involves the helping approach discussed in Chapter 2. This approach places the focus of counseling on the patient, allowing patients to participate in their own treatment and to decide for themselves what they need to know and what problems they need to overcome for the therapy to be most effective. It also allows the pharmacist to focus on the most important areas for that particular patient.

The pharmacist must also use good communication skills as discussed in Chapter 7. The pharmacist needs to establish conditions for effective communication, in particular, a helping relationship. The pharmacist must employ communication skills such as listening skills and skills to encourage the patient to identify his or her counseling needs and concerns. Above all, the pharmacist must allow the counseling session to be a two-way communication process, and interviewing skills will assist in doing this.

The pharmacist should also employ the appropriate educational approach as discussed in Chapter 6. The pharmacist should take into consideration adult educational principles and various factors such as the goals of the counseling session when selecting the specific educational methods for the patient. In addition, pharmacists should use an appropriate selection of the many counseling aids available, or develop ones to suit the individual patient's needs.

Attitude. The pharmacist's attitude toward counseling itself and toward individual patients will contribute further toward effective and efficient counseling when conducting the session. The pharmacist should maintain a professional but relaxed attitude, ensuring that he or she does not appear to be in a rush. Awareness of nonverbal language is important.[55] In the course of gathering information, an attentive attitude and posture that conveys interest and concern will be most likely to encourage the patient to talk.

If patients are to be willing to spend the time necessary for counseling with the pharmacist, they must be convinced that it is to their benefit. As discussed in Chapter 7, by maintaining an assertive attitude during the session, the pharmacist will indicate to the patient that it is important to listen and to understand.

The pharmacist should try to persuade patients that taking their medication is in their best interest, rather than to simply give orders to patients. As discussed in Chapter 4, the pharmacist should realize that it must be the patient's decision to follow a recommended course of therapy.

Pharmacists should also try to develop an attitude of confidence in their knowledge. Although they certainly must keep abreast of current pharmacology and therapeutics, they should also realize that, in most cases, they already possess a vast store of information that is likely to be sufficient for most counseling situations. Most questions from patients are fairly simple, and the majority of patients require quite basic information. Where more complex information is required, it is quite appropriate for the pharmacist to defer the answer to a later time, and consult a reference text or a drug-information center. It is important, of course, to arrange with the patient how and when the answer will be provided, and to make a point of following through.

Pharmacists who are anxious to provide patient-counseling services should be careful to avoid aggressiveness in their approach to counseling. They should remember that, in some situations, particularly those in which the patient is angry or upset, it may be counterproductive to proceed with the session at that time.

Motivating and Managing Resistance

A key element noted in the literature on organizational change is the need to manage resistance to change.[7] Sources of resistance can come from external and internal stakeholders.

External resisters are most likely to be other health professionals, but individual patients or the community also may not be prepared at first.[7] As discussed earlier, other health professionals may fear pharmacist encroachment on their professional roles or be concerned that patient care is not being handled as they wish. Patients may not be expecting pharmacy services and may not have time or the interest, awareness of the need, or faith in the pharmacist's ability. The community may be concerned about services such as provision of methadone to drug addicts or specialized services for patients with HIV or psychiatric illnesses. To deal with these external resisters, the pharmacist must identify decision makers and trendsetters, and build relationships with them. It is important to personally communicate with them about the services and advantages to patients. Where possible, the need should be demonstrated and the benefits shown, e.g., through individual cases or through presentation of studies conducted elsewhere.

Internally, pharmacy business owners or managers, and pharmacy staff may be resistant to change.[7] Internal resistance may come from staff, often because they do not see the benefits to themselves, and see the negatives of extra workload and stress. Some people may be unwilling or unable to make the necessary changes, because of age, personality, or lack of knowledge and personal resources. Not only must they be shown the benefits to themselves, but also whatever is necessary must be put in place to minimize extra work, stress, or overcome lack of knowledge. Simply adding on work will never be accepted or manageable.

Business owners and managers may fear the outlay of resources for little or no proven potential revenue. As best a business case as possible must be made. It should be pointed out that although implementing the services is a risk, there is also the risk of doing nothing in a time of changing health care management and cost containment so that the status quo may not be an option, as discussed in Chapter 1.

However, realistically, some people may never be convinced. If possible, these people must be allowed to opt out, and their choices should be respected. Staff should be given roles that need to be maintained, thus freeing up other staff to take on new challenges.[7]

The enthusiasm of those involved in implementing the services is very important in overcoming resistance.[7] This along with faith in the need for the services and for the change in the pharmacist's role are important in providing trial services to the point that resisters see the benefits and start to come on side.

Evaluating for Continual Improvement

Since implementing and providing counseling services is a large undertaking requiring a "global practice reorientation," it takes time and significant changes that need to be continually evaluated and modified as needed.[42,56] Pharmacists should practice their skills, but they must also reflect on their progress and receive feedback in order to improve.[56]

Practicing

For some pharmacists, it may be useful to practice patient counseling in order to feel more comfortable interacting with patients. One way to do this is to practice the dialogues suggested in Appendix A, using an audiotape or videotape recorder, or simply by practicing in front of a mirror. Practice can help the pharmacist learn the order of the protocol and the suggested wordings of, say, the introduction or the discussion of side effects.

Another form of practice that may be helpful is role-playing, where participants assume an identity other than their own and are asked to cope with hypothetical problems. Mistakes can be made and observed, and alternative responses can be tried, allowing for experimentation in relatively nonthreatening circumstances with different ways of handling a situation.[57]

Role-playing should ideally be carried out with at least two players and one observer. Roles may include pharmacist and patient, nurse, physician, pharmacy technician, supervisor, and so on.

Self-evaluation

Patient counseling and communication skills cannot be learned overnight or acquired through studying or reading a book. The pharmacist who implements and provides patient-counseling services is embarking on a gradual process of learning and self-development. Each new counseling experience will build on the previous one. And, even after many years of patient counseling, pharmacists will be faced with new situations that may require new approaches.

To learn from and to evolve through these experiences, pharmacists should evaluate their performances after each counseling situation, taking the following elements into consideration:

1. Identify what you are trying to improve and monitor improvement in that.
2. Focus on what went right and what went wrong, identifying strengths to build on, and weaknesses to work on.
3. Develop a checklist of aspects to monitor and score on a scale of one to five.
4. Evaluate the overall handling of the situation: Did the encounter end satisfactorily from the pharmacist's and patient's perspectives?
5. Evaluate whether the goal of counseling was accomplished, e.g., will it help the patient get the most benefit from his or her medication, were the patient's concerns or problems resolved or, alternatively, were arrangements made to deal with them later?
6. Evaluate each of the elements in the counseling session, e.g., gathering information, identifying drug-related problems, and identifying goals.
7. Evaluate outcomes of counseling, e.g., patient understanding of necessary information, improved adherence, and improved clinical outcomes.
8. Evaluate appropriate use of communications skills, e.g., interviewing skill and listening.

The only way to evaluate some of these aspects of counseling is of course through follow-up counseling and monitoring. Pharmacists can also self-assess by using videotape recordings to evaluate their tone of voice and nonverbal language, either in simulated, role-playing situations (as described above) or in real situations (with the permission of the patient).

SUMMARY

Understanding what counseling involves and the techniques to use is only half the battle. Pharmacists must find ways, in their individual practice situations, to implement patient counseling. This is accomplished by envisioning patient counseling as a pharmacy service and by practice reorientation. It may mean remodeling the pharmacy, extra staffing, extra learning, and new business skills. The critical element is the pharmacist's enthusiasm and willingness to work at expanding patient-counseling activities and skills at his or her own pace. The profession of pharmacy has been evolving over hundreds of years, and each pharmacist can evolve too, into a provider of effective and efficient patient-counseling services.

REFLECTIVE QUESTIONS

1. Pharmacist Richard, who owns a pharmacy in an urban community with elderly patients and young families, is considering offering patient-counseling services. What types of services could he consider offering?
2. What is a good way for Richard to decide what services to offer?
3. What kinds of challenges might Richard find to implementing patient-counseling services?
4. Richard employs a pharmacist who graduated 5 years ago and an older female clerk. What considerations and actions in regard to staffing will Richard need to make?
5. After deciding what services to offer, dealing with staffing issues, and making a number of other changes such as pharmacy design, Richard feels he is prepared to provide counseling services. What advice would you give Richard and his staff about getting ready to provide the services?

REFERENCES

1. Tomechko M, Strand L, Morley P, et al. Q and A from the pharmaceutical care project in Minnesota. Am Pharm. 1995;35(4):30–39.
2. Meade V. APhA survey looks at patient counseling. Am Pharm. 1992;32(4):27–29.
3. Anderson-Harper H, Berger B, Noel R. Pharmacists' predisposition to communicate, desire to counsel and job satisfaction. Am J Pharm Educ. 1992;56(Spring):252–258.
4. De Young M. A review of the research on pharmacists' patient-communication views and practices. Am J Pharm Educ. 1996;60(Spring):60–77.
5. Svarstad B, Bultman D, Mount J. Patient counseling provided in community pharmacies: Effects of state regulation, pharmacist age, and busyness. J Am Pharm Assoc. 2004;44(1):22–29.
6. Anonymous. Community Pharmacy Trends Report 1994-1999. Healthcare and Financial Publishing, Rogers Media, Toronto, Canada, 1999.

7. Dunphy D, Palmer I, Benrimoj S, et al. The Shape of our Future: Change management and community pharmacy project. Pharmacy Guild of Australia, 2003. Available at: www.guild.org.au/public/researchdocs/2003-06_change_finalreport.pdf (accessed June 2005).

8. Gossel TA. A pharmacist's perspective on improving patient communication. Guidelines to Professional Pharmacy. 1980:7(3):1, 4, 5.

9. Knapp DA. Challenges faced by pharmacists when attempting to maximize their contribution to society. Am J Pharm Educ. 1979:43(4):357–359.

10. Krska J, Kennedy E, Milne S, et al. Frequency of counselling on prescription medicines in community pharmacy. Int J Pharm Pract. 1995;3(July):178–185.

11. Ramaswamy-Krishnarajan J, Hill D. Designing success: Workflow and design processes that support pharmaceutical care. Can Pharm J. 2005;138(3):39–44.

12. Bennett J. Increasing interactions with patients in a busy pharmacy. Drug Topics. 1997;(June):130–139.

13. Bond C. Evolution and Change in Community Pharmacy. The Royal Pharmaceutical Society of Great Britain, London, UK, 2003.

14. Cohen J, Nahata M, Roche V, et al. Pharmaceutical care in the 21st century: From pockets of excellence to standard of care: Report of the 2003-04 Argus Commission. Am J Pharm Educ. 2004;68(3) Article S9:1–9.

15. Schommer J. Patients expectations and knowledge of patient counseling services that are available from pharmacists. Am J Pharm Educ. 1997;61(Winter):402–406.

16. Raisch D. Barriers to providing cognitive services. Am Pharm. 1993;33:54–58.

17. Schommer J, Wiederholt J. Pharmacists' perceptions of patients' needs for counseling. Am J Hosp Pharm. 1994;51:478–485.

18. Ortmeier B, Wolfgang A. Job-related stress: Perceptions of employee pharmacists. Am Pharm. 1991;NS31(9):27–31.

19. Chi J. How pharmacists feel about: Careers and workplace. Drug Topics. 1992;136(3):47, 51, 52, 57.

20. Janke K, Tobin C. Getting ready for pharmaceutical care. Pharm Pract. 1997;13(10):39–42, 44, 46.

21. Norwood G, Sleath B, Caiola S, et al. Costs of implementing pharmaceutical care in community pharmacies. J Am Pharm Assoc. 1998;38(6):755–761.

22. Kassam R, Farris K, Burback L, et al. Pharmaceutical care research and education project: Pharmacists' interventions. J Am Pharm Assoc. 2001;41(3):401–410.

23. Leggat S, Dwyer J. Improving hospital performance: Culture change is not the answer. Healthc Q. 2004;8(2):60–68.

24. Ewan E, Triska O. What is the pharmacist's role in the community? Can Pharm J. 2001;134(June):33–39.

25. Worley M, Schommer J. Pharmacist-patient relationships: Factors influencing quality and commitment. J Soc Admin Pharm. 1999;16(3/4):157–173.

26. Ranelli PL. The utility of nonverbal communication in the profession of pharmacy. Soc Sci Med. 1979;13A(6):1733–1736.

27. Anonymous. Schering Report XIV. Ky Pharm. 1992;(June):176–178.

28. Anonymous. NACDS study rates the value of some pharmacy services. Am Pharm. 1992;NS32(4):5.

29. Ramaswamy-Krishnarajan J, Hill D. Pharmaceutical care in Canada. An exploratory study of 81 community pharmacies. Can Pharm J. 2005;138(4):46–50.

30. Laurier C, Poston J. Perceived levels of patient counseling among Canadian pharmacists. J Soc Admin Pharm. 1992;9(3):104–113.

31. Polanski R, Polanski V. Environment for communication. Am Pharm. 1982;22(10):545–546.

32. Seifert P, Hickman D. Enhancing patient safety in a healing environment. Top Adv Pract Nurs J. 2005;5(1):1–11. Available at: www.medscape.com/viewarticle/499690.htm (accessed April 1, 2005).

33. Malone D, Rasciti K, Gagnon JP. Consumers' evaluation of value-added pharmacy services. Am Pharm. 1993;NS33(3):48–56.

34. Anonymous. Schering Report XIV, Improving patient compliance: Is there a pharmacist in the house? Schering Laboratories, Kenilworth, NJ, 1992.

35. Mackowiak JI, Manasse HR. Expectations for ambulatory services in traditional and office-practice pharmacies. Am J Hosp Pharm. 1984;4l:1140–1146.

36. Airaksinen M, Vainio K, Koistinen J, et al. Do the public and pharmacists share opinions about drug information. Int J Pharm. 1994;8(4):168–171.

37. Huyghebaert T, Farris K, Volume C. Implementing pharmaceutical care: Insights from Alberta community pharmacists. Can Pharm J. 1999;132(Feb):41–46.

38. Sellors J, Sellors C, Woodward C, et al. Expanded role pharmacists: Consulting in family physicians' offices—a highly acceptable program model. Can Pharm J. 2001;135(Sept):27–35.

39. Halpin P. Reading the numbers. Interaction. Improving physician–pharmacist communication. Pharm Pract. 1997;(Suppl):26.

40. Rinelli P, Biss J. Physicians' perceptions of communication with and responsibilities of pharmacists. J Am Pharm Assoc (Wash). 2000;40(5):625–630.

41. Hargie O, Morrow N, Woodman C. Pharmacists' evaluation of key communication skills in practice. Patient Educ Couns. 2000;39:61–70.

42. Janke K, Kennie N. Developing a "practice change" approach. Can Pharm J. 1996;29(2):48–49.

43. Ling C. Top 5 tips for setting up a successful cognitive services practice. Ont Pharmacist. 2004;62(June/July):12–13.

44. Stover K. Overcoming workplace barriers is key topic at APhA annual meeting. Pharm Today. 1996;2(4):15.

45. Weygman L. Time management. On Cont Pract. 1988:15(3):27–28.

46. Feegel K, Dix Smith M. Counseling and cognitive services for Medicaid patients under OBRA-90. Pharm Times. 1992;9(Suppl):1–9.

47. Whitehead P, Atkin P, Krass I, et al. Patient drug information and consumer choice of pharmacy. Int J Pharm Pract. 1999;7(June):71–79.

48. Heard B. The pharmacy setting in patient counseling. On Cont Pract. 1985;12(3):17–21.

49. Ball S. Technicians: Boon or bane to busy pharmacists? Drug Store News. 1991:1(8):23, 24, 26, 28.

50. Cataldo R. Obra'90 and your pharmacy computer system. Am Pharm. 1992;NS32(11):39–41.

51. Janke K. Better use of technicians. The Efficient Pharmacy. 1997;1(1):1, 4. Available at: www.efficientpharmacy.com/EPInewsletter.html (accessed July18, 2005).

52. Janke K. Maximizing your technician resource. The Efficient Pharmacy. 1997;1(2):2. Available at: www.efficientpharmacy.com/EPInewsletter.html (accessed July18, 2005).

53. Nelson M. Our guest for tonight is...Pharmacists and public speaking. Am Pharm. 1993;NS33(3):59–62.

54. Quiring V. Finding the Right Words. In: Peister S, Smiley T, eds., Operation M.E.T.C. How the Medical Expense Tax Credit Opens Doors to Bill for Service. Pharmacy Practice, Rogers Communications, Toronto, Canada, 2004, p. 19.

55. Samuelson K. Nonverbal messages can speak louder than words. Health Care. 1986:12–13.

56. Janke K. Initiating practice change: Assessing your pharmaceutical care skills. Can Pharm J. 1998;131(Feb):40–43.

57. Beardsley W, Knapp D. Developing role-playing scenarios. Am J Pharm Educ. 1980;44(2):162–167.

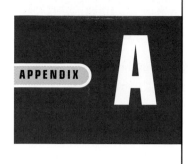

A Suggested Dialogues for Counseling

The following dialogues are provided to assist pharmacists in the patient-counseling discussion, in particular, ways to introduce topics and ways to word difficult concepts like side effects. Of course this is just a suggestion, and the pharmacist should use words with which he or she feels natural and comfortable. Please note also that, since this does not include patient dialogue, real-life counseling may result in a slightly different organization as discussed in Chapter 8.

COUNSELING FOR A NEW PRESCRIPTION

Opening Discussion

a. Personal introduction:
    "Hello, Mrs. Jones. I'm the pharmacist, Melanie."
b. Exchange pleasantries where appropriate:
    "Nice weather we're having today?"
c. Explain the purpose of the counseling session:
    "I'd just like to take a few minutes to discuss your prescription with you to make sure you get the most benefit from it."
d. Give written information if available:
    "Here is some information about your medication. Read it over when you get home, and if you have any questions, give us a call."

Discussion to Gather Information and Identify Needs

a. Medication history:
    • If the patient is new to the pharmacy, conduct a medication management consultation. See the dialogue in the Medication management consultation section.

- If the patient is already on record, confirm before embarking on counseling that he or she has not had this medication before and that the situation therefore requires new-prescription counseling.

b.   Patient's present knowledge:
  - Find out what the patient knows about the medication and the reason that he or she must take it:

    "What did the doctor tell you about the medication?"
  - If necessary, also ask:

    "How did the doctor say it would help?"

    "What did he or she say it was for?"

c.   Potential problems:
  - Identify potential problems. Ask:

    "Do you have any questions or concerns about anything at this point?"

Discussion to Develop Care Plan and Resolve Problems

a.   Summarize problems identified:

"I have a concern about..."

"I need to ask you more about..."

b.   Discuss problems and rank:

"First I think we need to..."

c.   Agree on alternatives:

"There are a few ways that I can help you with this..."

"What would you like to do?"

d.   Implement plan:

"We agree then that..."

e.   Discuss outcomes and monitoring:

"To make sure this is working you need to..."

"You can keep track of this by..."

"You should be feeling some relief of pain within 30 minutes of taking this medication. Let me or your doctor know if you are not finding relief. Hopefully by the time you have finished all these pills, you'll no longer be needing it."

Discussion to Provide Information and Educate

a.   Proceed to provide information as needed:
  - (i)   What the medication is called:

    "This medication is called _____."
  - (ii) What the medication is supposed to do (if the patient doesn't know):

    "They are pain killers, to relieve the pain in your back."
  - (iii) How and when to take the medication:

    "How did the doctor tell you to take it?"

If the patient doesn't know, tell him or her, for example:

"Take them every 3 to 4 hours, but only when you need them for the pain. It's best to take them with food or milk so that the aspirin won't upset your stomach."

(iv) Adherence discussion:

"Do you see any difficulties in taking what we have discussed?"

If suggestions seem necessary:

"You may find it easier to remember to take the pills if you always take them at meal times."

(v) Precautions or side effects:

"Sometimes along with the wanted effect of the drug, unexpected effects occur. Did the doctor mention anything about this?"

- Mention only the most common side effects and only those that are appropriate (e.g., warn against sun exposure only in summer or if the patient spends prolonged periods out of doors).

- Include instructions on how to minimize or avoid side effects:

  "Some people find that these pills make them drowsy, so see how they affect you before you drive or do anything that requires alertness."

(vi) Symptoms of adverse effects:

- Mention only the most common adverse effects, and put them into perspective by noting how rarely they occur. Describe the signs of adverse effects (do not give complicated names) and what to do if they arise. If data are available express this in numbers:

  "Very rarely (occasionally, frequently)/one in ten (hundred, thousand, etc.) people develop a reaction to this medication. This probably won't happen to you, but if you notice an unexplained fever or a rash, let your doctor or the pharmacist know about it right away."

(vii) Storage instructions, if any

(viii) Refill instructions:

"The doctor has written that you may get these pills again in 10 days if you still need them."

- If there are no refill instructions and it's a medication that would likely be refilled, find out if the doctor instructed the patient verbally:

  "Did the doctor tell you what to do after you finish these pills?"

b. Discuss outcomes and monitoring if not discussed under Care Plan development:

"Be sure and let me know about how the medication is working as we discussed earlier."

Closing Discussion

a. Recap important points:

"Remember, this medication may make you drowsy."

b. Get feedback:

- Make sure the patient understands:

  "Do you have any questions about this?"

- If the directions are complicated or if you doubt that the patient has understood them, ask the patient to repeat the directions back to you:

  "Just to make sure I've made myself clear, could you tell me now how you are going to take these pills?"

c. Encourage the patient to call if any questions or problems arise:

   "If you have any questions or problems, don't hesitate to call us."

d. Arrange follow-up:

   "Would you give me a call tomorrow to let me know how you are doing with the medication?"

   - Alternatively:

     "Can I call you tomorrow to see how you are doing with the medication? . . . What time would be convenient?"

REFILL PRESCRIPTION COUNSELING AND MEDICATION MONITORING/FOLLOW-UP

Opening Discussion

a. Personal introduction (including both the patient's name and your name if you're not already acquainted):

   "Hello, Mrs. Jones. I'm the pharmacist, _____."

b. Exchange pleasantries where appropriate:

   "Nice weather we're having today?"

c. Explain the purpose of the counseling session:

   "I'd just like to discuss your prescription with you for a few minutes to make sure you're getting the most benefit from it."

d. If this is a prearranged follow-up consultation, remind the patient why you are calling:

   "I'm calling to make sure you're getting the desired effect from the medication."

Discussion to Gather Information and Identify Needs

a. Medication history:

   - Check the patient record before counseling for any new medications that could cause problems in combination with this one (e.g., scheduling or drug interactions). To confirm that there are no changes ask the patient:

     "Are you on any new medications that were prescribed by a doctor or that you purchased yourself, since you were last here?"

b. General inquiry:

   - Ask the patient if he or she has any questions about or has had any problems with taking the medication:

     "Is there anything you'd like to discuss about this medication?"

c. Effectiveness:

   - Ask the patient if the medication is having the desired effect:

     "Are you finding it helps the symptom or condition being treated?"

d. Adherence:
- Ask the patient if he or she has any problems with taking the medication:
  "Are you finding any difficulty taking it?"
- Determine whether the patient is compliant by checking the date of the last refill and by asking how he or she takes the medication:
  "When during the day do you take the pills?"
- If you suspect nonadherence, probe further, without sounding judgmental:
  "It's sometimes difficult to find the time to take your medication. How often would you say you miss a dose?"

e. Side effects or adverse effects:
- Find out if the patient is experiencing any untoward effects:
  "Have you noticed anything unusual or out of the ordinary while taking this?"
- Be more specific, if necessary, naming possible symptoms of adverse effects or side effects:
  "Have you had an upset stomach at all while you've been taking this?"

Discussion to Prevent or Resolve Problems

Discuss problems identified regarding any adherence, or side effect problems detected, or other questions or problems mentioned by the patient:

"There seem to be a few things that you may need help with . . ."

"You may be experiencing an unwanted effect of the medication . . ."

Discussion to Provide Information and Educate

Give information about the illness and the drug where necessary, for example:

"You might find this medication less irritating to your stomach if you take it at meal times or with some food or milk."

or

"This medication is not intended to actually cure your back problems. It will just help relieve the pain."

or

"This medication may be more effective if you take it on a regular basis when your back is bothering you a lot, rather than waiting until the pain is extreme."

Closing Discussion

Same as for new prescription.

a. Recap important points or provide reassurance as needed.
b. Get feedback.
c. Encourage the patient to call if any questions or problems arise.
d. Arrange follow-up.

NONPRESCRIPTION DRUG COUNSELING

Opening Discussion

a. Personal introduction:
    "I'm the pharmacist, _____. Can I help you find something?"

b. Find out for whom the over-the-counter drug is intended:
    "Who is the medication for?"

c. Explain the purpose of the counseling session:
    "I'll just ask you a few questions to find out the best medication for you in this situation."

d. Provide print information, if available:
    "Here is some information about colds."

Discussion to Gather Information and Identify Needs

a. If the patient is not present, find out his or her age.

b. Medication history and chronic conditions:
    - If you have a patient record for this patient, check it before counseling to see whether the patient is currently taking any medications or has any conditions that might interfere with nonprescription medication use.
    - If the patient is new, conduct a brief medication history:
      "I need to ask you a few questions about your health."
      "Are you taking any other medications at the moment?"
      "Have you ever had a reaction to any drug that you've taken before?"
      "Do you have any medical conditions at the moment, such as diabetes, high blood pressure, heart condition, ulcer, and so on?"

c. Patient's present situation:
    - Find out if the patient has consulted a doctor or a pharmacist about this condition before:
      "Have you spoken to your doctor or a pharmacist about this before? . . . What did he tell you to do?"

d. History of condition:
    "How long have you had this?"
    "Have you ever had it before?"

e. Description of symptoms:
    "Is the cough dry and tickly? . . . Is it loose and rattling?"

f. Past treatment:
    "What have you taken already or in the past for this condition? . . . How well did it work?"

Discussion to Develop Care Plan and Resolve Problems

a. Summarize problems identified:

"*I believe you are experiencing symptoms indicating a viral infection . . .*"

"*I need to ask you more about . . .*"

b. Discuss problems and rank:

"*First I think we need to . . .*"

c. Agree on alternatives:

(i) If no medication is warranted or if it appears necessary to see the doctor, then recommend this:

"*It seems that the best thing for you would be to continue using the humidifier and the medication the doctor gave you already.*"

or

"*In your case, I think it's best not to take anything right now. I suggest you see your doctor as soon as possible.*"

(ii) If medication is needed:

"*There are a few ways that I can help you with this . . .*"

"*What would you like to do?*"

d. Implement plan:

"*We are agreed then that you should contact the doctor/take medication/try doing the following that I have suggested in addition to medication/before taking medication.*"

Discussion to Provide Information and Educate

a. Give information about the condition:

"*Your cough sounds like it's a tickly cough resulting from your cold and runny nose.*"

b. Suggest nondrug remedies if possible:

"*Try having frequent sips of juice or water, and try sucking cough candies to ease the tickle.*"

c. If appropriate, suggest a product to use:

"*This cough medicine may help dry up your runny nose and reduce your coughing.*"

d. Be supportive and encouraging:

"*It will probably improve as the cold gets better.*"

e. Product information:

● If a product is recommended, give information about the medication as described for prescription counseling: name, purpose, directions, side effects, precautions, and so on.

f. Discuss outcome and monitoring:

"*You should find the cough is reduced within an hour of taking the medication.*"

Whether a medication is recommended or not, suggest that the patient contact his or her physician if the condition persists:

"*If this continues on for _____ days, or seems to get worse _____ (give specific signs if appropriate, e.g., green sputum), then see your doctor.*"

Closing Discussion

a.   Recap important points:

b.   Get feedback:

- Make sure the patient understands:

     "Do you have any questions about this?"

c.   If the directions are complicated or if you doubt that the patient has understood them, ask him or her to repeat the directions:

"Just to make sure I've made myself clear, could you tell me now how you are going to take this cough medicine?"

d.   Encourage the patient to call if any questions or problems arise:

"If you have any questions or problems, don't hesitate to call us."

e.   Arrange follow-up: Same as for new prescription.

MEDICATION MANAGEMENT CONSULTATION

Opening Discussion

a.   Personal introduction:

"Hello, Mrs. Jones. I'm the pharmacist, _____."

b.   Exchanging pleasantries where appropriate:

"Nice weather we're having today?"

c.   Explain the purpose of the medication management consultation:

"In this pharmacy, we keep records about you and the medications you take to help ensure that you get the most benefit from them. I'd like to take a few minutes to ask you some questions."

d.   Ensure confidentiality:

"Of course, any information you give me will be strictly confidential and will be kept in the computer in your personal patient record."

e.   Get consent:

"Would it be all right for me to continue with this now?"

or

"I'd like to continue with this now."

Inquiry of Personal Information

a.   Introduce the section:

"First I need some information for our records about yourself."

b.   Ask personal questions:

"Sometimes your age or what you do for a living can affect your health and medication use so I need to ask you about these."

"What is your birth date?"

"Are you working at the moment? . . . Do you mind telling me what you do?"

Some comments following the patient's responses would help set a conversational tone, e.g., *"That's the same month as my birthday . . . That sounds like an interesting job."*

c. Use of health care professionals:

"Who is your family doctor? . . . How often do you see him or her?"

"Do you also see any specialists? . . . What is your dermatologist's name? . . . How often do you see him or her?"

d. Social support and cultural issues:

"Is there someone at home who helps you when you are not well?"

"Who makes the decisions about your health in your family?"

Discussion of Medical Conditions and Medication Use

a. Introduce the section:

"Now I'd like to ask about your medical conditions and medication use."

b. Ask about the condition currently being treated:

"First, what brought you to the doctor?"

c. About existing conditions in general:

"Do you have any medical conditions at the moment, such as diabetes, high blood pressure, heart condition, ulcer, and so on?"

d. Gather information about each condition and the medications associated with it before proceeding to the next condition.

- ● Ask about the duration of the condition:

  "Now I'd like to discuss each of your conditions. First, how long have you had diabetes?"

- ● Ask about medication used for the condition:

  "Are you taking any medication at the moment for your diabetes?"

- ● Ask details about each medication sequentially:

  1. Prescriber: *"Who prescribed this medication for you?"*
  2. Method of use: *"How do you take this medication?"*

- ● Probe for details, if necessary, to ascertain adherence:

  "How much do you take each time?"

  "When during the day do you take it?"

  "When do you take it in relation to meal times?"

  "How many days a week do you take it, on average?"

  3. Effectiveness: *"Do you find that these pills help you?"*
  4. Reasons for nonadherence (if nonadherence is detected):

  "Is there any particular reason that you don't take this every day?"

  or

  "I realize it's difficult to remember to take medications on a regular basis. Is that a problem for you?"

    5. Side effects and adverse effects:

       "Have you noticed anything unusual or out of the ordinary while taking this?"

- Be more specific, if necessary, naming possible symptoms of adverse effects or side effects:

       "Have you had an upset stomach at all while you've been taking this?"

e.   Repeat (1–5) for each medication.

f.   Past medications for the condition:

  "Have you been on any other medications for this condition in the past?"

  "Why were they discontinued?"

g.   Repeat (c–e) for each condition.

h.   Other prescribed medication use:

  "Other than the medications we've discussed, are there any other medications that you take?"

Nonprescription Drug Use, Herbals, Alternative Remedies Used

a.   Names of nonprescription drugs used:

  "Are there any medications that you take that you buy yourself without a prescription?"

  "Do you take any herbal or home remedies?"

- Probe if necessary:

  "Do you take anything for stomach upset? . . . What about for colds? . . . For headaches or pain?"

  "Do you get acupuncture, or other alternative treatments?"

b.   Method of use:

    1. Dosage:

      "How much do you take each time?"

    2. Frequency:

      "When do you take it during the day?"

    3. Duration:

      "Are you taking this at present?"

      "How often do you take this (most days?

      "How often have you used this in the past few weeks?

    4. Side effects or adverse effects:

- Find out if the patient is experiencing any untoward effects:

  "Have you noticed anything unusual or out of the ordinary while taking this?"

- Be more specific, if necessary, naming only possible symptoms of adverse effects or side effects:

  "Have you had an upset stomach at all while you've been taking this?"

Discussion of Alcohol and Tobacco Use

a. Introduce the topic:

"Now, I need to ask you about alcohol and tobacco use. This is important for me to know since alcohol and tobacco can affect your conditions and your medications."

b. Proceed with a question about smoking:

"Do you smoke at all? How many cigarettes do you smoke in a day?"

c. Ask about alcohol use:

"Many people have a glass of wine or beer with their meals or in the evenings. How often do you have an alcoholic beverage? ... Do you alter the way you take your medication when you are planning to have a drink?"

Discussion of Allergies or Drug Sensitivities

a. Ask about allergies:

"Are you allergic to any medication that you know of?"

b. If the answer is yes, ask the patient to describe the reaction:

"What happened when you took _____?"

c. Ask if the present physician is aware of this:

"Does Dr. _____ know about this?"

d. Ask about any previous problems with drug use:

"Have you ever had an unpleasant or untoward effect from a medication?"

e. If the answer is yes, repeat (b) and (c).

Discussion to Develop Care Plan and Resolve Problems (May Occur at a Later Time)

"When we talked ... (earlier, yesterday, last week, etc.) ... I asked you quite a few questions about your health and medication use. I've thought it over and there's a few things I'd like to discuss with you that might help you get more benefit from your medications."

a. Summarize problems identified:

"I have a concern about..."

"I need to ask you more about..."

b. Discuss problems and rank:

"First I think we need to..."

c. Agree on alternatives:

"There are a few ways that I can help you with this..."

"What would you like to do?"

d. Implement plan:

"We are agreed then that..."

e.   Discuss outcomes and monitoring:

"To make sure this is working you need to..."

"You can keep track of this by..."

f.   Arrange for further consultations to educate or monitor as needed:

"I'd like to talk to you further, to explain about your condition/medications. Perhaps we can arrange a time to do this. When would be convenient for you?"

g.   Get permission to contact physician if necessary:

"I need to let your doctor know about the things we've discussed today. With your permission I will send him a report/speak to him."

Closing Discussion

a.   Ask if there is any other information the patient thinks you should know:

"We're just about finished now. Is there any other information you think I should know?"

b.   Tell the patient what will be done with the information:

"I'll be keeping this information on your medication record for future reference."

or

"I'll be looking this over and will probably meet with you again when you are discharged from the hospital."

c.   Provide documentation:

"Here is a summary of the things we have discussed."

d.   Thank the patient for his or her time:

"Thank you for your time and help."

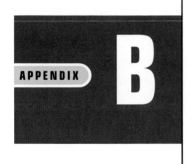

APPENDIX

B

Forms to Assist in Patient Counseling

MEDICATION MANAGEMENT CONSULTATION FORM

When conducting a medication management consultation, it is helpful for the pharmacist to use a medication-history interview form to gather data. This form can also be used to document the history-taking activity and to note any interventions that the pharmacist decides to make as follow-up to the interview.

PATIENT QUESTIONNAIRE

In order to save time during information gathering, a patient questionnaire can be used. The pharmacist should explain the purpose of gathering the information, then ask the patient to complete the form while, he or she waits for the prescription to be prepared. When it is complete, the pharmacist can then review the information on it with the patient, asking questions where more detailed information is needed.

NONPRESCRIPTION COUNSELING RECORDING FORM

When counseling patients regarding nonprescription drugs, it is useful to have a form to record information gathered during the discussion with the patient. It can also serve as documentation of the counseling encounter for the pharmacist's records and, if necessary, to send to the patient's physician.

One part of the form listing the pharmacist's suggestions for treatment can also be separated and given to the patient for his or her future reference.

HEALTH CARE PROFESSIONAL COMMUNICATION REPORT

In order to communicate and share information with other members of the health care team, pharmacists need to document their interactions with shared patients. It should follow the SOAP format (subjective, objective, assessment, plan) but should also explain the pharmacist's involvement with the patient. This should be preceded or followed-up by verbal communication whenever possible.

PATIENT CONSULTATION REPORT

It is useful to provide a written summary following a consultation with a patient in which medication-related problems are identified and actions recommended. This will provide similar information to that in the Health Care Professional Communication Report, but should be presented in more patient-friendly language.

MEDICATION MANAGEMENT CONSULTATION FORM

Patient Name:_____ Date: _____

Address:_____ Phone: _____

Birth Date:_____ Drug Plan:_____

Physicians: _____

1. Conditions (*duration*): Primary concern today:_____

  ● Kidney disease _____   ● Heart disease _____   ● Diabetes _____
  ● Liver disease _____   ● High blood pressure _____   ● Thyroid disease _____
  ● Stomach or duodenal ulcer _____   ● Asthma, bronchitis _____
  ● Epilepsy _____   ● Hay fever or other allergies _____
  ● Other: _____

2. **Medications currently used for each condition:**
Condition # 1

Drug Name	Dose	Freq/day	Duration	Effectiveness	ADR

Condition # 2

Drug Name	Dose	Freq/day	Duration	Effectiveness	ADR

Condition #3

Drug Name	Dose	Freq/day	Duration	Effectiveness	ADR

3. **Over-the-counter/Herbal/Homeopathic/Home Remedies:**

Drug Name	Dose	Freq/day	Duration	Effectiveness	ADR

4. **Adverse Effects:**

DrugName	Effects

5. **Drug-related Problems and Recommendations:**

Problem	Recommendations

6. **Interventions:**
Patient counseled: _____   Physician contacted: _____
Other:

PATIENT QUESTIONNAIRE

Patient Name:_____ Date: _____
Address:_____ Phone: _____
Birth Date:_____ Drug Plan:_____
Physicians: _____

Note: All information given in this questionnaire will be kept strictly confidential.

This pharmacy keeps records about you and the medication you take to help ensure that you get the most benefit from your medication. The pharmacist will spend some time with you to discuss the use of your medication in confidence. To allow the pharmacist to accurately assess your medications, please answer the following questions:

1. Do you have any chronic illnesses? (*If yes, please check below*) yes _____ no _____
   - Kidney disease_____
   - Heart disease_____
   - Diabetes_____
   - Liver disease_____
   - High blood pressure_____
   - Thyroid disease_____
   - Stomach or duodenal ulcer_____
   - Asthma, bronchitis_____
   - Seizures_____
   - Hay fever or other allergies_____
   - Other:_____

2. What medications are you currently taking on a regular basis, including drugs prescribed by a physician and those you take yourself (such as vitamins, nonprescription products, herbal or home remedies)? How much are you taking per day?

Prescription drugs	Dose	Freq/day	Physician

Nonprescription, Vitamins, Herbal, or Home Remedies:

	Purpose	Dose	Frequency
Laxative			
Stomach/antacid			
Pain medication			
Cold/allergy			
Other			

3. Have you ever experienced any ill effects from medications? yes _____ no _____
   If yes, please describe:

Drug	Ill Effects

NONPRESCRIPTION COUNSELING RECORDING FORM

Patient Name:_____ Date: _____

Age:_____ Address:_____

Phone:_____

Medication History

Illness Conditions: See patient record _____ or form attached _____

Physician's Name: _____ Consulted: yes____ no_____

Presenting Complaint

Location: _____

Quality: _____

Severity: _____

Modifying factors: _____

Timing: _____

Associated symptoms: _____

Previous treatment: _____

Recommended time for follow-up: _____

Copy and tear here for the patient

Pharmacist's Suggestions for Treatment

Patient's name: _____

Contact physician: _____

Nonmedication recommendations: _____

Nonprescription medication: _____

Information provided (as per label): _____

Additional information: _____

If the condition worsens or does not improve within _____
contact the pharmacist or your physician.

Pharmacist: _____ Date: _____

Source: Srnka Q. Implementing a Self-care-consulting Practice. Am Pharm. 1993:NS33(1):61–70.

Health Care Professional Communication Report
Rantucci Medical Dispensary, 1399 King Street, Buffalo, New York

April 4, 2005
Re: Jason Philbrook

Dr. R. Fulton
233 Queen Street
Buffalo, New York

Dear Dr. Fulton,

Jason is a 10-year-old boy who has been taking medication for asthma for approximately 2 years. As prescribed by you, he has been receiving salbutamol inhaler and budesonide turbuhaler approximately monthly from a previous pharmacy for the last year. He also started receiving salmeterol, 1 puff twice daily two months ago.

In speaking with his mother, Susan Philbrook, on April 4, 2005, it came to my attention that Jason has been experiencing more frequent episodes of shortness of breath and wheezing (approximately 3 times daily), for which he is using the salbutamol. I reviewed his method of use of medications and discovered that he has discontinued use of the budesonide as his mother thought the salmeterol was replacing it. In addition, the family has recently acquired a new pet rabbit which Jason handles frequently.

I have explained the use of all the medications and retrained Jason and his mother on appropriate use and technique for administration, and cautioned that the rabbit may be exacerbating Jason's condition. I have recommended that an appointment be scheduled with you to review his asthma condition and therapy. I would also recommend that Jason undergo allergy testing to determine if the rabbit and possibly other environmental factors are contributing to his condition and that a spirometer be utilized regularly and results charted by Jason in order to get a clear picture of treatment effectiveness. I can provide instructions about this and a regular asthma monitoring consultation service if you and Mrs. Philbrook wish. There will be a pharmacy service fee for this consultation (possibly covered by Mrs. Philbrook's third party drug coverage).

Please contact me if you need additional information or to arrange for the above services.

Sincerely,

Melanie Rantucci,
Pharmacist, Rantucci Medical Pharmacy

cc: Mrs. Susan Philbrook

Source: Fitzgerald, Jr, W. Documenting Drug Use Review Activities. In: Ed. Canaday B. OBRA'90 A Practical Guide to Effecting Pharmaceutical Care. APhA, Washington, 1994.

Patient Consultation Report
Rantucci Medical Dispensary, 1399 King Street, Buffalo, New York

Date: April 4, 2005

Patient: Jason Philbrook   Age: 10 years

Current Conditions and Medications:
    Asthma for approximately 2 years.
- Salbutamol inhaler and budesonide turbuhaler approximately monthly for the last year.
- Salmeterol, 1 puff twice daily for 2 months.

Problem:
1. Jason has been experiencing more frequent episodes of shortness of breath and wheezing (approximately 3 times daily), for which he is using the salbutamol.
2. He has discontinued use of the budesonide.
3. The family has recently acquired a new pet rabbit which Jason handles frequently.

Service:
- Counseled on the use of all the medication.
- Retrained on appropriate use and technique for administration.
- Cautioned that the rabbit may be exacerbating Jason's condition.

Recommendations:
- Schedule an appointment with physician to review asthma condition and therapy.
- Arrange for allergy testing to determine if the rabbit and possibly other environmental factors are contributing to his condition.
- Use a spirometer regularly and keep a chart of results to get a clear picture of treatment effectiveness.

Future Service Recommended:
- Instructions about spiromenter use and charting—half-an-hour consultation.
- Regular asthma monitoring consultation service—half-an-hour consultation.

As extra time is needed with the pharmacist, there will be a pharmacy service fee for these additional future recommended services. (It may be covered by third party drug coverage.)

Thank you for your time. Please contact me if you need additional information or to arrange for the above services.

Sincerely,

Melanie Rantucci,
Pharmacist, Rantucci Medical Pharmacy

Note: Page numbers in italics indicate figures; page numbers followed by t indicate tables.